QUALITY AND SAFETY IN ANESTHESIA AND PERIOPERATIVE CARE

T0323564

QUALITY AND SAFETY IN ANESTHESIA AND PERIOPERATIVE CARE

EDITED BY

KEITH J. RUSKIN, MD
Professor of Anesthesia and Critical Care
University of Chicago
Chicago, Illinois

MARJORIE P. STIEGLER, MD
Associate Professor of Anesthesiology
University of North Carolina
Chapel Hill, North Carolina

STANLEY H. ROSENBAUM, MD
Professor of Anesthesiology, Medicine, and Surgery
Yale University School of Medicine
New Haven, Connecticut

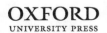
OXFORD
UNIVERSITY PRESS

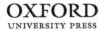

OXFORD
UNIVERSITY PRESS

Oxford University Press is a department of the University of Oxford. It furthers
the University's objective of excellence in research, scholarship, and education
by publishing worldwide. Oxford is a registered trade mark of Oxford University
Press in the UK and certain other countries.

Published in the United States of America by Oxford University Press
198 Madison Avenue, New York, NY 10016, United States of America.

Library of Congress Cataloging-in-Publication Data
Names: Ruskin, Keith., editor. | Stiegler, Marjorie P., editor. | Rosenbaum, Stanley H., editor.
Title: Quality and safety in anesthesia and perioperative care /
edited by Keith J. Ruskin, Marjorie P. Stiegler, Stanley H. Rosenbaum.
Description: Oxford ; New York : Oxford University Press, [2016] |
Includes bibliographical references and index.
Identifiers: LCCN 2016006863 (print) | LCCN 2016007645 (ebook) | ISBN 9780199366149 (alk. paper) |
ISBN 9780199366156 (e-book) | ISBN 9780199366163 (e-book) | ISBN 9780199366170 (online)
Subjects: | MESH: Medical Errors—prevention & control | Patient Safety—standards |
Anesthesiology—standards | Perioperative Care—standards | Patient Care Team—standards
Classification: LCC RD82 (print) | LCC RD82 (ebook) | NLM WX 153 | DDC 617.9/60289—dc23
LC record available at http://lccn.loc.gov/2016006863

9 8 7 6 5 4 3 2 1

Printed by WebCom, Inc., Canada

In memory of Lloyd Leon Ruskin

הכרבל ונורכיז

CONTENTS

FOREWORD

Although safety issues confront many industries, the most complex challenges—by far—lie in patient safety. As Lewis Thomas[1] pointed out, nineteenth-century physicians could influence the outcome of illness only modestly at best. Advances in medical science and technology now enable extraordinary interventions that can dramatically improve patients' lives. On the other hand, highly specialized procedures that are designed to intervene precisely in intricate physiological processes are inherently vulnerable to adverse events and are terribly unforgiving of errors. Moreover, patients who seek medical care often have multiple disease processes, further increasing their vulnerability to mishap.

Modern healthcare systems are extremely complex, involving many individual professionals with different kinds of expertise who must work together as teams. Diverse organizational factors influence how effectively individuals and teams are able to do their work. Every action in the extended healthcare process provides opportunities for things to go wrong, adversely affecting patient outcome. By the time the Institute of Medicine's 1999 report, *To Err Is Human*,[2] galvanized public awareness of the extent of iatrogenic harm, anesthesiologists had already established themselves as leaders in the medical community's search for ways to improve patient safety.

As part of that search, the medical community has examined ways in which other industries have improved their safety, and this has led to collaboration with the human factors community. Human factors is an applied discipline that draws upon the cognitive, social, physiological, and engineering sciences to understand the conditions that affect human performance and to devise ways to enhance and protect that performance. Medical safety researchers have particularly drawn on the contributions that human factors science has made to commercial aviation safety, through concepts such as situation awareness, crew resource management, threat and error management, high-reliability organizations, and safety culture. Procedures such as checklists and explicit practices for data monitoring have also emerged from aviation, as have principles for designing equipment interfaces such as the visual displays in modern airline cockpits that help pilots maintain situation awareness. These concepts, procedures, and design principles can be adapted to improve patient safety.

Human factors science has also improved safety in many industries by chipping away at long-standing but misleading concepts of the nature of the errors made by expert professionals. For many years, it was assumed that if a well-trained professional could normally perform some task without difficulty, then errors in the performance of that task in an accident sequence must be the "cause" of that accident. This philosophy implies that the professional who made the error is deficient in some way. But in reality, accidents almost always involve the confluence of many factors, and the interaction of those factors is partly a matter of chance. Errors are only part of this confluence, and indeed are themselves consequences of other underlying causes. Unfortunately, investigators have too often lacked normative data on routine operations in which no accident occurred—data that sometimes show the same errors and procedural deviations taking place fairly frequently, but without producing mishap. Without this normative data, it is all too easy to draw simplistic conclusions about the causes of error and the interacting roles of many factors in accident sequences.

In recent years a more sophisticated understanding of both errors and accident causality has emerged. It is now generally accepted that any errors made by human operators should be used as a starting point of an accident investigation, not the endpoint. Errors made by skilled experts (as opposed to novices) are not root causes in themselves, but rather manifestations of the flaws and inherent limitations of the overall sociotechnical system in which these experts work.

The causes of experts' errors are intimately related to the cognitive mechanisms that enable experts to skillfully perform tasks that do not allow 100% reliability. Both correct and incorrect performance must be understood in the context of the experience, training, and goals of the individual; the characteristics of the tasks performed; human-machine interfaces; both routine and unanticipated events; interactions with other humans in the system; and organizational aspects. These aspects include both the explicit and implicit manifestations of the organization's culture and goals, the inherent tensions between safety and production, and institutional reward structures, policies and procedures. Organizations whose leaders formally endorse high safety practices all too often fail to realize that their reward structure encourages individuals to take actions that are unsafe.

As the authors of several chapters in this book point out, iatrogenic error is only one of many issues that affect patient outcome. Practices that reduce vulnerability to error and enable trapping of errors before harm is done allow medical practitioners and institutions to identify and correct broader systemic problems that lead to the errors that cause harm. Further, these practices can also help identify factors affecting patient outcome, even when professional error is not involved. For example, incident-reporting systems can identify systemic issues such as the lack of timely availability of critical resources for dealing with emergencies in operating rooms.

Although concepts and practices from domains such as aviation can be brought to bear in medicine to good effect, simply importing these concepts and practices and plopping them down in medical settings will not be effective and may cause harm. Any intervention must be tuned to the specific setting. For example, aviation checklists, which have saved many lives, are integrated into the flow of cockpit tasks in ways that do not distract the pilots or interfere with performing other essential duties. This integration did not happen overnight; it is an ongoing process still being refined and tailored to the needs of individual airlines. The value of checklists in medical practice has been established,[3] but considerable work is still required to design their content and integrate their use into settings such as operating rooms in ways that are easy to use and that do not impose additional cognitive workload on practitioners.

Introducing new concepts into medical practice requires expert analysis of the specific settings in which they are to be used, including the flow of tasks among members of the team, the information each team member has and needs, the roles and responsibilities of each team member, the level of workload, the arrangement of equipment, and the culture in which the team works. This analysis is best accomplished through extensive collaboration between medical professionals and human factors experts. The chapters of this book illustrate the benefits of this kind of collaboration. The authors, all leading experts in their respective fields, have worked across disciplinary lines to good effect. Anesthesiologists with extensive expertise in patient safety demonstrate a thorough understanding of human factors issues, and the chapters by human factors experts show solid understanding of the medical issues.

When human factors concepts such as crew resource management were introduced to the aviation industry in the early 1980s, not all parties welcomed the changes. Many senior airline captains felt threatened and worried that their command authority would be undermined. Acceptance was gradual, but was consistently supported by airline management and regulatory authorities, and over time pilots learned that these concepts could help them avoid errors and make good decisions. The concepts continue to evolve, but today few in the airline industry question the value of these concepts when applied appropriately.

A similar situation exists today in medicine—not all medical practitioners are enthusiastic about the pathways suggested in this book. (An entire field of study, implementation science, has sprung up to address cultural, economic, and management bottlenecks impeding implementation of healthcare improvements.)

This book offers clearly written chapters based on accepted safety, human performance, and quality management science that will help to ameliorate this resistance. Beyond that, we must understand that cultural change is almost always difficult and slow. Regulatory and organizational support is of course crucial, but in the long run, the effectiveness of the changes proposed in this book will determine acceptance. Business managers who discover a long-term cost benefit will become advocates, as will senior surgeons and anesthesiologists who avoid a mishap because a team member was empowered to speak up. In spite of sometimes conflicting pressures, every healthcare professional wants to improve patient outcome.

This book lays a solid scientific foundation for understanding the challenges that must be addressed to substantially improve patient safety and outcome. It also provides explicit guidance on practical ways to initiate reform at all levels, from operating room practices to institutional procedures. Although the book focuses on anesthesiology and perioperative care, it provides a foundation that can be a model for all areas of medicine.

REFERENCES

1. Thomas L. *The Medusa and the Snail: More Notes of a Biology Watcher*. New York: Viking Press; 1974.
2. Institute of Medicine. *To Err Is Human: Building a Safer Health System*. Washington, DC: National Academy Press; 1999.
3. Gawande A. *The Checklist Manifesto*. New York: Metropolitan Books; 2010.

R. Key Dismukes, PhD
Chief Scientist for Aerospace
Human Factors (Retired)
NASA Ames Research Center
Moffett Field, California

PREFACE

Perioperative medicine is characterized by many factors that can cause patient harm. Care is delivered by multispecialty teams with varying levels of expertise and mutual familiarity, while patients present in various states of preexisting health and optimization for procedures that impart significant physiologic stresses and surgical insults. Patient care in this environment requires a high level of coordination and communication among team members, management of large quantities of information, and effective interfaces between humans and sophisticated technology. Hundreds of thousands of adverse events and near misses occur throughout the United States annually. At any time, one or more factors, including patient illness, the surgical procedure, team dynamics and communication, or equipment malfunction, may combine to cause a life-threatening condition. Creating a safe environment requires a coordinated strategy that reduces the number of errors while simultaneously decreasing the harm that an error can cause. As part of this, conditions that foster or allow error must be minimized, while systems for earlier identification and rescue from errors must be robust.

Anesthesiologists were among the first to recognize that teamwork training, safety culture, and quality management were essential components of clinical care, and *Quality and Safety in Anesthesia and Perioperative Care* expands on this knowledge. Chapters in this book emphasize strategies that can be used in community practice as well as major academic medical centers. Part I of the book provides an overview of the scientific foundations of human factors science. Chapters in this section explore causes of errors and violations, threat and error management, team training, and the essentials of a culture of safety. Part II offers practical organizational suggestions for improving quality of care and patient safety in the perioperative setting and for the growing number of procedures that take place in remote locations, including change management, quality measurement, safety regulation, optimizing team and technology interactions, and managing clinicians who are disruptive or impaired, whether by fatigue, substance abuse, or the aftermath of an adverse event. Chapters are concisely written, with illustrations that highlight key points.

Quality and Safety in Anesthesia and Perioperative Care offers a depth of information on this topic that cannot be found in a single chapter in an anesthesiology textbook. Although this book was written primarily for anesthesia clinicians, fellows, and residents, nearly all of the content is applicable to operating room personnel, hospital administrators, and medical risk managers. The book provides critical information for the anesthesiologist in academic or private practice, as well as physicians who manage a training program and are looking for a structured method of teaching safety and quality. Physician executives can also use this book to guide quality and safety programs throughout a healthcare institution. Indeed, the content of this text is applicable to

any healthcare setting or discipline, because
the concepts of error prevention, risk mitigation, safety culture, and quality improvement
are the same. It is our sincere hope that readers
of this book will be better equipped to improve
patient outcomes.

Keith J. Ruskin, MD
Marjorie P. Stiegler, MD
Stanley H. Rosenbaum, MD

ACKNOWLEDGMENTS

Successfully completing a project of this magnitude is impossible without the support of many people. The editors would first like to thank Rebecca Suzan and Andrea Knobloch for their insights and guidance. We would like to thank our chapter authors, who provided well-written, highly informative chapters and kept us on schedule. We thank the many residents and faculty of our respective institutions, who read and commented on the manuscript. Most important, we thank our families for their constant support and encouragement. Keith J. Ruskin would like to thank Anna Ruskin, MD, and Daniel Ruskin, and dedicates the book to the memory of his father, Lloyd Leon Ruskin. Marjorie P. Stiegler would like to thank James Stiegler for his unwavering support, and Henry and Juliet Stiegler for their resilience. Stanley H. Rosenbaum would like to thank Judith and Adina Rosenbaum for their loving support, and always treasures the memory of Paula E. Hyman.

CONTRIBUTORS

Keith Baker, MD, PhD
Associate Professor of Anaesthesia
Harvard Medical School
Massachusetts General Hospital
Boston, Massachusetts

David J. Birnbach, MD, MPH
Miller Professor and Vice Provost
Senior Associate Dean for Quality,
    Safety, and Risk
Director, UM-JMH Center for Patient Safety
University of Miami Miller School of
    Medicine
Miami, Florida

Amanda R. Burden, MD
Associate Professor of Anesthesiology
Director Clinical Skills and Simulation
    Cooper Medical School of Rowan
    University
Cooper University Hospital
Camden, New Jersey

Thomas R. Chidester, PhD
Federal Aviation Administration
Civil Aerospace Medical Institute
Oklahoma City, Oklahoma

Stephan Cohn, MD
Assistant Professor of Anesthesia
    and Critical Care
University of Chicago
Chicago, Illinois

Jeffrey B. Cooper, PhD
Professor of Anesthesia
Harvard Medical School
Executive Director, Center for Medical
    Simulation
Massachusetts General Hospital
Boston, Massachusetts

**Martin Culwick, MB, ChB, BSc,
FANZCA, MIT**
Medical Director
Australian and New Zealand Tripartite
    Anaesthetic Data Committee
Senior Specialist
Royal Brisbane and Women's Hospital
Brisbane, Australia

Christine A. Doyle, MD
Anesthesiology Partner, CEP America
San Jose, California

Frank A. Drews, PhD
Professor Cognitive Psychology
Director of the Human Factors
    Certificate Program
Department of Psychology
University of Utah
Salt Lake City, Utah

Richard P. Dutton, MD, MBA
Chief Quality Officer
US Anesthesia Partners
Anesthesiologist, Baylor University
  Medical Center
Dallas, Texas

David M. Gaba, MD
Professor of Anesthesiology,
  Perioperative and Pain Medicine
Stanford University School of Medicine
Stanford, California

Samuel Grodofsky, MD
Department of Anesthesiology
  and Critical Care
The Hospital of the University
  of Pennsylvania
Philadelphia, Pennsylvania

Patrick J. Guffey, MD
Assistant Professor of Anesthesiology
University of Colorado
Children's Hospital Colorado
Aurora, Colorado

Elizabeth Harry, MD
Instructor in Medicine
Harvard Medical School
Brigham and Women's Hospital
Boston, Massachusetts

Michael Keane, BMBS FANZCA
Adjunct Associate Professor
Centre for Human Psychopharmacology
Swinburne University
Adjunct Lecturer in Public Health
Monash University
Melbourne, Australia

Sheri A. Keitz, MD, PhD
Chief, Division General Internal Medicine
Vice Chair for Clinical Affairs Department
  of Medicine
UMass Memorial Health Care
University of Massachusetts Medical School
Worcester, Massachusetts

P. Allan Klock, Jr., MD
Professor of Anesthesia and Critical Care
University of Chicago
Chicago, Illinois

Viji Kurup, MD
Associate Professor of Anesthesiology
Yale University School of Medicine
New Haven, Connecticut

Robert S. Lagasse, MD
Professor and Vice Chair, Quality
  Management and Regulatory Affairs
Department of Anesthesiology
Yale University School of Medicine
New Haven, Connecticut

Meghan Lane-Fall, MD, MSHP
Assistant Professor of Anesthesiology
  and Critical Care
The Hospital of the University of Pennsylvania
Perelman School of Medicine
University of Pennsylvania
Philadelphia, Pennsylvania

Alex Macario, MD, MBA
Professor of Anesthesiology, Perioperative
  and Pain Medicine
Stanford University Medical Center
Stanford, California

**Alan F. Merry, FANZCA, FFPMANZCA,
FRCA, FRSNZ**
Professor and Head of School of Medicine
The University of Auckland
Specialist Anesthesiologist
Auckland City Hospital
Auckland, New Zealand

Michael J. Murray, MD, PhD
Professor of Anesthesiology
Mayo Clinic
Phoenix, Arizona

Loren Riskin, MD
Clinical Instructor in Anesthesiology,
  Perioperative and Pain Medicine
Stanford University School of Medicine
Stanford, California

Christian M. Schulz, MD
Department of Anesthesiology
Klinikum rechts der Isar
Technische Universität München
Munich, Germany

Sven Staender, MD
Past-Chairman ESA Patient Safety & Quality
  Committee
Vice-Chairman European Patient Safety
  Foundation
Department of Anesthesia and Intensive
  Care Medicine
Regional Hospital
Männedorf, Switzerland

Robert K. Stoelting, MD
President, Anesthesia Patient Safety
  Foundation
Emeritus Professor of Anesthesia
Indiana University School of Medicine
Indianapolis, Indiana

John Sweller, PhD
Emeritus Professor of Educational Psychology
School of Education
University of New South Wales
Sydney, Australia

Mark S. Weiss, MD
Assistant Professor of Clinical
  Anesthesiology and Critical Care
The Hospital of the University
  of Pennsylvania
Perelman School of Medicine
University of Pennsylvania
Philadelphia, Pennsylvania

Jonathan R. Zadra, PhD
Adjunct Assistant Professor of Psychology
University of Utah
Salt Lake City, Utah

PART I

Scientific Foundations

1

Patient Safety

A Brief History

ROBERT K. STOELTING

INTRODUCTION

Patient safety is a new and distinct healthcare discipline that emphasizes the reporting, analysis, and prevention of medical error that often leads to adverse healthcare events.[1,2]

Hippocrates recognized the potential for injuries that arise from the well-intentioned actions of healers. Greek healers in the fourth century BCE drafted the Hippocratic Oath and pledged to "prescribe regimens for the good of my patients according to my ability and my judgment and never do harm to anyone." Since then, the directive *primum non nocere* ("first do no harm") has become a central tenet of contemporary medicine. However, despite an increasing emphasis on the scientific basis of medical practice in Europe and the United States in the late nineteenth century, data on adverse outcomes were hard to come by, and the various studies commissioned collected mostly anecdotal events.[2]

The modern history of patient safety can be traced to the late 1970s and early 1980s and reflects initially the activities of the American medical specialty of anesthesiology.[3] Anesthesiology, via its professional society, the American Society of Anesthesiologists (ASA), was the first medical specialty to champion patient safety as a specific focus.[4] An early driving force to address the causes of anesthesia accidents was the spiraling cost of professional liability insurance for anesthesiologists. Anesthesiologists constituted 3% of physicians and generated 3% of malpractice claims, but those claims accounted for a disproportionately high 12% of medical liability insurance

payout. The relationship of patient safety to malpractice insurance premiums was easy to predict: if patients were not injured, they would not sue, the payouts would be reduced, and insurance rates would follow.

The creation of the ASA Committee on Patient Safety and Risk Management in 1983 represented the first time a professional medical society independently addressed patient safety as a specific focus, with the goal of determining the cause of anesthetic accidents.[4] Subsequently, the formation of the Anesthesia Patient Safety Foundation (APSF) in 1985 marked the first use of the term *patient safety* in the name of a professional reviewing organization.[3-8] Likewise, in Australia, the Australian Patient Safety Foundation was founded in 1989 for anesthesia error monitoring.[2]

Today, the specialty of anesthesiology is widely recognized as the pioneering leader in patient safety efforts. It has been stated that the "discovery" of anesthesia in the 1840s was a uniquely American contribution to the world of medicine. The legitimization and recognition of *patient safety* as an important concept was again a uniquely American contribution to the world of medicine.

THE EARLY HISTORY OF THE ASA AS A PIONEER IN SAFETY

Serendipitous Coincidences

As with most important historical developments, coincidence was prominent in the creation of the APSF.[4] Several factors came together to facilitate the development of an idea ("vision") held by Ellison C. Pierce, Jr., MD, who was then the chair of anesthesia at the New England Deaconess Hospital in the Harvard Medical School system. Dr. Pierce's interest in patient safety was originally stimulated in 1962 when, as a junior faculty member, he was assigned to give a lecture to the residents on "anesthesia accidents." After that he sustained his interest in this topic, keeping files, notes, and newspaper clippings regarding adverse anesthesia events that harmed patients, especially unrecognized esophageal intubation.

In April 1982 the ABC television program *20/20* aired a segment entitled "The Deep Sleep: 6,000 Will Die or Suffer Brain Damage."[9] The segment opened with the statement, "If you are going to go into anesthesia, you are going on a long trip and you should not do it, if you can avoid it in any way. General anesthesia is safe most of the time, but there are dangers from human error, carelessness and a critical shortage of anesthesiologists. This year, 6,000 patients will die or suffer brain damage." Following scenes of patients who had suffered anesthesia mishaps, the program went on to

say, "The people you have just seen are tragic victims of a danger they never knew existed—mistakes in administering anesthesia." In another example, a patient was left in a coma following the anesthesiologist's error in turning off oxygen rather than nitrous oxide at the end of an anesthetic (Figure 1.1).

This watershed presentation provoked public concern about the safety of anesthesia. Dr. Pierce transformed this potential problem for the specialty into an opportunity to take positive, proactive measures. Taking advantage of his position as first vice president of ASA in October 1983, he convinced the society's leaders to create the Committee on Patient Safety and Risk Management.

Another important event was the groundbreaking research led by Jeffrey B. Cooper, PhD, a bioengineer in the Department of Anesthesia at the Massachusetts General Hospital.[10] Dr. Cooper had focused on revealing how human errors were a major and fundamental cause of preventable anesthesia accidents. He and his colleagues adopted the techniques of *critical incident analysis*, used in the study of aviation accidents, to study analogous events that were occurring in anesthesia. Based on Cooper's work, Richard J. Kitz,

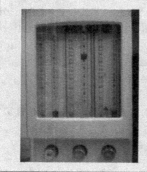

"If you are going to go into anesthesia, you are going on a long trip and you should not do it, if you can avoid it in any way. General anesthesia is safe most of the time, but there are dangers from human error, carelessness and a critical shortage of anesthesiologists. This year, 6,000 patients will die or suffer brain damage.... The people you have just seen are tragic victims of a danger they never knew existed—mistakes in administering anesthesia."

Excerpts from *"The Deep Sleep: 6,000 Will Die or Suffer Brain Damage,"* aired on the ABC television show *20/20* in April 22, 1982. They reported an error by an anesthesiologist in which the nitrous oxide was turned up and the oxygen was turned off at the end of the case, causing severe brain damage in the patient. The public concern provoked by this show provided an opportunity for Dr. Ellison C. Pierce, Jr., soon to be ASA president, and with a strong interest in anesthesia accidents, to direct ASA's organizational efforts around patient safety research and education.

FIGURE 1.1: Driving forces behind the creation of the Anesthesia Patient Safety Foundation.

From Eichhorn JH. The APSF at 25: pioneering success in safety, but challenges remain. *APSF Newsletter* 2010;25:21–44 (http://www.apsf.org/newsletters/pdf/summer_2010.pdf). Reproduced with permission of the Anesthesia Patient Safety Foundation.

MD, then chair of Cooper's department, lectured on the topic to the Royal College of Anesthetists. The esteemed Professor T. Cecil Gray was in the audience and suggested that an international meeting be convened to further understand and discuss preventable anesthesia injuries.

Dr. Kitz brought the idea of an international meeting on anesthesia safety to Dr. Pierce, who by this time was president of ASA. The three collaborated to organize and host in Boston the International Symposium on Preventable Anesthesia Mortality and Morbidity. The 50 invited participants expressed enthusiastic support for some sort of action to make anesthesia safer. After the close of the meeting, a small group stayed behind, and Dr. Pierce outlined his proposal to create an independent foundation dedicated solely to improving the safety of anesthesia care, with the vision that "no patient shall be harmed by anesthesia." When it came to naming the foundation, Dr. Cooper suggested the "Anesthesia Patient Safety Foundation."[4]

Creation of the Anesthesia Patient Safety Foundation

The APSF (www.apsf.org) was launched in late 1985 as an independent (allowing organizational agility and the freedom to tackle openly the sensitive issue of anesthesia accidents) nonprofit corporation with the vision that "no patient shall be harmed by anesthesia" (Figure 1.2).[3-8] The APSF "mission" is to improve continually the safety of patients during anesthesia care by

- sponsoring investigations that will provide a better understanding of preventable anesthetic injuries;
- encouraging programs that will reduce the number of anesthetic injuries;
- promoting national and international communication of information and ideas about the causes and prevention of anesthetic injuries;
- establishing a complimentary information newsletter for all anesthesia professionals.

Initial financial support came from the ASA and several corporate sponsors. Members of the APSF Board of Directors represent a broad spectrum of stakeholders, including anesthesiologists, nurse anesthetists, nurses, manufacturers of equipment and drugs, regulators, risk managers, attorneys, insurers, and engineers. The APSF is unique in that it brings together all stakeholders in patient safety under a neutral umbrella that facilitates open communication about the sensitive issues of anesthesia accidents. Today, the APSF persists in pursuit of its mission of zero tolerance for injury to patients. It serves as a model for pioneering collaboration and commitment of the entire constellation of anesthesia-related professions to the common goal of patient safety.

Public Recognition

Recognition of the safety efforts and leadership came to the APSF in the landmark 1999 report from the Institute of Medicine (IOM) on errors in medical care.[11] The APSF was the only organization mentioned as one that had made a demonstrable and positive impact on patient safety. In 2005, the *Wall Street Journal* carried a front-page article about the successful efforts of anesthesiologists, the ASA, and the APSF to improve patient safety, rather than focusing specifically on tort reform.[12]

Culture of Safety

In the long term, the most important contribution of anesthesiology to patient safety may be the institutionalization and legitimization of patient safety as a topic of professional concern.[3-8] In this regard, the creation of the APSF was a landmark achievement. Unlike professional societies such as the ASA, the APSF can bring together many constituencies in healthcare that may well disagree on economic (e.g., industry competitors) or political issues, but that all agree on the goal of patient safety.

ANESTHESIA IS NOW SAFER

It is widely believed that anesthesia is safer today (at least for healthy patients) than it was 25 to 50 years ago, although the extent of and reasons for the improvements are debatable.[2]

Anesthesia Patient Safety Foundation
NEWSLETTER

Volume 1, No. 1, pp 1-8   March, 1986

Safety Foundation Organized

Statement of Purpose

This is the first *Newsletter* of the Anesthesia Patient Safety Foundation, which was incorporated on September 30, 1985. The mission of the APSF is clear and simple—to encourage activities that will prevent patients from being harmed by the effects of anesthesia. Why such a foundation? What activities shall it promote to fulfill its mission? What resources will support those activities? What can you do to help?

It is generally agreed that anesthesia is safer than it has ever been, but that it still isn't safe enough. In the United States, annually some several thousand patients die or are seriously injured at least in part by their anesthetic experience. There is strong evidence that more than half of these adverse outcomes are preventable by applying known precepts of anesthesia management. Yet, the causes of preventable deaths and injuries are diverse and complicated. There is no one evil and no simple cure.

The first step toward improvement is creating awareness that a problem exists. Education, training, application of current and developing technologies and acquiring new knowledge about the causes and prevention of mishaps are components of a solution matrix.

Anesthesia mortality is everybody's problem. Most people will be exposed to the risk several times in their life. When a bad outcome occurs, it affects not only the patient, but has a lasting impact on the family, the anesthetist, and the anesthetist's colleagues as well. It is also a problem for many other constituencies—the manufacturer and designer of equipment that is involved or implicated in an accident and the hospital administrator in whose operating room an accident occurred. For the companies that provide liability insurance, there is the clear and present danger that the malpractice crisis, caused at least in part by preventable inju-

ries, may severely damage or cripple the viability of their organizations. That this crisis puts the entire health care system in jeopardy makes this a problem for the federal government also.

Because there has been no place that these constituencies can join forces to promote change, the Anesthesia Patient Safety Foundation was formed. Its goals are:

*To foster investigations that will provide a better understanding of preventable anesthetic injuries;

*To encourage programs that will reduce the number of anesthetic injuries; and

*To promote national and international communication of information and ideas about the causes and prevention of anesthetic injuries.

During the first year, the Foundation's aims are to start a communication vehicle (this newsletter) and to establish a research fund, awarding several grants. Committees have been created to implement these activities.

Who is the APSF? Its 30-member Board of Directors includes representatives from anesthesiology, nurse anesthesia, device and pharmaceutical manufacturing, the insurance industry, hospitals,

biomedical engineering, and the FDA (see page 5 of this newsletter for a complete list of the Board and committees). Membership in the APSF is open to any individual contributing at least $25 and any corporation contributing at least $500. Contributions will go toward funding the cost of producing and distributing this newsletter to the approximately 45,000 people who have a stake in preventing anesthesia injuries and toward the support of safety-related research activities.

You won't have to be a member of the APSF to benefit from its efforts but, yes, you will receive a certificate of membership if you join. The real reason to contribute $25 or more is because you want to make anesthesia safer. Because it can be. Because it should be. We think that some improvements, through increasing awareness and through implementing some new technologies, can be had in the short term—a few years. But, the ultimate goal of near-absolutely injury-free anesthesia will take longer because the impact of training, of education, and of innovative ideas derived from research take time to percolate through a culture. But, it can be done. We need your help.

Jeffrey B. Cooper, Ph.D.
Ellison C. Pierce, M.D.
For the Executive Committee

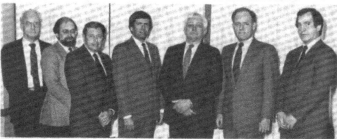

THE APSF EXECUTIVE COMMITTEE recently met in Atlanta, GA. Left to right: Dr. J.S. Gravenstein, Dr. J.B. Cooper, Dr. E.S. Siker (Secretary), Mr. J.F. Holzer, Dr. E.C. Pierce (President), Mr. B.A. Dole (Treasurer), and Mr. W.D. Rountree (Vice President).

Grant Applications Sought—Pg. 3

FIGURE 1.2: Front page of the March 1986 inaugural issue of the APSF Newsletter. Members of the APSF Executive Committee, left to right: J. S. Gravenstein, MD; Jeffrey B. Cooper, PhD; E. S. (Rick) Siker, MD (Secretary); Mr. James E. Holzer; Ellison C (Jeep) Pierce, Jr., MD (President); Mr. Burton A. Dole (Treasurer); and Mr. Dekle Rountree (Vice President).

From *APSF Newsletter* 1986;1:1. http://www.apsf.org/newsletters/html/1986/spring. Reproduced with permission of the Anesthesia Patient Safety Foundation.

Traditional epidemiological studies on the incidence of adverse anesthesia events often cannot be compared because of different analysis techniques and inconsistent definitions of adverse events. An important result of this problem is the emergence of investigative techniques that do not focus on the incidence of an event but rather on the underlying characteristics of mishaps (root cause analysis) and the attempt to improve subsequent patient care so that similar accidents do not recur. Examples of this approach include critical incident analysis and the analysis of closed malpractice claims by the ASA.[13] These approaches analyze only a small proportion of events that occur, but nevertheless attempt to extract the maximum amount of valuable information.

Technological Improvements

In the early 1980s, important advances in technology became available. Electronic monitoring (inspired oxygen concentrations, pulse oximetry, capnography) that extended the human senses facilitated reliable, real-time, and continuous monitoring of oxygen delivery and patient oxygenation and ventilation. Although these monitors are believed to improve safety, no study has demonstrated improved outcomes from the use of these technologies.

Standards and Guidelines

In the early 1980s, a committee at the Harvard Hospitals proposed the first standards of practice for minimum intra-operative monitoring, which became the forerunner of the ASA Standards for Basic Anesthetic Monitoring that were adopted in 1986.[14,15] Subsequent revisions of the standards have included the addition of audible alarms on pulse oximetry and capnography. The intention of standards is to codify and institutionalize specific practices that constitute safety monitoring as a strategy to prevent anesthesia accidents. The ASA is nationally recognized as a leader among medical specialty societies in the development of standards to improve patient safety. Additional ASA standards and guidelines (recommendations, consensus statements, and practice advisories) have been developed. The American Association of Nurse Anesthetists (AANA) has also promoted patient safety efforts to its members through the development and publication of standards.

Closed Claims Project

In the mid-1980s, amid professional liability insurance concerns, the ASA instituted the Closed Claims Project, which continues today under the direction of the Anesthesia Quality Institute (www.aqihq.org) as an ongoing project to yield important information through the study of anesthesia mishaps.[13] The Closed Claims Project is a standardized collection of malpractice claims against anesthesiologists, created by the ASA Committee on Professional Liability. The goal of the Closed Claims Project is to discover unappreciated patterns of anesthesia care that may have contributed to patient injury and subsequent litigation. This goal is based on the philosophy that the prevention of adverse outcomes is the best method for controlling the costs of professional liability insurance.

In the late 1980s, analysis of the claims in the database revealed that respiratory-related events were the most frequently cited source of anesthesia liability.[16] The reviewers also determined that most of these events could have been prevented if there had been better monitoring. These findings compelled the ASA to develop standards and guidelines relating to pulse oximetry, capnography, and management of the difficult airway.

Safety Research

The APSF awards research grants for projects that study patient safety–related issues. When the first APSF grants were awarded in 1987, funds for patient safety research in anesthesia were nonexistent. The most important outcome of the grant awards may not be the knowledge created and disseminated, but rather the new cadre of investigators and scholars that the grants have helped to develop by providing a funding source and an intellectual home for individuals who devote their careers to patient safety.

Simulation

In the late 1980s, supported by APSF grant funding, realistic patient simulators were introduced into anesthesiology.[17] Anesthesiology became the leader in the application and adoption of simulators that provide realistic patient safety experience through education (resident learning new skills for the first time on a mannequin), training (teamwork, critical event management), and research (human performance). Use of realistic simulators has now become common in other medical specialties.

Systems-Based Response to Error

In 1987, David M. Gaba, MD, introduced the concept of "normal accident theory" to the anesthesia literature.[18] Drs. Gaba and Cooper, along with others, advanced the principles of a systems-based (rather that individual-based) response to error. A 1991 conference on "human error in anesthesia," sponsored by the APSF and the US Food and Drug Administration, resulted in a better understanding of the role of human error in anesthesia and in the organizational theory of safety in healthcare, in particular the idea of learning from high-risk environments such as aviation and nuclear power (high reliability organizations).[3]

Advantageous Alliances

In early 2000, the APSF created the Data Dictionary Task Force (DDTF; http://www.apsf.org/initiatives.php?id=1), with members from clinical medicine and industry, to develop a common terminology in clinical anesthesia practice that would allow computerized records and information systems to generate compatible and comparable data with standard definitions.[20] By 2003, the membership of the DDTF included representatives from the anesthesia and informatics communities in the United Kingdom, the Netherlands, and Canada. In order to reflect its international membership, the DDTF adopted as its the name the International Organization for Terminologies in Anesthesia (IOTA).

An alliance with the Society for Pediatric Anesthesia that included funding from the APSF helped launch the "Wake Up Safe" initiative, which is a network of pediatric hospitals with the goal of creating an incident-reporting system and event-analysis paradigm. In 2007, the APSF partnered with the International Anesthesia Research Society to create a patient safety section in the journal *Anesthesia and Analgesia.*

APSF-sponsored consensus conferences reflect efforts to maintain momentum for safety initiatives, with the ultimate goal of anesthesia professional associations creating best practice policies based on these consensus conferences. Recently, the APSF has produced and placed on the APSF website (www.apsf.org) videos on anesthesia patient safety issues (fire safety in the operating room, medication safety, continuous electronic monitoring of patients receiving postoperative opioids, perioperative visual loss, simulated informed consent scenarios for patients at risk for perioperative visual loss) that can also be requested as complimentary copies.

EVIDENCED-BASED MEDICINE MEETS PATIENT SAFETY

As in aviation, many of the accepted and proposed safety changes in anesthesia lack evidence-based support, but the common theme is that they make sense and are the right thing to do (monitoring standards, audible information, automated information systems). Evidence from randomized trials is important, but it is neither sufficient nor necessary for the acceptance of safety practices.[21] There will never be complete evidence for everything that needs to be done in medicine. The prudent alternative is to make reasonable judgments based on the best available evidence. The perceived decrease in anesthesia morbidity and mortality over the past 3 decades is not attributable to any single practice or the development of new anesthetic drugs, but rather to the application of a broad array of changes in process, equipment, organization, supervision, training, and teamwork. These safety advances have been achieved through the application of a host of changes that made sense; all were based on sound principles, technical theory, or experience, and addressed real-life issues. Anesthesiology showed that safety is doing a lot of little things that, in the aggregate, make a big difference. Indeed, recent studies into checklists and their impact on the reduction of adverse events have not been randomized trials.[19,20,22,23]

Nevertheless, rigorous empirical evidence (not necessarily from randomized controlled trials) may be needed for many of the interventions intended for improving patient safety.[2,24] A key point is that interventions to improve patient safety should be based on sound theoretical construct, and the possibility of unintended consequences should be clearly defined.[25]

PATIENT SAFETY IN SURGERY

Anesthesia and surgery are inextricably linked, and the recognition of the importance of teamwork, communication, and collaboration among members of the perioperative team has been pivotal to advancing the safety of patients undergoing surgery.[2]

Traditionally, surgeons have viewed patient safety as safety from preventable errors (wrong site surgery, retained foreign bodies, medication errors, accidents in care in and out of the operating room). The 1999 Institute of Medicine (IOM) report focused attention on these types of errors and cast patient safety in terms of safety from iatrogenic injury.[11] This influential healthcare publication created a major concern about patient safety and prompted a wide array of constituencies in healthcare to conduct research and engage in efforts to improve patient safety. The IOM report set a goal of 50% reduction in error-related deaths over 5 years. Although evidence to support a reduction in error-related deaths is not available, laudable efforts have been expended in anesthesia and surgery to achieve this goal.[26] In this regard, the US Department of Veterans Affairs, through its Center for Patient Safety, has developed very specific guidelines to avoid surgery on the wrong patient, wrong site, and wrong side, and has mandated a "time out" before any surgical incision, wherein the entire surgical team is briefed on the details of the intended surgical procedure.

The American College of Surgeons (ACS), much like the APSF, has expanded and renewed its efforts to improve patient safety in surgery. A result of these efforts is a publication by the ACS detailing the state of patient safety in surgery, including a conceptual framework of surgeons and the clinical guidelines advocated for safety of the surgical patient.[27]

The development of the National Surgical Quality Improvement Program (NSQIP), first in the Veterans Administration System and then in the private sector, has provided surgeons with new tools to assess and improve the quality of surgical care. Several years of experience with the NSQIP has provided new insight on patient safety in surgery and has stimulated the surgical community to view patient safety in surgery in a different conceptual framework.

The National Surgical Quality Improvement Program

NSQIP is a validated state-of-the art system for the comparative measurement and continuous improvement of the quality of major surgery nationwide.[28] The comparative metric used is a risk-adjusted outcome that focuses initially on risk-adjusted 30-day morbidity and mortality. Continuous improvement is achieved through feedback to providers of comparative data that include patient risk factors and risk-adjusted outcomes.

NSQIP originated in the Veterans Health Administration and was prompted by a 1987 congressional mandate that had been issued because of concern about perceived poor outcomes of surgery in the Veterans Administration (VA). NSQIP was initiated in 1994 after the conclusion of a large observational VA study that validated the use of risk-adjusted outcomes as measures of the quality of surgical care.[29]

To ascertain the applicability of NSQIP to the private sector, a NSQIP Private Sector Initiative was begun in 1998, utilizing three academic non-VA surgical departments. The subsequent data showed that the processes, methodology, and 30-day outcome predictive models developed by the VA NSQIP were fully applicable to the private sector, at least in general and vascular surgery.[29, 30]

Knowledge gained from NSQIP and numerous observational studies has resulted in a view of surgical patient safety that is different from the framework that was popularized in the IOM report.[11] This view is based on three important patient-safety-related observations made by NSQIP.[8]

- *Safety is indistinguishable from overall quality of surgical care and should not be addressed independent of surgical quality.* Whether it is preventable or not, an adverse outcome compromises patient safety. NSQIP has demonstrated, through its day-to-day operation and in several observational studies, that rates of adverse outcomes, properly measured and risk-adjusted, can reflect the quality of surgical care. Improved quality of surgical care reduces the incidence of adverse outcomes and improves patient safety. Within this rubric, the prevention of errors is synonymous with a reduction of adverse outcomes and, as such, can be a reliable quality measure.
- *During an episode of surgical care, adverse outcomes, and hence patient safety, are primarily determined by quality of systems care.* Invariably, structures or processes are found to be problematic at high-outlier hospitals, which reflect deficiencies in systems of care. Errors in these hospitals, although sometimes committed by specific providers, are more likely to be system errors rather than provider incompetence. The providers are important in the sense that they contribute to the system. The clear message is that adequate communication, coordination, and teamwork are critical to achieve quality surgical care.
- *Reliable comparative outcome data are imperative for the identification of system problems and the assurance of patient safety from adverse outcomes.* Although iatrogenic and accidental provider errors can be easily detected utilizing local monitoring systems, the subtler system errors that lead to a much larger body of adverse outcomes cannot be adequately appreciated or recognized without comparative data with other institutions and peer groups.[25] Deficiencies and errors within a system of care can result in adverse outcome rates that might be considered acceptable by the local provider community. It is only when these rates are compared with similarly risk-adjusted rates at other institutions that the providers appreciate the increased adversity at their center, and are thus prompted to investigate and improve the quality of the adversity-related processes and structures.

NSQIP data have documented that the most important determinant of decreased postoperative survival over an 8-year follow-up period is the occurrence, within 30 days postoperatively, of any one of 22 types of complications followed in the NSQIP protocol.[31] Independent of preoperative patient risk, the occurrence of a 30-day complication reduces median patient survival by 69%. A specific adverse event such as a pulmonary complication reduces median survival by 87%, and a wound infection decreases median survival by 42%. The adverse effect of a complication on patient survival is also influenced by the operation type.

There is accumulating evidence that in-hospital and intra-operative management of patients by anesthesiologists and surgeons can influence the long-term safety of these patients, although the underlying mechanisms for these relationships are poorly understood. The perioperative inflammatory and immune response may be a potential biological link to long-term outcomes after anesthesia and surgery.[32] It is conceivable that the inflammatory response to surgery may amplify the pro-inflammatory mechanisms of certain disease states such as coronary artery disease and thus may contribute to disease acceleration and adverse perioperative events.

US-BASED SAFETY ORGANIZATIONS

National Patient Safety Foundation

The success of the anesthesia patient safety movement was recognized in 1996 when the American Medical Association and corporate partners founded the National Patient Safety Foundation (NPSF; www.npsf.org), which was based on the APSF model. NPSF's vision is to create a world where patients and those who care for them are free from harm. NPSF provides a voice for patient safety and partners with patients and the healthcare community and key stakeholders to advance patient safety and healthcare workforce safety and to disseminate strategies to prevent harm. NPSF follows a collaborative approach, offering a portfolio of programs targeted to diverse stakeholders across the health care industry.

VA Center for National Patient Safety Anesthesia Quality Institute

The VA National Center for Patient Safety (http://www.patientsafety.va.gov) was established in 1999 to develop and nurture a culture of safety throughout the Veterans Health Administration. The center is part of the VA Office of Quality, Safety, and Value. The center's goal is the nationwide reduction and prevention of inadvertent harm to patients as a result of their care.

Leapfrog Group

The Leapfrog Group (http://www.leapfrog-group.org) was launched in November 2000 as an employer-based coalition advocating for improved transparency, quality, and safety in hospitals. Its mission is "to trigger giant leaps forward in the safety, quality and affordability of health care by (1) supporting informed healthcare decisions by those who use and pay for health care; and, (2) promoting high-value health care through incentives and rewards."

The Leapfrog Group is a voluntary program aimed at mobilizing employer purchasing power to alert the US health industry that big leaps in healthcare safety, quality, and customer value will be recognized and rewarded. The Leapfrog

Hospital Survey is the gold standard for comparing hospitals' performance on the national standards of safety, quality, and efficiency that are most relevant to consumers and purchasers of care.

Patient Safety Organizations

The Patient Safety and Quality Improvement Act of 2005 (Patient Safety Act) authorized the creation of patient safety organizations (PSOs; (http://www.pso.ahrq.gov) to improve the quality and safety of US healthcare delivery. The Patient Safety Act encourages clinicians and healthcare organizations to voluntarily report and share quality and patient safety information without fear of legal discovery. The Agency for Healthcare Research and Quality (AHRQ) administers the provisions of the Patient Safety Act and the Patient Safety Rule dealing with PSO operations.

The stimulus to create PSOs was the 1999 Institute of Medicine (IOM) report entitled, *To Err Is Human: Building a Safer Health System.*[11] This report highlighted critical areas of research and activities needed to improve the safety and quality of healthcare delivery, including the need for the reporting and analysis of data on adverse events.

PSOs are organizations that share the goal of improving the quality and safety of healthcare delivery. Organizations that are eligible to become PSOs include public or private entities, profit or not-for-profit entities, provider entities such as hospital chains, and other entities that establish special components to serve as PSOs.

By providing both privilege and confidentiality, PSOs create a secure environment where clinicians and healthcare organizations can collect, aggregate, and analyze data, thereby improving quality by identifying and reducing the risks and hazards associated with patient care.

Council on Surgical and Perioperative Safety

The Council on Surgical and Perioperative Safety (CSPS; http://www.cspsteam.org) was created in 2007 and includes seven professional organizations representing the "surgical team" (American College of Surgeons, American Society of Anesthesiologists, American Association of Nurse Anesthetists, Association of periOperative Registered Nurses, American Association of Surgical Physician Assistants, American Society of PeriAnesthesia Nurses, Association of Surgical Technologists). CSPS's mission is to "promote excellence in the surgical and perioperative environment" provided by an integrated team of dedicated professionals. The goal is to establish partnerships (regulatory, private, research agencies) that improve patient safety.

The Joint Commission Center for Transforming Healthcare

Created in 2008, the Joint Commission Center for Transforming Healthcare (http://www.centerfortransforminghealthcare.org) aims to solve healthcare's most critical safety and quality problems. The Center's participants—some of the nation's leading hospitals and health systems—use a systematic approach to analyze specific breakdowns in care and discover their underlying causes in order to develop targeted solutions that solve these complex problems. In keeping with its objective to transform healthcare into a high-reliability industry, the Joint Commission shares these proven effective solutions with the more than 20,000 healthcare organizations it accredits and certifies. Hospitals have made significant advances in quality— even better results are now achievable. Hospitals and the Joint Commission are working together to improve systems and processes of care.

ABMS Patient Safety Foundations

The ABMS Patient Safety Foundation (http://www.abms.org/Products_and_Publications/pdf/ABMS_PS_Foundations.pdf) is a Web-based self-assessment that covers patient safety curriculum in four topics:

- Epidemiology of Safety and Harm
- Systems Approach to Improving Patient Safety
- Communication
- Safety Culture.

Participating physicians earn AMA PRA Category 1 credits that count toward the ABMS Maintenance of Certification. The goal is to provide the foundation for acquiring the knowledge and skills to assess the safety of patient care and to make that care safer.

Anesthesia Quality Institute

The Anesthesia Quality Institute (AQI; http://www.aqihq.org/about-us.aspx) was established by the American Society of Anesthesiologists in October 2008 with the vision "to become the primary source of information for quality improvement in the clinical practice of anesthesiology." The mission is to "develop and maintain an ongoing registry (NACOR) of case data that will become the primary source for anesthesiologists looking to assess and improve patient care." AQI helps hospitals and practices answer important questions about the care they deliver by gathering, analyzing, and providing the data the providers need. AQI is accredited as a PSO by the Department of Health and Human Services.

US-BASED PATIENT SAFETY ORGANIZATIONS OUTSIDE ORGANIZED MEDICINE

A number of "patient safety organizations" have been created by patients and/or their families following medical errors (not unlike Mothers Against Drunk Drivers). The common theme of these foundations is to advocate for patient safety by creating patient and caregiver awareness and lobbying for changes intended to reduce the likely recurrence or a similar injury in another patient.

Medically Induced Trauma Support Services

Medically Induced Trauma Support Services (MITSS; http://www.mitss.org) is a nonprofit organization founded in June 2002 whose mission is "to support healing and restore hope" to patients, families, and clinicians who have been affected by an adverse medical event.

MITSS provides education to the healthcare community on the uniqueness of medically induced trauma, the broad scope of its impact, and the crucial need for support services through participation in and sponsorship of forums, local and national conferences, and through the media.

In October 2005, APSF sponsored a conference that included presentations by patients and families impacted by adverse medical events (http://www.apsf.org/newsletters/pdf/winter2006.pdf). A major recurrent theme of the conference was the failure of communication with the patient/family at the time of the catastrophic event and thereafter. The overall concept of trying to shift from a "culture of blame" to a "culture of learning" certainly applies. It was agreed that, in the spirit of "the patient's bill of rights," there should be an expectation by the patient/family of open communication and full disclosure (even to the point that the surgical/anesthesia consent forms should specify that after any event, prompt full disclosure will be made). The expected concerns about risk management and the potential legal liability implications of apologies and full disclosure were expressed, but reference was then made to the study from the VA system demonstrating a significant reduction in liability costs associated with prompt full disclosure after an event.

For many, the need is to "understand what happened" and have some assurance that steps to prevent a similar error in the future will be taken. When adverse medical events occur, the patient and his or her family are not alone in being "victims," as serious psychological issues are also likely to confront the caregivers.

Leah's Legacy

Leah's Legacy (http://leahslegacy.org) is a nonprofit organization working to achieve zero preventable deaths from medical error though prevention, education, and advocacy, and to make continuous postoperative monitoring the law (Leah's Law). The organization was created following the death of the founder's daughter owing to undetected opioid-induced respiratory depression in the postoperative period.

Mothers Against Medical Error

Mothers Against Medical Error (http://www.mamemomsonline.org) is a group of parents

whose mission is to promote safety in the medical system by providing support for victims of medical harm. Its founder, Helen Haskell, became a patient safety advocate after her 15-year-old son died from a medical error in 2000. She successfully worked for passage of the Lewis Blackman Hospital Safety Act in 2005 in honor of her son. The law requires all doctors to wear identification tags, so patients will know if a doctor or medical resident is attending a patient.

Louise G. Batz Patient Safety Foundation

The mission of the Louise H. Batz Patient Safety Foundation (http://www.louisebatz.org/Home.aspx) is to help prevent medical errors by ensuring that patients and families have the "knowledge" they need to promote a safe hospital experience for their loved ones, and to support innovative advancements in patient safety. The goal of the Foundation is to open the pathways of communication between patients, doctors, nurses, and hospitals in an effort to enhance hospital safety and prevent adverse events. It is important to empower the patient and family with knowledge about the type of care they will receive in order to make informed decisions. It is vital to create awareness through literature that is accessible and easy for the patient to understand. It takes teamwork to ensure that patients, families, doctors, nurses, and hospitals are safe, informed, and protected.

Promise to Amanda Foundation

The mission of the Promise to Amanda Foundation (http://www.promisetoamanda.org) is to raise awareness of respiratory depression so that it becomes mandatory to continuously electronically monitor all patients using capnography and pulse oximetry. The stimulus to form the foundation was the death in 2010 of 18-year-old "Amanda" who experienced undetected respiratory depression while receiving postoperative pain management utilizing patient-controlled analgesia.

Patient Safety Movement

The Patient Safety Movement (http://patientsafetymovement.org) is connecting people, ideas, and technology to confront the large-scale problem of over 200,000 preventable patient deaths in US hospitals each year by providing actionable ideas and innovations that can transform the process of care, dramatically improve patient safety, and help eliminate preventable deaths. The movement is dedicated to breaking down silos between hospitals, medical technology companies, patient advocates, patients, the government, and all the stakeholders affected in healthcare.

INTERNATIONAL PATIENT SAFETY ORGANIZATIONS

Australian Patient Safety Foundation

The Australian Patient Safety Foundation (AusPSF; http://www.apsf.net.au) is an independent organization dedicated to anesthesia patient safety.[2] Inspired by developments in the United States, Dr. William B. Runciman was instrumental in creating the vision and momentum for formation of a foundation in 1987 to promote anesthesia patient safety and, more ambitiously, throughout healthcare. An early initiative developed a voluntary national incident reporting system for anesthesia known as the Australian Incident Monitoring System (AIMS). Adverse medical events, both sentinel events (patient death and injury) and near misses (medical errors with potential harm), are reported and analyzed through the foundation's subsidiary, Patient Safety International (PSI). These data, along with ASA Closed Claims Project data, established the utility of pulse oximetry and capnography in anesthesia and influenced the promulgation of the International Standards for a Safe Practice of Anesthesia, which were endorsed by the World Federation of Societies of Anesthesiologists (WFSA).[2]

Canadian Patient Safety Institute

The Canadian Patient Safety Institute (CPSI; http://www.patientsafetyinstitute.ca) was created in 2003 as an independent corporation to promote solutions and collaboration among governments and stakeholders to improve patient safety. Areas of improvement are education, system innovation, communication, regulatory affairs, and research.

World Health Organization

The World Health Organization (WHO; http://www.who.int/patientsafety/safesurgery/tools_resources/SSSL_Checklist_finalJun08.pdf) has undertaken a number of global and regional initiatives to address surgical safety, including the Second Global Patient Safety Challenge: Safe Surgery Saves Lives. The resulting Surgical Safety Checklist list identifies three distinct phases of an operation, each corresponding to a specific period in the normal flow of work: (1) before the induction of anesthesia, (2) before the incision of the skin, and (3) before the patient leaves the operating facility.[33] The intention of such a checklist is to systematically and efficiently ensure that all conditions are optimum for patient safety, and that all staff are identifiable and accountable, and errors in patient identity, site, and type of procedure are avoided completely. By following a few critical steps, healthcare professionals can minimize the most common and avoidable risks endangering the lives and well-being of surgical patients. A result of the Surgical Safety Checklist was the advancement of the Global Oximetry project, which is now known as the Lifebox project.[34]

SUMMARY

Patient safety is not a fad. It is not a preoccupation of the past. It is not an objective that has been fulfilled or a reflection of a problem that has been solved. Patient safety is an ongoing necessity. It must be sustained by research, training, and daily application in the workplace.

ELLISON C. PIERCE, JR., MD
(Founding President, Anesthesia Patient Safety Foundation)[4]

REFERENCES

1. Patient safety. From *Wikipedia, the Free Encyclopedia*. en.wikipedia.org/wiki/Patient_safety.
2. Runciman WB, Merry AF. A brief history of the patient safety movement in anaesthesia. In: Eger EI, Saidman LJ, Westhorpe RN, eds. *The Wondrous Story of Anesthesia*. New York: Springer; 2014:541–556.
3. Gaba DM. Anaesthesiology as a model for patient safety in health care. *BMJ*. 2000:320:785–788.
4. Pierce EC, Jr. The 34th Rovenstine Lecture: 40 years behind the mask: safety revisited. *Anesthesiology*. 1996;84:965–975

5. Eichhorn JH. The APSF at 25: pioneering success in safety, but challenges remain. *APSF Newsletter*. 2010;25:21–44. http://www.apsf.org/newsletters/pdf/summer_2010.pdf.

6. Eichhorn JH. Anesthesia patient safety foundation turns 25, savors success, targets future. *ASA Newsletter*. 2011;16–21 (25th anniversary edition).

7. Stoelting RK. A historical review of the origin and contributions of the Anesthesia Patient Safety Foundation. *ASA Newsletter* (Special Commemorative Issue 1905–2005) 2005:*25–27*. www.asahq.org/newsletters/2005.

8. Stoelting RK, Khuri SF. Past accomplishments and future directions: risk prevention in anesthesia and surgery. *Anes Clin NA*. 2006;24:235–253.

9. Tomlin J. *The Deep Sleep: 6,000 Will Die or Suffer Brain Damage*. Chicago: WLS TV, 20/20, April 22, 1982.

10. Cooper JB, Newbower RS, Long CD, McPeek B. Preventable anesthesia mishaps: a study of human factors. *Anesthesiology*. 1978;49: 381–383.

11. Kohn L, Corrigan JH, Donaldson M, eds. *To Err Is Human: Building a Safer Health Care System*. Washington, DC: National Academy Press; 2000.

12. Hallinan JT. Heal thyself: once seen as risky, one group of doctors changes its ways. *Wall Street Journal*, June 21, 2005, p. 1.

13. Solazzi RW, Ward RJ. Analysis of anesthetic mishaps: the spectrum of medical liability cases. *Int Anesthesiol Clin*. 1984;22:43–59.

14. Eichhorn JH, Cooper JB, Cullen DJ et al. Standards for patient monitoring during anesthesia at Harvard Medical School. *JAMA*. 1986;256:1017–1020.

15. Standards for basic anesthetic monitoring. American Society of Anesthesiologists. www.asahq.org.

16. Caplan RA, Posner KL, Ward RJ, et al. Adverse respiratory events in anesthesia: a closed claims analysis. *Anesthesiology*. 1990;72:828–833.

17. Gaba DM, Howard SK, Fish K, et al. Simulation-based training in anesthesia crisis resource management (ACRM): a decade of experience. *Simulat Gaming*. 2001;32:175–193.

18. Gaba DM, Maxwell M. DeAnda A. Anesthetic mishaps: breaking the chain of accident evolution. *Anesthesiology*. 1987;66:670–676.

19. Cooper JB, Gaba DM. A strategy for preventing anesthesia accidents. *Int Anesthesiol Clin*. 1989;27:148–152.

20. Stoelting RK. Data dictionary task force (DDTF) launches initiative. *APSF Newsletter* (Summer) 2002;17:2. http://www.apsf.org/newsletters/html/2002/summer/01ddtf.htm.

21. Leape LL, Berwick DM, Bates DW. What practices will most improve safety? Evidence-based medicine meets patient safety. *JAMA*. 2002;208:501–507.

22. Haynes AB, Weiser TG, Berry WR, et al: A surgical safety checklist to reduce morbidity and mortality in a global population. *N Engl J Med*. 2009;360:491–499.

23. Birkmeyer JD. Strategies for improving surgical quality-checklists and beyond. *N Engl J Med*. 2010;363:1963–1965.

24. Shekelle PG, Pronovost PJ, Wachter RM, et al. Advancing the science of patient safety. *Ann Intern Med*. 2011;154:693–696.

25. Tenner EW. Why things bite back: technology and the revenge of unintended consequences. New York: Vintage Books; 1997.

26. Brennan TA, Gawande A, Thomas E, et al. Accidental deaths, saved lives, and improved quality. *N Engl J Med*. 2005;353:1405–1409.

27. Manuel BM, Nora PF, eds. Surgical patient safety: essential information for surgeons in today's environment. Chicago: American College of Surgeons; 2004.

28. Khuri SF. The NSQIP: a new frontier in surgery. *Surgery*. 2005;138:19–25.

29. Daley J, Khuri SF, Henderson W. et al. Risk adjustment of the postoperative morbidity rate for the comparative assessment of the quality of surgical care: results of the National VA Surgical Risk Study. *J Am Coll Surg*. 1997;185:328–340.

30. Neumayer L, Mastin M. Vanderhoof L, et al. Using the Veterans Administration National Surgical Quality Improvement Program to improve patient outcomes. *J Surg Res*. 2000;88:58–61.

31. Khuri SF, Henderson WG, DePalma RG, et al. Determinants of long-term survival after major surgery and the adverse effect of postoperative complications. *Ann Surg*. 2005:242:326–343.

32. Meiler SE, Monk TG, Mayfield JB, et al. Can we alter long-term outcome? The role of inflammation and immunity in the perioperative period (Part II). *APSF Newsletter* (Spring) 2004;19:1. http://www.apsf.org/newsletters/pdf/spring2004.pdf.

33. Gawande A. *The Checklist Manifesto*. New York: Metropolitan Books Henry Holt; 2010.

34. Merry AF, Eichhorn JH, Wilson IH. Extending the WHO "Safe Surgery Saves Lives" project through Global Oximetry. *Anaesthesia*. 2009;64:1045–1058.

2

Cognitive Load Theory and Patient Safety

ELIZABETH HARRY AND JOHN SWELLER

INTRODUCTION

Safe patient care depends, in part, upon being able to learn new information, store it for future use, and retrieve it when needed. Clinical care delivery, particularly in perioperative and intensive care settings, requires that physicians turn knowledge into action. Taking the correct action depends upon several factors, which include having the proper knowledge, being able to appropriately identify which knowledge is needed in a given situation, and retrieving that information. Factors that impair the ability to acquire new, patient-related information can therefore have a negative impact on clinical performance and can decrease safety.

Resource theory posits that there is a limited pool of resources available for attention, which imposes limits on cognitive information processing abilities.[1,2] *Cognitive load theory* has built upon this concept, looking specifically at the process of knowledge acquisition and how humans process information. Cognitive load theory describes working memory, which is the short-term, limited-capacity structure that everyone possesses in order to integrate new information or retrieve stored information for action. Working memory is the space where cognitive processing occurs. The cognitive load of the clinician is a critical consideration in patient safety and system design, because the cognitive system of a clinician who is "overloaded" will be compromised.[3] The function of cognitive load theory is to provide techniques that facilitate understanding and learning. The theory is based on an understanding of human mental processes and has been used to generate

a variety of new procedures for presenting information.[4]

Cognitive load theory and the cognitive architecture that is described in this chapter apply to knowledge classified as *secondary knowledge* that requires explicit education (e.g., medical knowledge), in contrast to primary knowledge that can be naturally acquired (e.g., language acquisition or recognizing faces).[5-7] The cognitive architecture associated with the acquisition of secondary knowledge is central to cognitive load theory.[4,5,8,9,10] Understanding how clinicians process information is critical to designing techniques for presenting information that complement and augment information integration. That natural information-processing system—the system responsible for knowledge acquisition and subsequent retrieval—can be described by considering five basic principles: the *information store* principle, the *borrowing and reorganizing* principle, the *randomness as genesis* principle, the *narrow limits of change* principle, and the *environmental linking and organizing* principle.

THE NATURAL INFORMATION-PROCESSING SYSTEM

The *information store* principle deals with human *long-term memory*. Long-term memory is a physician's repository of medical knowledge and situation-specific knowledge. Everything that is learned is stored in long-term memory which is immeasurably large in capacity. If a given piece of information is not stored in long-term memory, then it is not retained because no other cognitive structure permanently stores information. Cognitive load theory assumes that the primary goal of presenting information is to help a person to store domain-specific information in long-term memory for subsequent retrieval and action.

Most information stored in long-term memory is acquired via the *borrowing and reorganizing* principle. Humans are intensely social animals, and we "borrow" information from the long-term memories of other people by imitating what they do, listening to what they say, and reading what they write. The majority of our medical knowledge stored in long-term memory, particularly early in our career, comes from things that we have seen, heard, or read. This process is how expertise is created.

Although the bulk of information held in long-term memory is borrowed from other people, that information must have been created at some point. The *randomness as genesis* principle deals with how individuals create novel information while solving a problem. If there is no preexisting knowledge that suggests which action should be attempted, there is no alternative other than to randomly choose a move and test whether it brings us closer to our goal. A randomly created strategy is then followed by tests of effectiveness. Although this theory applies to novel research or spontaneous problem-solving, there is ideally some knowledge present in long-term memory that helps to limit the range of possible actions.

If preexisting knowledge cannot sufficiently limit the range of possible responses to a novel situation, an alternative mechanism, the *narrow limits of change* principle, prevents information overload. This fundamental principle is related to the concept of resource theory and asserts that there is a limited amount of working memory that is available to process novel information. If we do not have sufficient expertise and stored information to respond to a given situation (for example, an unexpected patient complication), we are quickly overwhelmed by the data we are being presented with. The limited capacity and duration of working memory prevents us from developing an impossibly large combination of moves. In other words, if we are faced with a situation in which we have little expertise

or stored knowledge, inherent limitations in data-processing bandwidth force us to indiscriminately filter or narrow data input from the environment that can be used to decide on our next action. This random filtering increases the possibility of an error because potentially important information might not be processed.

Finally, the *environmental linking and organizing* principle provides the ultimate justification for our cognitive machinery. Environmental signals can trigger the transfer of unlimited amounts of stored, organized information from long-term to working memory in order to generate an appropriate series of actions. This process is best exemplified by observing well-established routines, or habits, all of which are stored in long-term memory. Once a routine or habit has been established, the behavior is governed by that stored information. Although working memory is limited when dealing with novel information (i.e., narrow limits of change principle), it has no known limits when dealing with familiar information that has been stored in long-term memory. In that sense, this principle links with the information store principle and indicates that organized information held in long-term memory determines how we interact with our environment. A crucial part of this principle relies on a person's ability to identify the appropriate trigger in the environment that allows him or her to retrieve and then apply the correct stored information. This need to link an appropriate trigger to a given piece of stored information implies that there must be a high signal-to-noise ratio surrounding the trigger.

Cognitive load theory uses this cognitive architecture to devise procedures that facilitate the assimilation of clinically relevant information to long-term memory through limited working memory and then to use that information to provide effective patient care. The aim of presenting information to clinicians, based on the information store and the environmental linking and organizing principles is to accumulate knowledge in long-term memory that permits us to care for patients at a later time. In an acute clinical setting, that knowledge is best acquired from other people, using the borrowing and reorganizing principle, via mentors, educators, textbooks and journal articles, or point-of-care references. In some situations, however, this information is not present in long-term memory, in which case new knowledge must be created via the randomness as genesis principle, or by trial and error. In either case, according to the narrow limits of change principle, the presentation of information must be organized so as to reduce the load placed on working memory.

TYPES OF LOAD PLACED ON WORKING MEMORY

Three factors affect the level of demand that is placed on working memory at any given time and thus determine the ability to process data and identify the correct stored knowledge that will guide behavior. The three types of cognitive load are referred to as *intrinsic load, extraneous load*, and *germane load*. Designing an optimal environment for clinicians to perform high-stakes cognitive tasks requires a clear understanding of these factors.

- *Intrinsic cognitive load* is determined by the inherent characteristics or the degree of difficulty of the material being processed. Highly complex information that requires multiple elements to be processed simultaneously leads to a high intrinsic cognitive load, imposing greater stress on working memory. Anesthesia and surgery, for example, impose a high intrinsic load because they require the physician to coordinate the planning of next moves while simultaneously making contingency plans and sometimes requiring motor coordination.
- *Extraneous cognitive load* is determined by the way in which novel information is presented but is independent of the complexity of the information. Information that is presented in a disorganized and nonstandardized form increases the amount of working memory required to process it.[8] For example, any change in the equipment, the layout of the OR, or the preoperative routine increases the extraneous cognitive load on the healthcare professional, who must then use free working memory to process these new modes of organization. Standardization allows these tasks to become routine more quickly, which allows habits to form, shifting information to unlimited long-term working memory. Routines, checklists, and standardization free up working memory by reducing the extraneous use of working memory, allowing physicians to focus on complex, high intrinsic load tasks.
- *Germane cognitive load* is created by tasks or information that help to reduce extraneous load. It can be viewed as an investment that permits the management of a greater intrinsic load by directing the limited working memory to new information instead of extraneous factors. Mental models of disease processes are examples of how germane working memory resources are used to allow a clinician to more easily pick out salient triggers for long-term memory information retrieval. The use of checklists, which brings salient information to the forefront of attention, is another example of how germane working memory increases the signal-to-noise ratio.

STRATEGIES TO MINIMIZE EXTRANEOUS COGNITIVE LOAD

Intrinsic cognitive load cannot be altered, except by changing either the information itself or the knowledge level of the recipients of that information. In contrast, extraneous cognitive load is determined by the manner in which the information is presented or by altering the activities required of the people receiving the information. Strategies that reduce cognitive load include minimizing extraneous load by organizing and standardizing information delivery while maximizing germane load by facilitating transfer of the most pertinent information to clinicians. A reduction in extraneous cognitive load permits more working memory to manage the intrinsic cognitive load that is essential to learning and performance. Information presented to the clinician should therefore increase the use of working memory resources that are germane to dealing with intrinsic cognitive load while decreasing the extraneous cognitive load. This in turn maximizes the transfer of information to long-term memory.

Two cognitive load effects are associated with a reduction in extraneous cognitive load: the *split-attention effect* and the *redundancy effect*. The *split-attention effect* occurs when a clinician is faced with multiple sources of information, all of which are essential to understanding the content. Consider, for example, a clinician who is evaluating glycemic control in a hospitalized patient. If blood glucose levels are stored in one record, insulin orders in another, drug administration records in a third, and home insulin dosing in a fourth, an extraneous cognitive load is imposed by the split-attention effect. All of this information must be integrated before it can be understood, which requires the commitment of working memory to deal with an extraneous cognitive load. Those cognitive resources will therefore be unavailable for other tasks. An alternative presentation of a "glucose report" brings all of the germane information to one location and facilitates mental integration of these data. This decreases the amount of integration required and frees working memory resources for other tasks.

The *redundancy effect* occurs when additional, unnecessary sources of information are added to essential information. Consider again the clinician evaluating glycemic control in a hospitalized patient. Instead of presenting distinct data points that are essential for understanding the patient's overall glycemic picture, some electronic health records present multiple forms of the same information. For example, there might be a graph of glucose trends shown next to a flow sheet of the same information. These are then coupled to patient notes and nursing pages that discuss the same data points. In this situation, four presentations of the same information require clinicians to process redundant data modalities using working memory. This point should be considered by patient safety leaders, because redundancy is generally considered to be a protective feature that helps to avoid errors. Although presenting the same information in multiple ways seems intuitive to ensure at least one modality is processed correctly, redundant presentations of the same information impose a greater cognitive load. Clinicians must always process the additional information before determining they do not need it. Working memory resources that should be allocated to decision-making are therefore wasted if the information is indeed redundant. Randomized controlled trials in a variety of contexts overwhelmingly support the hypothesis that the presentation of redundant information has negative rather than positive effects.[4] There is, therefore, a balance between notifying clinicians of information "just in case" and overloading cognitive processing abilities.

THE EFFECT OF STRESS ON WORKING MEMORY

The emotional and physiological states of the clinician directly impact the total resources available for working memory. In a review of the main theories of abilities of attention under stress,[11] Chajut and Algom found that (1) stress decreases resources available for attention (n.b., the allocation of working memory resources is synonymous with the allocation of attention); (2) with these narrowed resources, people will attend indiscriminately to what is proximal, accessible, or automatic (capacity resource theory); and (3) thought suppression, or the focus on what one should *not* attend to, occupies a greater degree of working memory. These effects of stress result in decreased availability of working memory, increased extraneous load, and thus less dedicated attention to intrinsically important information.

The practical implications of these findings occur throughout the clinical environment. Increased stress can be caused by factors ranging from unintended outcomes to high patient load. This increased stress decreases clinicians' attention and working memory resources. This produces an enhanced focus on central cues while potentially disregarding more peripheral information, resulting in cognitive processing errors such as anchor and confirmation bias because not all information is being equally considered. Finally, excessive focus on extraneous aspects of the information (those aspects that are not central to the clinical problem) caused by thought suppression further deplete precious working memory resources.

Environmental factors impact attentional resources as well. The effect of noise on breadth of attention has been extensively studied; noise produces a similar "attention tunneling" effect, diminishing the capacity or resources available for attention or working memory.[12] Noise affects information processing by decreasing signal detection (i.e., the sensitivity of clinical acumen), increasing inefficiency and subsequently error rates, and causing selective attention. Most clinicians are fully aware that noise is a prominent component of the operative and perioperative space with stimuli that include alarms, music, conversations, and possibly other patients. In this sense, noise is an unnecessary source of information that imposes an extraneous cognitive load due to redundancy and that decreases available working memory via attention tunneling.

LOAD SHEDDING

The ability to obtain new information, store that information, and subsequently retrieve it is a critical component of safe and effective patient care. The structure with which information is presented directly affects the efficacy of this process. Information structure includes, in part, the load imparted by the complexity of the information itself, the complexity of the presentation of this information, and the ability to apply order to the information either through internal knowledge, or through external models such as checklists. The environment and the physiological and psychological states of the clinician directly affect the resources that he or she can use to deal with these loads. Modern-day clinical settings include highly complex clinical information, combined with complex and nonstandardized presentation of data to overworked clinicians in noisy and distracting environments.

This high intrinsic/extraneous load is met with degraded resources for working memory caused by stress and environmental effects, often imposing a greater load than the clinician can effectively manage. Excessive cognitive load requires information shedding, intentionally or unintentionally, when the load overwhelms the resources of working memory. Load shedding is an adaptive response and begins in a logical manner with less critical information being shed, but as the level of stress rises, further decreasing working memory resources, shedding becomes more erratic and illogical, ultimately increasing the possibility that critical information is lost.[13]

An alternative strategy is to acknowledge that load shedding occurs, and proactively make a decision to shed less valuable information. This can be facilitated by checklists or delegation, or by deferring less critical tasks. This behavior is often observed in the critical care setting or during cardiac arrests, where less critical tasks are postponed in order to attend to a potentially life-threatening event. Recognizing and formalizing this process, however, can ensure that shedding is a conscious process that minimizes the loss of critical information.

HEALTHCARE AND COGNITIVE LOAD

In comparison to other high-risk industries, such as aviation, healthcare is just beginning to consider concepts such as cognitive load. These concepts are critical, however, as the amount and complexity of information germane to healthcare delivery increases. Understanding the factors that impact data acquisition, cognition, and subsequent performance are key to building systems that facilitate maximal clinician performance. Accepting the facts that physicians have limited attention resources, that those resources are used more aggressively if information presentation is disorganized and nonstandardized, and that fewer resources are available in times of physiologic or psychologic stress is critical to the design of systems that support the most effective critical thinking and thus patient care.

Cognitive load theory suggests that certain clinical environments can create more favorable load-distribution profiles to optimize information acquisition, storage, and integration—key factors in decision-making, learning, and performance. In addition, attention to the environment in which clinicians practice is critical for maximal cognitive performance. This attention must range from the mode and organization of data presentation to the degree of stress imposed on front-line professionals. Cognitive load theory also explains why checklists, routines, and standardization improve patient care by decreasing extraneous load and ensuring the processing of critical information at risk of being lost during unconscious load-shedding activities.

REFERENCES

1. Kahneman D. Attention and effort. *The American Journal of Psychology* 1973;88. doi:10.2307/1421603.
2. Hamilton, V, Warburton DM, Mandler G. Human stress and cognition: an information processing approach. In: Hamilton, Warburton DM, eds. *Thought Processes, Consciousness, and Stress*. New York: John Wiley & Sons; 1979:179–201.
3. Brookhuis KA, de Waard D. The use of psychophysiology to assess driver status. *Ergonomics*. 1993;36(9):1099–1110. doi:10.1080/00140139308967981.
4. Sweller J, Ayres P, Kalyuga S. *Cognitive Load Theory*. 2011;1. doi:10.1007/978-1-4419-8126-4.
5. Sweller J. Human cognitive architecture: why some instructional procedures work and others do not. In: *APA Educational Psychology Handbook, Vol 1: Theories, Constructs, and Critical Issues.*; 2012:295–325. doi:10.1037/13273-011.
6. Geary DC. *The Origin of Mind: Evolution of Brain, Cognition, and General Intelligence*. 2005:307–337. doi:10.1037/10871-009.
7. Geary DC. An evolutionarily informed education science. *Educ Psychol*. 2008;43(February 2014):179–195. doi:10.1080/00461520802392133.
8. Sweller J. Element interactivity and intrinsic, extraneous, and germane cognitive load. *Educ Psychol Rev*. 2010;22(2):123–138. doi:10.1007/s10648-010-9128-5.
9. Sweller J, Sweller S. Natural information processing systems. *Evol Psychol*. 2006;4:434–458.
10. Sweller J. Cognitive load theory. In: Ross B, Mestre J, eds. *The Psychology of Learning and Motivation: Cognition in Education*. Oxford: Academic Press; 2011:37–76.
11. Chajut E, Algom D. Selective attention improves under stress: implications for theories of social cognition. *J Pers Soc Psychol*. 2003;85(2):231–248. doi:10.1037/0022-3514.85.2.231.
12. Broadbent DE. The current state of noise research: reply to Poulton. *Psychol Bull*. 1978;85(C):1052–1067. doi:10.1037/0033-2909.85.5.1052.
13. Staal MA. Stress, cognition, and human performance: a literature review and conceptual framework [Internet]. NASA Technical Memorandum. 2004. http://human-factors.arc.nasa.gov/flightcognition/Publications/IH_054_Staal.pdf\npapers3://publication/uuid/E92DA994-B825-40CA-9E74-A94101F33496.

3

Errors and Violations

ALAN F. MERRY

INTRODUCTION

Civil aviation is often cited as an example of how a systems-based approach within a just culture can lead to high levels of reliability (and therefore safety) in a large-scale, complex undertaking. Contrasts are often drawn between aviation and healthcare, especially in the context of anesthesia. Healthcare, it is often suggested, is characterized by a person-oriented approach and a culture that responds to accidents by focusing on blame rather than learning.

There is some justification for these views, but great strides have been made in recent years within many healthcare organizations toward a just culture[1] committed to systems-based continuous improvement. The impressive reductions in the rates of central line–associated bacteremia that have been achieved, repeatedly, through challenging the status quo and implementing systems-based initiatives to standardize and ensure good practice are but one example.[2,3] Conversely, the airline industry is still prone to failures, albeit infrequently, and these failures typically have much in common with accidents that harm patients in healthcare.

AIR FRANCE FLIGHT 447

This is certainly true of Air France Flight 447, which crashed en route from Rio de Janeiro to Paris, on June 1, 2009.[4] The aircraft was an Airbus A330, designed for a two-pilot crew, but this was to be a 13-hour flight, so a third pilot was on board to comply with crew rest requirements. One of the copilots took the first rest break, and the captain took the second. Apparently, he made a comment indicating that he had had too little sleep on the preceding night. The timing of these shifts meant that this change occurred shortly before the aircraft entered an area of turbulence. The pilot flying the airplane began a climb, presumably to get above the turbulence, although there was no collective decision to do this.

The A330 is designed to "fly by wire" with a high reliance on computers. This approach is intended to improve safety by reducing dependence on human performance. Unfortunately, it seems that the aircraft's pitot tubes (devices used in measuring airspeed) were briefly occluded by ice crystals, which led to an inaccurate airspeed indication, and this caused the autopilot system to disconnect. Pilots usually fly an A330 manually only while taking off or landing, and seldom at high altitude, particularly with airspeed sensors prone to intermittent malfunction because of icing. This was, therefore, an unfamiliar situation. The pilots took over flying in manual mode (so called "alternate law"), but they may not have been fully alert to the possibility that in this mode the aircraft was able to accept control inputs that could cause the wings to stop flying; in normal mode, this would have been impossible. It seems that the two pilots did not coordinate their efforts to manage the situation. In the A330, side stick controls take the place of conventional joysticks, but they do not move together (as joysticks on a Boeing do), so there is little if any visual or tactile feedback from one pilot to the other. It seems that both pilots were active on their sticks at the same time, the one in the left-hand seat trying to exit the stall, and the other pilot still trying to lift the airplane's nose. Under these circumstances, the inputs from the two sticks are summed algebraically, which presumably meant that one input negated the other. An alarm is sounded, but there were several audible alarms over this period, which would have been confusing.

The captain was called back to the cockpit. He did not take over the controls, but instead sat in a second-row seat to oversee the situation. This is consistent with current teaching, as it is with anesthesiologists in crisis management in the operating room (OR). The leader, or coordinator, of a crisis is taught to stand back and reduce cognitive load by allocating practical tasks to others, in order to maintain "situation awareness."

Thus, an essentially functional aircraft had stalled and was falling from the sky while the entire crew tried to figure out what was happening and how to regain control. They each had the necessary technical skills—the primary problem was their failure to understand their situation. In this particular situation, there would have been no sense of falling, and there was an overload of potentially confusing information from their instruments and warning systems. Chillingly, the last recorded words spoken by the captain were, "Damn it, we're going to crash. . . . This can't be happening!" Seconds later, 228 people died.

The principles underlying this disaster are typical of those that often underlie failures in the delivery of health services in general and anesthesia in particular. Years ago, Perrow made the point that in complex systems, failures are, ultimately, inevitable.[5,6] Understanding *how* decisions are made is the key to understanding how such failures occur. The wider context is also relevant: in complex systems, actions can have far-reaching and often unpredictable consequences.

This chapter therefore starts with a discussion of healthcare as a system. Error is intrinsic to human cognitive processes, so error is discussed next and contrasted with violation to introduce the concept of a just culture. The chapter ends with a consideration of general approaches to making healthcare safer.

(Chapter 17 of this volume deals with medication safety, informed by the general principles dealt with in this chapter.)

HARM IN HEALTHCARE

When a commercial airplane crashes, the substantial human and financial loss is self-evident. Jet airliners are expensive, and many lives are lost at once. A prolonged period of adverse publicity follows the accident, with consequent loss of reputation and business for the airline company.

In contrast, the death of a single ill patient in a bed at the back of a hospital ward may not seem unexpected, especially if the patient is sick or elderly: the possibility that the proximal cause of death might be an error may not even be considered. It takes determined advocacy to capture the public's attention, and this is usually a response to clusters of failure—as happened in the Mid Staffordshire Trust Hospital in the United Kingdom.[7] Even if an episode of poor care is recognized as such, patients and their families may be reluctant to complain: after all, they are often vulnerable, dependent upon the system, and lacking in choice. It is only through studies based on the systematic review of large, randomly selected samples of patient charts that the extent of *iatrogenic* harm (harm caused by the healthcare actually intended to help patients) has been appreciated (Table 3.1). It has been suggested that between 50,000 and 98,000 Americans die every year from errors in healthcare,[8] equivalent to three jumbo jets full of passengers crashing every two days.[9]

There are differences in estimates between studies, but these probably relate primarily to the methodological challenges associated with this type of research.[10] Even when an error is identified, its contribution to the patient's outcome is often uncertain. This issue was examined in a study in which board-certified, trained internists reviewed 111 active-care hospital deaths at seven Department of Veterans Affairs medical centers. Almost a quarter of the deaths were rated as at least possibly preventable by optimal care, but it was judged that only 0.5% of these patients would have lived 3 months or more in good cognitive health if care had been

TABLE 3.1. ADVERSE EVENT RATES FROM MEDICAL RECORD REVIEWS

Country in Which the Study Was Done	No. of Records Studied	Adverse Events % of Admissions	Permanent Harm and Death % of Admissions
Australia	14,179	10.6	2.0
America[16]	30,121	3.7	0.5
America	14,565	~10.0	2.0
Canada	3,745	7.5	1.6
Denmark	1,097	9.0	0.4
England	1,014	11.7	1.5
New Zealand	6,579	12.9	1.9

Reproduced and modified with permission from Runciman B, Merry A, Walton M. *Safety and Ethics in Healthcare: A Guide to Getting It Right.* Aldershot, UK: Ashgate; 2007.

optimal. It seems that errors may often accelerate deaths that would have occurred soon, rather than cause deaths in patients expected to recover.[11] These deaths still matter, but in the interest of rigor and objectivity, the jumbo jet analogy should "be qualified by the notion that the passengers would nearly all be of the sort who might be on their way to Lourdes for a 'miracle cure.'"[12] Nevertheless, the words *nearly all* are important. In anesthesia there is a particular risk of unexpected deaths of patients who are young and (essentially) healthy.[13] Also, in contrast to many other deaths in a hospital, attribution tends to seem obvious—in a fatal drug error[14] or a scenario of "can't intubate can't oxygenate" (CICO),[13,15] for example, the anesthesiologist is likely to be seen as directly responsible for the death. The overall message is clear: far too many patients are harmed by the healthcare intended to help them.[16]

Despite the Institute of Medicine's call for a 50% reduction in iatrogenic harm in hospitals in the United States, there have been only sporadic and isolated improvements.[17] Anesthesiologists have been leaders in the advancement of patient safety,[18] with initiatives that have included (among others) the early adoption of "Normal Accident Theory,"[19] reporting and learning from incidents,[20,21] simulation in teaching and research,[22–25] and the establishment of the Anesthesia Patient Safety Foundation (APSF) in 1985[26] with the mission to "ensure that no patient is harmed by anesthesia."

If we are to achieve this mission, we need to know not only how often things go wrong

in healthcare, but also why. Our primary aim is the safety of our patients, but justice is also important. Blame should not unreasonably be assigned to competent practitioners trying to do the right thing simply because the outcome was both unexpected and tragic.[1,27,28]

SAFETY I, SAFETY II, OR SAFETY^N?

Many anesthesiologists must, by now, know the basic categories of error outlined by James Reason[29] and the *Swiss Cheese* model of accidental harm.[30] More recently, less emphasis has been placed on understanding failure and more on learning from examples of success (the terms "Safety I" and "Safety II" have been used in this context).[31,32] To the extent possible, it is obviously better to anticipate and prevent accidents (e.g., with approaches such as *failure mode effect analysis*) than to rely on analyzing what went wrong after the event.

In reality, however, the problem of iatrogenic harm is not homogenous, and the challenge of improving safety in healthcare is substantial. For example, drug administration errors by anesthesiologists are quite different from failures by psychiatrists in the prediction of which patients are going to commit suicide. Even in the operating room, the way in which a cardiac surgeon might inadvertently tear an aorta differs from the way in which an anesthesiologist might accidentally (and unknowingly) contribute to postoperative infection of the surgical site.[33] The solutions are not the same, and top-down global initiatives are unlikely to be effective. Instead, the need is for every healthcare professional to work with his or her immediate colleagues on improving their particular area of responsibility, using all available approaches. Reviewing and learning from mistakes is necessary,[34,35] and so is proactive analysis leading to initiatives to maximize desired outcomes safely.[32] Perhaps one should call for "Safety"—a multifaceted approach to improvement in a very large number of contexts.

Measurement and the Goal of the Perioperative Team

Measurement is widely held to be essential for the improvement of quality in healthcare (and other activities), and the generic framework of structure, process, and outcome is well known.[36] It can, however, be difficult to know precisely what to measure. Safety II advocates have a good point: in surgery and anesthesia, it is arguable that the primary aim should not be the reduction of error, or even safety, although both are important: it should be to work within a team toward the common goal of achieving a satisfactory outcome for as many patients as possible from the conditions for which surgery and the associated perioperative care are offered.

One important form of error is to undertake operations in patients for whom the operation is, on balance, not indicated. This is called *overutilization*. Overutilization implies treatment that is inherently ineffective or that fails to adequately address a significant problem for the patient.[37] Overutilization represents an opportunity cost, which, because of limited healthcare resources, may limit services available for other patients.[38] It also represents an unnecessary risk: if an error results in avoidable harm during an unnecessary procedure, then the primary cause of that harm is the decision to provide the unwarranted treatment.

Another form of error is to deny or unreasonably delay operations in patients for whom effective surgery is needed and wanted. This is called *underutilization*, and it is a major problem,[39,40] with many healthcare services overwhelmed by sick or injured patients. Many of these need surgery, for which they also need safe anesthesia.[41] Even in high-income regions,

unreasonable delays in surgery can create risk or prevent the best outcome. Ensuring adequate and timely access to anesthesia and surgery should not, however, be accomplished by taking shortcuts or compromising safety.

There may be an optimal point in a complex function relating benefit to the competing demands for resources. This function would have several potentially measurable outputs, of which the primary would be the number of patients returned to the community with an improved quality of life.[42] Minimizing mortality from anesthesia is very important, but for many operations, mortality rates are too low to compare institutions or monitor progress over time. Moreover, the effect of differences in case-mix can be difficult to eliminate. Mortality rates of certain relatively standardized and high-risk operations (e.g., coronary artery bypass grafting), however, can sometimes be used as an index of overall quality and safety.[32,43] There is increasing evidence that smaller adverse events also matter,[44] but measuring their rate is difficult and expensive.[32] Furthermore, excessive concern over eliminating error may be counterproductive.

Consider, for example, a patient with dissection of the aorta who requires emergency surgery. It is probably impossible to treat such a person without any errors because there are too many challenges and significant time pressure. The goal is to end up with a live patient who has a repaired aorta and an intact central nervous system and (ideally) working kidneys and who can go home and continue to lead a useful life. If the aorta is accidentally torn, but successfully repaired, or an incorrect drug is given but the mistake identified and addressed, these errors only matter to the extent that they make the goal somewhat harder to achieve.[44] Greater harm would result if the surgeon were inappropriately reluctant to do the operation, or if the anesthesiologist were too preoccupied with errors to administer drugs when they were needed. Decisions must be made, often under limitations of time and other resources, and a mix of expertise, skill, judgment, courage, and care is required.

Part of the required judgment lies in allocating patients between alternative management options, which may include surgery, stenting, or perhaps no intervention at all. Errors in decisions at this level are important, so the denominator should include all patients who present with the problem, not just those who are treated surgically.

The Triple Aim and the Elements of Quality in Healthcare

In the United States, The Institute of Healthcare Improvement has articulated a "Triple Aim" for healthcare:[45,46] improving the patient experience (including safety, quality, and satisfaction); improving the health of the population; and reducing the per capita cost of healthcare. In order to achieve these three goals simultaneously, it is necessary to do things right the first time and to do the right things. The latter requires evidence, which is often missing or difficult to interpret. The recent emphasis in anesthesiology on large trials that provide reliable guidance on simple and important aspects of practice are therefore important contributions to safety.[47–49]

Traditional views on what constitutes harm to patients may have been too limited.[37] In the United States, the Institute of Medicine has defined quality in healthcare as depending not just on safety but also on timeliness, efficiency, efficacy, equitability, and patient-centeredness (represented by the acronym STEEEP).[50] It seems artificial to isolate safety from any of the other elements of quality in healthcare. For example, care that is not efficacious or timely cannot be considered to be safe.

Variation in the Provision of Healthcare

There is substantial variation in the healthcare provided to patients both within countries (including the United States)[51–53] and between countries.[54] The value of standardization in improving reliability and safety has long been recognized in other industries, notably aviation. Standardization of practice in anesthesia does not imply "dumbing down" or imposing a "cookbook" mentality. Variation is appropriate in response to differing needs of individual patients with differing combinations of medical problems (i.e., comorbidities) and differing wants and values. Much of the variation in healthcare, however, is driven by differences between practitioners and institutions in their beliefs and approaches to common problems, rather than by differences between patients.

Fisher and Wennberg[55] identify three categories of medical services. *Effective care* should be received by all patients, but underutilization is common in this category. Although countries differ in their resources, in wealthy countries (including the United States), the best patient outcomes are not always associated with the highest levels of healthcare expenditure. *Preference-sensitive* care is characteristic of treatments of uncertain value, and requires individual judgment. Patients wish to be well informed and to exercise choice in regard to such treatments, but choices typically reflect the preferences of physicians, rather than those of patients.[56] *Supply-sensitive* care includes newly introduced technology. Patients may be harmed during the learning curves associated with the introduction of new treatments, and treatments may be widely adopted before there is sufficient evidence of value.[57] This often reflects undue enthusiasm and optimism bias (see discussion later in this chapter) by physicians and is often associated with overutilization.

SYSTEMS AND COMPLEXITY

Perrow describes systems as having two dimensions.[5] *Coupling* describes the relationship between an action and its consequences. Many aspects of anesthesia are tightly coupled with outcome (see Chapter 17, Box 17.2), while in other aspects the coupling is looser.

Complexity is the second dimension. Processes and systems can be simple, complicated, or complex.[58] It is possible to describe the steps involved in both simple and complicated processes and to provide a prescription for successfully completing the process. After the process has been described successfully, the same approach can be relied upon to produce success again and again unless error intervenes. It is arguable that flying an airplane from Rio de Janeiro to Paris is a complicated process that occurs within a complex system.

It is not possible to describe a complex process in a way that will reliably produce repeatable results. Raising children is an example of a complex process: an approach that has succeeded with one child may not work with another. According to Perrow, the combination of complexity with tight coupling makes accidents ultimately inevitable, so he coined the term "normal accidents."[5]

The concept of *normal accidents* requires consideration of the balance between the extent of harm if an accident happens and the value placed on the activity by society. The fact that patients are human and infinitely variable places the process of anesthesia in the "high complexity, high coupling" quadrant of the two-dimensional grid representing these considerations. For an individual patient, the potential consequences of an accident are catastrophic, but the social value of anesthesia is high. In the past, accidents were accepted as a cost of the benefits of anesthesia, and did not necessarily imply negligence on the part of the anesthesiologist. The imperative to make anesthesia as safe as possible is very high, however, and serious accidents are now so infrequent that they are no longer viewed as "normal." In fact, they still are, and notwithstanding that the worthy aim of the APSF should be pursued vigorously, it is impossible to eliminate all accidents.

Webster has defined *a system* as "any collection of two or more interacting parts, and as complex if the number of possible interactions is such that predicting its long term behavior on the basis of knowledge of its component parts becomes difficult or impossible."[59]

Complex systems are often referred to as chaotic. This does not imply that they are random, but rather that their behavior cannot be predicted more than a short time into the future. For example, weather predictions are often fairly accurate for a day or two, but after that it is necessary to make new predictions with a renewed set of baseline data. Healthcare is a complex system, and anesthesia is a complex process within healthcare. With a complex process or in a complex system such as anesthesia, it is necessary to repeatedly re-evaluate the situation and reset the direction of travel. The way humans respond to their environment and make decisions is superbly adapted to success in managing complexity, but these human strengths also lead, occasionally, to error.

THE NATURE OF ERRORS
Flight 447 illustrates the key attributes of human errors perfectly.

Errors Are Unintentional
The first attribute of errors is that they are unintentional, and do not represent carelessness. This is the fundamental distinction between errors and violations (see discussion later in this chapter). It is reasonable to assume, for example, that the pilots of Flight 447 intended to do the right things and cared very much about their decisions and actions. Yet they made mistakes. It follows that the threat of punishment is unlikely to deter people from making errors: if the prospect of crashing into the ocean and dying cannot do so, neither will threats of legal consequences.

Errors and Outcome Are Not Related
The process of making and acting on a decision (consciously or unconsciously) should not be judged on the basis of its outcome. Failure can follow a sound decision, while many errors have little impact, and some even result in a better outcome than would otherwise have occurred (Box 3.2).

Unfortunately, the tendency for outcome to drive the judgment of process is almost overwhelming. For example, many drug errors are without consequence,[60] but occasionally the consequences may be catastrophic. There is no cognitive or moral difference between harmless drug errors and harmful ones; differences in outcome are usually attributable to chance. The tendency, however, is to respond punitively (sometimes by criminal prosecution[61]) to those with bad outcomes and to do little or nothing about the others. It is the outcome rather than the decision or the act that is being used to determine culpability. Had the pilots of Flight 447 managed to regain control before crashing, it is unlikely that errors made before saving the situation would have been subject to the same level of investigation as they were after 228 lives had been lost.

BOX 3.1   INFORMATION AVAILABLE TO AN ANESTHESIOLOGIST MAKING A DECISION ABOUT A PATIENT: THE POTENTIAL KNOWLEDGE BASE

(A) Information contemporaneously available
    (I) Information in the mind of others
        The mind of the patient
        The minds of the patient's family and other supporters
        The minds of other members of the operating room team (and other colleagues)
    (II) Information in the world
        Physical—the patient's physical signs and other information in the environment (the anesthesia machine and the drug trolley, for example) that can be examined or inspected
        Written or recorded—in various printed and electronic resources (notably, patient records, databases, reference books or websites)
(B) Information stored in the anesthesiologists' mind, previously acquired through training, study, and experience—the anesthesiologists' *expert knowledge*

Note: This list is illustrative rather than exhaustive.

Reprinted by permission from Information available to the health professional. In Runciman B, Merry A, Walton M, Safety and Ethics in Healthcare: A Guide to Getting it Right. *Farnham: Ashgate, 2007, p. 113.*

All errors, including harmless errors, should be reviewed, as should "near misses" - errors that were almost made, but were "caught" in time. The airline industry is more proactive in reporting and learning from events of this type than is the healthcare industry. Notwithstanding the pioneering work of Cooper[62] and Runciman[63] on promoting incident reporting for learning in anesthesia, it is unusual in healthcare for errors that cause little or no harm to be reported or investigated. Even serious events are unlikely to be investigated as thoroughly as an airline accident, although some programs in healthcare have been established that at least seek to report such events openly, and to learn from them.

Definition of Error

An *error* occurs "when someone is trying to do the right thing, but actually does the wrong thing." A more formal definition of error is "the unintentional use of a wrong plan to achieve an aim, or failure to carry out a planned action as intended".[64] Others have provided different definitions of *error*,[29] which may be nuanced, and may reflect different contexts. The definition given here has the advantage of explicitly

stating that error is unintentional, and of focusing on processes (decisions and actions) rather than outcomes—important points in the context of promoting a just culture.

Decisions and Actions

If errors do not represent carelessness, then why do they occur? Errors are manifested through actions. In this context, inaction (e.g., failing to take a necessary action) can be construed as a type of action. Actions are, in general, the manifestation of human decisions, which may be conscious or unconscious. An understanding of how humans make decisions is, therefore, the key to understanding errors.

"FAST" AND "SLOW" THINKING: SYSTEM I AND SYSTEM II

The way humans make decisions is thought to involve two systems, or types, of cognitive process: System I is fast and automatic and operates primarily through pattern recognition, while System II is slow and effortful and seeks to work things out logically[65–68] (see Table 3.2). Humans default to System I thinking but have

TABLE 3.2. THE TWO SYSTEMS BY WHICH WE THINK

System I Fast and Automatic	System II Slow and Reflective
• Effortless	• Effortful
• Fast	• Slow
• Associative and interactional	• Deductive and analytical
• Unconscious	• Self-aware
• Rule-based—in the sense of rules stored in memory as schemata	• Knowledge-based (but uses rules)
• Feedforward	• Feedback
• Acquisition by biology, exposure and personal experience	• Acquisition by cultural and formal tuition

Modified from Kahneman D. *Thinking, Fast and Slow.* London: Penguin Books; 2011.
With reference also to Thaler and Sunstein 2008,[56] Stanovich and West 2000,[67] Klein 1999,[68] and Reason.[29]

the capacity to monitor and moderate System I thinking by System II thinking. For example, anesthesiologists work in a complex and dynamic context, and must make a series of related decisions in quick succession. Many of these decisions involve System I thinking, but these decisions are typically monitored and moderated using System II thinking, in real time. It is probably more helpful to think about a continuum than a dichotomous divide, with each decision involving elements of each system of thinking to a varying degree.

Klein[68] has provided important insights into how decisions are made in crises by taking his research out of the laboratory into the field. System I thinking tends to predominate in the heat of a crisis. This makes sense, because there is little time for slow, methodical thinking. Successful decisions under intense time pressure are characterized by experts' capacity to recognize certain key elements in a situation and then match these to conceptually equivalent situations that were seen before. Their response is then informed by that previous experience, for example, by knowing that a particular approach did or did not work on that occasion. This implies that there is no substitute for experience in occupations that involve crises (including anesthesia). One of the paradoxes of anesthesia is that many hours of monitoring routine cases do not build up experience in dealing with rare crises. Reason has described this as "the catch-22 of human

supervisory control."[29] Thus in making decisions, even in crises, many anesthesiologists must call on education, training (including simulation-based training), and logical reasoning as well as experience, and their experience of similar crises may be very limited. Few anesthesiologists, for example, have gained real-life experience in obtaining an emergency surgical airway in a CICO situation: if a CICO situation does occur, it is likely to be the first time for the anesthesiologist concerned (as the situation was for the pilots on Flight 447). Thus simulation is particularly important in training anesthesiologists (as it is for pilots) because it can go a considerable distance toward providing an effective substitute for actual experiences of rare crises.

MENTAL MODELS, SCHEMATA, AND FRAMES OF REFERENCE

All decisions are made on the basis of one's *understanding* of a given situation. People gather information by seeing, feeling, smelling, and hearing; by speaking with other people; or by reviewing written or recorded material. They then integrate this contemporaneously acquired information with their *expert knowledge*, previously gained through various forms of learning, including context-relevant experience, to create conceptual *mental models* of their situation. Any decisions (i.e., whether and how to act) are made on the basis of these mental models.

The idea of mental models is broadly consistent with those of *schemata*[29] and *frames of reference*,[69] both of which are discussed in the following text. These terms are all used to convey the point that humans interpret their surroundings, and their interactions with others, through mental representations that are conceptual and interpretive in nature.

Bounded Rationality

Many sources of information are available from which to develop a mental model to use in making a decision (Box 3.1). However, it would be unusual for all available knowledge to be accessed accurately at the time that it was needed, particularly in a dynamic context such as the practice of anesthesia. There are typically gaps in knowledge, which may, or may not, be important for making the right decision.

This phenomenon is known as "bounded rationality."[29] This concept is best explained by an analogy. A blackboard in a dark room has a coherent message printed in letters arranged in several rows. Shining a flashlight on the board might illuminate a circular area including segments of two or three consecutive rows, revealing a subset of letters that do not typically convey the overall meaning of the message. There might be enough information to make a good guess, or there might not be. The illuminated letters might be completely uninformative, or they might, through coincidence, suggest a meaning that is misleading. As more of the blackboard is revealed, more information is obtained, increasing the chance of interpreting the message correctly.

Filtration and Interpretation: Signals and Noise

Humans are continuously bombarded with an overwhelming number of sensory inputs. Much of the available information contributes little to actual meaning, so this mass of inputs must be filtered and interpreted. For example, the exact number of people listening to a lecture is usually of little importance to the lecturer, as is the color of the wallpaper, the structure of the ceiling, and many other details. What matters is that there is an audience, that the attendees are listening to the lecture, that time is running short, and so on. The approximate size of the audience may be relevant and is easily judged and incorporated into a mental model. If the lecturer suddenly needed to know the exact number of people for some reason, he or she could easily count them because this information is readily available "in the world." It can be accessed if needed, but is usually not necessary. Details of this type are like interference, or "noise," in a signal. The underlying pattern is important and must be recognized within an overall pattern. Filtration and interpretation must therefore be used to develop a mental model. Perrow has provided graphic examples of how incomplete or imperfect mental models have sometimes contributed to collisions between ships at sea that would otherwise seem inexplicable.[6]

The Knowledge Base

Information that is accessed in a particular situation can be thought of as the *knowledge base* from which a decision is made. A mental model differs from the knowledge base in that the former is an interpretation of the latter.

Ironic Effects of the Mental Control of Action

Even when a person's expert knowledge includes the requisite information, it may or may not be accessed when a decision is made. It is not always possible to recall every fact at the precise moment it is needed. For example, some people tend to "block" when introducing an acquaintance; they may be completely unable to recall a name when they need to. This does not necessarily mean that they don't know their acquaintance's name. Later, when they have relaxed and moved on to other matters, the name may be recalled spontaneously.

Blocking in this way is part of a wider problem—the "ironic effects of the mental control of action."[70] Wegner et al. have conducted experiments that show, in essence, that strict instructions to avoid a particular outcome (overshooting the hole on a golf putt, for example) may actually make that outcome more likely, particularly under conditions of mental loading. These observations add support to the fundamental point that it is not possible to avoid errors simply by trying harder.

Swiss Cheese

The well-known *Swiss cheese model*, described by James Reason,[30] indicates that most systems have multiple defenses, depicted as slices of cheese. Each defense typically has several weaknesses, called latent factors, depicted as holes in the slices of cheese. In this model, accidents develop along a trajectory that traverses these defenses by penetrating their weaknesses. Even if some defenses are breached, others will usually interrupt the process of the accident before serious harm occurs. Occasionally, however, the holes line up, and the trajectory of the accident traverses all defenses and causes harm.

The Influence of Quantity and Stress on Error

Rudolph and Repenning have added a further insight into the genesis of disasters (see Figure 3.1).[71] Managing a dynamic process in a complex system, such as anesthetizing a patient in an OR within a hospital, often requires responses to a stream of interruptions, a few of which may be novel in nature. However, even non-novel interruptions vary in their urgency, importance, and complexity. Rudolph and Repenning propose a stock of pending interruptions. Its size depends upon the balance between the rates at which new interruptions are added and existing ones are resolved. Many individual interruptions could be dealt with by System I thinking, but ongoing resolution of the stream of interruptions requires three types of processes: attention processes to decide which interruptions warrant a response, activation processes to mobilize the knowledge required to respond to them, and strategic processes to prioritize the issues. In short, at least some degree of System II thinking is required to monitor and moderate System I responses to the interruptions. The arrival of a novel interruption increases the requirement of System II thinking because it would not be possible to have a stored response in memory for automatic application, learned from prior experience.

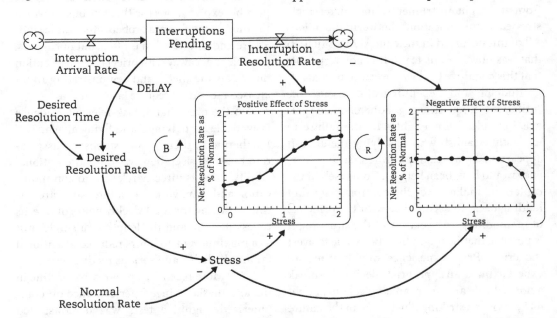

FIGURE 3.1: The role of quantity in relation to interruptions in the genesis of a disaster: in a dynamic situation, a stream of interruptions contributes to a stock of issues pending resolution at a rate influenced by stress; see text for a fuller explanation.

Reprinted from Rudolph JW, Repenning NP, Disaster dynamics: understanding the role of quantity in organizational collapse. *Adm Sci Q.* 2002;47:1–30, p. 11, with permission of SAGE Publications.

The Yerkes-Dodson curve[72] depicts the relationship between stress and performance. It suggests that increasing levels of stress initially improve performance, but after a certain point this effect plateaus, and thereafter further increases in stress impair performance. As the rate of interruptions increases, therefore, the initial response might be an improvement in performance that permits an increased rate of resolution of interruptions. The stock of interruptions pending attention may be maintained at an acceptable limit, or even may be decreased. At a certain point, however, increasing stress causes a possibly precipitous decrease in performance, and the rate of resolution will decrease. At this point, the system may suddenly become irretrievably unstable because of the combination of increasing demands and diminishing capability to deal with them.

The descriptions of the events in the cockpit of Flight 447 suggest exactly this type of scenario. Over a short period of time (the descent took less than 4 minutes), multiple interruptions included turbulence, various warnings that came on and went off, confusing information from the flight instruments, and increasingly stressed communications between the pilots. All of this occurred in the context of a situation that was novel to this team. It is not surprising that this cognitive load was overwhelming.

Rudolph and Repenning also discuss the "utility of unquestioning adherence to pre-existing rules." On Flight 447, the failure to explicitly establish who was flying the aircraft appears to be an example where such adherence would have been helpful. Conversely, if the captain had taken over the controls instead of holding back, in accordance with the principle of maintaining an overview of the situation, it is possible that he might have been able to avert the crisis. Prior experience might prime an expert to make an appropriate decision to break a normal rule and apply an atypical one. Flight 447 provides a striking illustration of the nature of a crisis: in effect, a crisis is a situation in which one has run out of effective rules and does not have the time to work things out using System II cognitive processes. Anesthesiologists faced with CICO situations will readily understand this point: these situations require rapid, pre-learned, rule-based responses.

The Role of Fatigue

It is generally accepted that fatigue impairs performance. Members of the public recognize this, and when surveyed, have indicated that they would request a different doctor if their surgeon had been awake for more than 24 hours.[73] Impairment equivalent to that seen with a blood alcohol of 0.05% has been demonstrated after just 17 hours of wakefulness.[74] Various healthcare organizations have implemented policies or statements on fatigue.[75,76] In this context, however, performance is often measured using vigilance tests, such as the psychomotor vigilance task (PVT), which may not be relevant to the practice of anesthesia or surgery, particularly in the presence of stimulants that include endogenous epinephrine as well as caffeine and other drugs.[77] In simulation-based research, 25 hours of wakefulness were associated with no difference in the clinical performance of anesthesia residents despite impairment in PVT, mood, and subjective sleepiness.[78] There are several possible explanations for this finding, of which the most compelling is probably that these studies are underpowered. It is often, but not always, possible to get away with brief lapses in attention during an anesthetic, and demonstrating an increased risk might require larger studies.

On the other hand, task-relevant evidence is available for driving[79] and flying airplanes.[80] Furthermore, there is an established association between sleep deprivation and emotional lability[81] that is directly relevant to communication and teamwork. In an intensive care setting, reducing the total weekly hours of interns to less than 80 and the length of a single shift to a maximum of 16 hours reduced attentional failures by half[82] and serious medical errors by 35.9%.[83] More recently, a progressive decline in the anesthesia trainees' performance on computerized cognitive tests was demonstrated over a week of successive night shifts.[84] There are also risks to physicians themselves associated with fatigue, in relation to the potential for road traffic accidents[85] and a decline in overall health.[86]

Managing fatigue is difficult. Factors such as circadian phase, prior sleep duration, and general ill health influence performance,[87] while curtailing work hours may adversely affect continuity of care and the acquisition and maintenance of expertise.[88] The aviation industry is far more sophisticated than most anesthesia practices; work hours are regulated, and scheduled napping is commonly used as a fatigue counter-measure.[89,90]

Although there were three pilots aboard Flight 447 and the idea of rest breaks was reasonable, the decision of the captain to leave the flight deck just before the airplane entered an area of severe turbulence, leaving the airplane to the two more junior pilots, might be thought to raise questions about judgment. Furthermore, it seems that he may have had inadequate sleep on the preceding night.[91] This phenomenon is not unknown among junior medical staff. Sleep loss away from work due to social activities or family responsibilities is common and may offset initiatives to limit work hours. Senior physicians often work excessively long hours. It is not possible to give firm rules, but there are situations (managing a long and difficult acute case, for example) where continuing to work when fatigued may be justified and other, more routine, situations when it is not.

Mental Models and Teams

Perioperative care is provided by teams who must coordinate their actions in order to achieve a desirable outcome. This requires that the mental models of the individual members overlap to some extent. In the OR, the mental models of the surgeon, the anesthesiologist, the scrub nurse, and the circulating nurse may be considered as partially overlapping circles. It is unreasonable to expect all the circles to overlap completely, but each individual's mental model must contain the key facts needed for completing the team's agreed-upon objective successfully. Furthermore, there should be the same understanding of those facts—the mental models need to be shared, at least to some extent, and certainly with respect to a common objective. For some facts, it may suffice if the partial intersects of certain combinations of individuals contain

the key points that they need to know (e.g., the surgeon and the anesthesiologist must know which antibiotic should be given and when, or the surgeon, scrub nurse, and circulating nurse must know which instruments will be needed).

An important source of error in the OR is a deficiency in the information base (and hence the mental model) of a single team member (e.g., the surgeon) that could have been addressed through communication with another member. In the setting of wrong-site surgery, for example, someone is commonly found to have recognized this mistake as it was evolving. It is important to foster a culture in which communication is seen as everyone's responsibility and in which all members of the team feel free to speak up if concerned.

Frames of Reference and Emotions

The emotional response to a colleague's action or words will also reflect the interpretation (or mental model) of what has been said rather than what was actually said, or was intended to be said (all three may be different). An understanding of the other person's *frame of reference*, in effect the mental model from which he or she acted or spoke, may completely change one's emotional response to the personal interaction in addition to the understanding of the situation.[69]

Talking "at cross-purposes" because of differences in mental models is itself a type of error and is very important in teamwork. A team member who becomes upset or angry because of a misunderstanding may tunnel his or her attention, lose situation awareness, and ultimately experience a reduction in capacity to function.

Pattern Recognition, Thinking, and Decisions

James Reason has provided a thorough exposition of the ways in which errors are made.[29,30,92] In essence, he emphasized that humans are avid pattern recognizers. They excel at extracting the key features of a situation from a mass of facts (many of which are just "noise"), formulating a pattern, and then matching it to stored patterns (schemata) of situations that they have encountered in the past. Humans also store responses (as schemata) to situations encountered in the past, which have been successful or unsuccessful to varying degrees.

For example, a man might put on a shoe, and recognize that the laces need to be tied. The process of tying the laces would typically be stored in its entirety, as a single, moderately complicated, schema. Most men can put on their shoes and tie the shoelaces unconsciously, perhaps having a conversation or thinking about the day's schedule while doing this task. If asked subsequently, they may have difficulty recalling either the decision to tie the laces or the act of tying them. If interrupted during the process, they would probably have to start again from the beginning. Experts drive cars in this way, automatically, even in traffic—often listening to the radio and having a conversation at the same time. These stored responses may be simple or complicated. They are mostly learned, but some are primarily instinctive (Box 3.2), and can be modified through experience or training.

CLASSIFYING ERRORS

There are several approaches to the classification of errors. In his *general error modeling system*, Reason distinguishes between *slips, lapses*, and *mistakes*.[29] He divides mistakes into *rule-based* errors and *knowledge-based* errors.

Slips and Lapses: Distractions at Decision Nodes

Slips and lapses[29] occur during automatic behavior (like tying shoelaces or driving a car). They are particularly likely when one makes a change from a well-established routine. Classic examples come from everyday things like giving up sugar in one's tea; the chances of adding sugar inadvertently at least once over the ensuing days are so high as to make this error almost inevitable (see also Box 3.3). Errors are not random—they are predictable, at least statistically.

Slips and lapses typically occur at decision nodes in complex patterns of activity. For example, consider an anesthesiologist who has worked at one hospital for many years and then moves to another. The route is mostly the same, but two-thirds of the way there a new turn must

be made, and a new route is then followed for the rest of the trip. For many years she has driven to work on "automatic," not thinking about where to turn. By concentrating, she successfully drives to the new hospital for several days. Then she begins to relax. One morning she reverts to automatic mode, which works well for the first two-thirds of the journey (the most familiar two-thirds). When she comes to the critical intersection (the decision node) she is distracted, either momentarily by some external event, or more generally by ongoing preoccupation—perhaps with listening to the radio, talking to a passenger, or just inner thoughts. She ends up following the old route "on automatic" and arriving at her former place of work, puzzled, not knowing how she got there. It is easy to see that similar things can occur during the administration of an anesthetic. For example, many doses of prophylactic antibiotic will have been forgotten because of distractions at the critical time in relatively routine anesthetics (see Box 3.4).

Understanding the nature of slips and lapses facilitates the design of initiatives to decrease their likelihood. One example would be the use of the World Health Organization Safe Surgery Checklist (SSC) to ensure that antibiotics have been given before the incision is made (Box 3.4). It is the forced break in the automatic behavior that is important—for the Checklist to work, everyone needs to stop following his or her automatic pattern of System I thinking and engage System II thinking on the itemized matters.

Rule-Based Errors

Rule-based errors[29] occur during System I thinking, which involves the fast, effortless, feed-forward pattern-recognition processes that humans strongly prefer. Most decisions are primarily rule based, particularly in an activity such as anesthesia, which requires that decisions be made rapidly, under pressure of time.

Errors of this type occur in several ways, and many are the result of poor rules. Poor rules may have a variety of causes. For example, they may have been learned from experience through *frequency gambling*. Frequency

BOX 3.2   TO RUN OR NOT TO RUN: DECISIONS AND OUTCOMES

The instinctive response for most people, on encountering a lion in the wild (as one might when visiting certain game parks in Africa), could be summarized by one word: "run."

This would be a simple rule-based response.

Apparently running is not a good idea: it increases the likelihood of being identified as escaping food, which, given that lions can sprint faster than humans, will tend to promote a bad outcome. Running would therefore be a rule-based error, reflecting a poor rule.

On entering a game park, one might be instructed not to run on encountering a lion, but to freeze. Additional advice (available from multiple sources online) includes shouting loudly, trying to make yourself look bigger than you are, and being prepared to hit the lion with whatever you have to hand if it actually charges you.

Armed with this information, and confronted by a lion, the "run" rule would, in all probability, still come to the fore, through System I, as "strong." The recently acquired information would now allow it to be identified as "wrong" via System II. Some tension might be involved in moderating the intuitive, automatic, and strong desire to run. There would be a fair chance that the strong rule would simply overwhelm System II thinking. Alternatively, one might decide, consciously, to back one's primal instincts—after all, how much weight should one give to advice untested in personal experience? On a particular occasion, running might just work out well, and freezing might not.

An expert, a game ranger perhaps, through many formal and informal (e.g., conversations) educational experiences, and perhaps several actual experiences in which the rule worked, might in the end completely replace the old rule with the new one. For the expert, recognizing a lion would then produce the System I response: "freeze," more or less automatically. Any System II thinking would simply reinforce the System I rule. This would be a good decision, predominantly but not entirely rule-based.

Expertise is largely about building up an extensive store of learned situations linked to good responses to those situations and, ideally, backed up with theoretical constructs supported by empirical data. Reliable empirical evidence is not always available. In relation to lion encounters, published, peer-reviewed data seem to be sparse, and randomized controlled trials completely absent.

Unfortunately many rules are not totally reliable. The ranger might eventually end up being eaten. That does not mean that it was an error to "freeze." The test is, if a person reviewing the tragedy had been placed in the same circumstances without the benefit of hindsight, would his or her recommendation have been to freeze rather than to run? This is also called the substitution test (see Figure 3.2). Freezing is not a mistake—it just doesn't work on every occasion. Also, when reviewing a disaster of this type, it must be remembered that the ranger might have been eaten either way: lions in the wild are very dangerous, and the most important rule is to avoid them.

Many comparable situations arise in anesthesia. For example, a common and terrifying situation of "can't intubate can't oxygenate" can arise after inducing anesthesia and attempting to establish spontaneous ventilation. Intuitively, and even on first principles, letting the patient awaken may well seem to be the safest option. It turns out, empirically, that this is often unsuccessful, and that a better strategy is to administer a short-acting muscle relaxant to provide optimal conditions for face-mask ventilation of the lungs and for intubation of the trachea.[93] This will not always save the day, but it usually will. Giving a short-acting relaxant in these circumstances should not be construed as an error even if the outcome is bad—the empirical data and expert consensus support this as the course of action most likely to succeed. Conversely, to choose to let the patient awaken should now generally be construed as a mistake, even if this decision happens to works out well on a particular occasion.

Unfortunately, it is hard to argue with success, and difficult to justify failure, so clear thinking is required if actions are to be evaluated on their merit rather than on the strength of their consequences.

BOX 3.3   LAPSES AND DEFICIENCIES IN THE KNOWLEDGE BASE

On a recent overseas flight, I placed a tube of sunscreen together with toothpaste in a tube of similar appearance in the small plastic bag required for airport security checks, and subsequently, in my hotel with my mind on other matters, used it to brush my teeth—at least until stopped short by the cue of the unexpected and unpleasant flavor.

This error had classic features of a lapse—it involved distraction during an automatic activity that was completely unconscious. However, a major factor was the similarity of appearance of the two tubes. In other words, there was nothing wrong with the decision to brush my teeth but the knowledge base used (unconsciously) in selecting the toothpaste was flawed. One tends to see what one expects to see. This is in contrast to the classic error of putting sugar into tea after giving up this practice. In these lapses, the right substance is chosen (there is no deficit in the knowledge base), but the fundamental decision to use the substance is no longer appropriate.

Many drug errors are slips or lapses. Placing "look-alike sound-alike" drugs in close proximity to each other makes a drug administration error (equivalent to the toothpaste error) much more likely. Removing the visual and tactile cues of conventional yokes in an airline cockpit may also create risk an unconscious error in which the fundamental problem is actually in the knowledge base (on Flight 447, each pilot was probably unaware that the other was using the side stick, notwithstanding the alarm, which might well have been misinterpreted because several other alarms were sounding).

The systems-based solution to errors of this type lies in providing better clues or technology (it should not be possible to use both side sticks at the same time). At a personal level (systems are hard to change), it is helpful to separate substances of similar appearance.

---

gambling is sometimes encouraged in medical training, through aphorisms like "hoof sounds are more likely to indicate a horse than a zebra." This technique usually works, which tends to reinforce the rule; repeated positive experiences decrease concern over the remote possibility that a "zebra" might eventually turn up. Failing to eliminate less frequent but potentially lethal options in a crisis may result in a fatal outcome. More rational, algorithmic approaches are needed, which require System II thinking.

Rules tend to be perceived as *strong* if the experiences associated with them were emotionally charged and/or recent, and humans are emotive rather than Boolean in their approach to making decisions. For example, a personal experience of an anaphylactic reaction

---

BOX 3.4   A CHECKLIST THAT FAILED TO STOP A LAPSE

A small single-specialty hospital chose not to include the check that antibiotics had been given in their local implementation of the WHO SSC because the vast majority of the procedures done in this institution do not require antibiotics. One day, a cochlear implant, for which prophylactic antibiotics are required, was scheduled. At the time the antibiotic should have been given, however, all concerned (including the anesthesiologist) were distracted and reverted to the familiar routine in that hospital. This was a classic lapse. The SSC failed to prevent it because the requisite check had been removed. No harm ensued, but the incident was reported and reviewed, and a decision was made to reinstate this check. No further failures of this type have been reported. It would be more logical to remove this check in ORs where every patient receives an antibiotic because universal administration of antibiotics does not require a reminder.

to rocuronium might make one reluctant to use the same agent again, even though the risk of doing so is unchanged. It is very difficult to understand risk when small numbers are involved; risks of 1 in 1000 and 1 in 1,000,000 both seem remote. These difficulties are compounded by the fact that accurate data on infrequent risks are hard to come by, but even when data are available, figures do not tend to influence the adoption of a rule to the extent that a recent frightening experience would. Rules are much preferred to thinking from first principles, stories are more compelling than statistics, and personal experience is more compelling still.

Bias

Bias is defined as "prejudice in favor of or against one thing, person, or group compared with another." Biases are typically unconscious and contribute to errors, notably but not only rule-based errors. Common biases include racism, sexism, and heightism.[65,66] The strength of a rule is a specific form of bias, but most people have more general biases. Biases important to anesthesiologists include *confirmation bias* (the tendency to interpret new information as confirming one's established view of a situation, which can be very dangerous in a crisis). *Optimism bias* is the belief that one is better than average at various things like driving a car or giving an anesthetic, and tends to be held by a substantial majority of people. Optimism bias is also the belief that a particular case will work out well, even when objective analysis suggests that this is unlikely.

Knowledge-Based Errors

Knowledge-based errors[29] are errors made in thinking from first principles. The name suggests that the underlying deficiency consists of missing or incorrect elements within the knowledge base, but the differentiating characteristic of decisions involved in knowledge-based errors is that they involve System II thinking—effortful, conscious thought. The term *deliberative errors* has been suggested to make this clearer,[27] but this may be taken as implying that the error was deliberate (which is not the case), so it may be better just to say *errors in thinking from first principles*.

Expertise, Education, and Continuous Professional Development

It should be clear by now that the *knowledge base* on which a decision is made is distinct from an anesthesiologist's *expert knowledge*. The knowledge base is brought into play, at the time of making a decision, by accessing some, not all, of the *potential knowledge base*, which includes all of the sources listed in Box 3.1.

The term *expertise* is commonly defined as embracing expert knowledge and expert skills. Expert skills include (a) the sort involved in airway management or central line insertion; (b) the sort used in acquiring and/or interpreting images, such as reading a radiograph or acquiring and interpreting ultrasound images; and (c) the sort required for effective communication and teamwork. A division of skills into technical and non-technical realms has been proposed,[94] but, arguably, all skills, even communication, include technical elements. For example, structured techniques can improve communication within teams.[95] Skills such as interpreting images depend upon schemata stored in memory, both for interpretation (largely a matter of pattern recognition) and for acquiring them. Once one has become an expert in acquiring images with ultrasound, for example, this becomes a largely automatic activity. Inserting a central line or a brachial plexus block using ultrasound and evaluating the heart using transesophageal echocardiography (TEE) are integrated activities; the acquisition and interpretation of images go hand in hand. The corrective strategy for an error in acquiring an image is, however, different from the corrective strategy for an error in interpreting an image. The intraoperative use of TEE involves interaction with surgeons and other members of the OR team and therefore incorporates communication skills. Attitudes are also relevant—reflecting, for example, whether an anesthesiologist will insist that all relevant information is available before determining the state of a heart valve, or before starting an anesthetic, or whether he or she will begin a procedure even when there are gaps in the information, assuming that they probably will not matter (a form of frequency gambling). There is no universal answer as to where lines of this sort should be drawn; the circumstances and detail are important in deciding how much information is enough, requiring expert judgment.

Expertise encompasses each of these components. It is developed through activities such as reading, attendance at didactic lectures, informal discussions with colleagues, participation in simulation-based training, team-training, and experience. There is no substitute for clinical experience in the formation of expertise, but its value is greatly enhanced when it is supported by other forms of learning. Interestingly, the balance has shifted over recent decades from an abundance of experience and somewhat limited formal instruction during training to an abundance of formal instruction with some difficulty in gaining adequate experience.

More on Classification of Errors

A precise understanding of the nature of an error is required to devise strategies that reduce the likelihood of recurrence and to determine whether an individual should be blamed. The cognitive processes associated with error fall on a spectrum from System I thinking to System II thinking, with one extreme represented by unconscious, automatic thinking (slips and lapses) and the other by conscious, effortful thinking from first principles (mistakes).

Reason has identified the importance of latent factors in the system (see the section on the Swiss cheese model), and one purpose of analyzing an error is to identify latent factors and then address them. Another is to provide insight into how highly motivated people can make errors and to assist in differentiating blameworthy from non-blameworthy actions. It is important to realize, therefore, that the outcome of the error will depend on the error itself, the context in which it is made, and chance. The best way to improve safety might also be to design initiatives that mitigate the consequences of unpreventable, predictable errors; airbags in motorcars are an example of this strategy.

A Proposed Outline for Evaluating Errors During Anesthesia

An approach has been outlined previously that is designed to facilitate identification of the origins of a particular error in a way that can inform an appropriate response, both to improve safety and to promote accountability.[12] The following is a modification of this outline. The numbers refer to those in Figure 3.2.

Few accidents involve a pure error. Many involve more than one of the 10 variations on error outlined in the following, and one or more violations may also be a factor. Attitude and bias may also play a role in the accident.

1. *Errors arising from deficiencies in information available in the world.* Often there are important gaps or mistakes in the available information. (e.g., an incomplete patient record).
2. *Errors in acquisition of information.* Even if the required information is available, there may be a failure to acquire it, including through a failure of communication between members of the OR team (i.e., a failure to share their mental models).
3. *Errors in perception.* The information may be acquired, but misunderstood. One word may be mistaken for another, or instructions may be incorrectly heard. People tend to see and hear what they expect to see and hear.
4. *Errors in interpretation.* The process of filtering and interpreting the overwhelming flood of information may go wrong. Bias is an important factor here (notably confirmation bias).
5. *Errors in expert knowledge stored as schemata.* These include situations in which expert knowledge (a) has never been stored; (b) has been stored but cannot be recalled at the time it is needed; (c) has been stored but has been forgotten; or (d) has been stored but is incorrect.
6. *Errors in knowledge stored as rules.* Subdivided as for 5, and see discussion of 8.
7. *Slips and lapses.* These have been called skill-based errors, but there may be very little substantive difference between

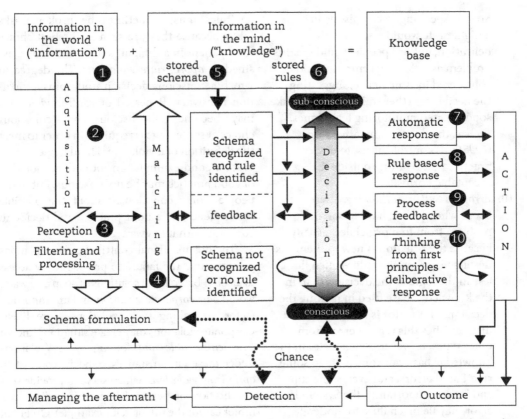

FIGURE 3.2: Schematic representation of the processes involved in making and carrying out a plan and ways (1–10: see text) in which failure can occur in these processes.

Reprinted with permission from Schematic of processes in making and carrying out plans. In: Runciman B, Merry A, Walton M, *Safety and Ethics in Healthcare: A Guide to Getting it Right.* Farnham, UK: Ashgate, 2007, p. 114.

some slips and lapses and some rule-based errors (see discussion of 8).

8. *Errors in choice of rule.* Using System I thinking, a rule that would work in a slightly different situation is applied in the wrong context. For example, starting an inotrope in response to hypotension when weaning from cardiopulmonary bypass after a mitral valve repair without remembering to first check for systolic anterior motion of the anterior mitral valve leaflet (SAM). This action (or lack of action) may represent an error of type 6 (the anesthesiologist did not know about SAM), or it may reflect "absent-mindedness"—simply forgetting to think of SAM, perhaps because of distraction. This would be a lapse.

9. *Technical errors.* These errors represent "mismatches between the skill and ability of the practitioner and the challenge posed by the task in the prevailing circumstances."[12] They are best thought of in normative terms. A minimum level of competence is expected of every anesthesiologist. Procedures such as insertion of epidural catheters, central venous lines, and endotracheal tubes may be more difficult to do in some patients than in others, and some practitioners are more skilled than others. A certain, low rate of failure is inevitable. For example, in competent hands, a rare dural puncture would seem to meet the definition of an error because it would be "a failure to carry out a planned action as intended."

Strictly speaking, each episode in a higher rate would also meet this definition, but few people would see this problem as reflecting error: it would be considered incompetence, suggesting the need for further training. It may take sophisticated monitoring techniques, such as the use of cumulative sum (CUSUM) control charts, to detect practice that is falling outside the acceptable norms.[96]

10. *Errors in System II thinking.* These occur when people have to solve a problem from first principles, usually because the situation is new to them. As discussed earlier, the failure often lies less in the logic of the decision than in the knowledge base used in making the decision. This factor is not the one that distinguishes this type of error from other types, however. Deficiencies in the knowledge base can contribute to some rule-based errors, and even some slips and lapses. Importantly, the System II error may lie in a failure to moderate a System I decision, or in incorrectly moderating a System I decision (see Table 3.2).

Violations

A simple English definition of violation is "an act that knowingly incurs a risk." More formally, "a violation is a deliberate—but not necessarily reprehensible—deviation from safe operating procedures, standards, or rules."[64] A person committing a violation has no intent to harm (that would be sabotage), but there is a conscious decision to take a risk that is not in the interests of the patient, in the hope (and usually the conviction) that one will "get away with it." The problem is that violations tend to increase the likelihood of an error and the severity of its consequences. For example, it would be an error to break the speed limit unintentionally, but intentionally speeding would be a violation. Not all violations are equal. Using the same analogy, intentionally exceeding the speed limit by 50% is, in general, much more serious than intentionally exceeding the speed limit by 5%.

Rules must sometimes be broken: risks taken because they are seen as the best choice for a patient in a difficult situation can be classified as *appropriate violations*. The degree to which a conscious decision underpins a violation may vary. Repeated or *routine violations* may become subconscious, but conscious choice at some stage is required in order to meet the definition of a violation. Hand hygiene provides a good example: an individual violation of good practice may be unconscious, but many people worry consciously about the possible consequences of a poor practice and decide to continue with it anyway.

The organizational contribution to violations is important. The failure to provide ready access to alcohol-based hand solutions or soap and water would be a *corporate violation* and an important factor in making such violations more likely. Corporate violations may create situations known as *systems double-binds* for employees. Violations under these circumstances stand in contrast to *optimizing violations*, which serve to provide self-gratification or personal benefit (speeding in a motor car for the fun of it, for example). On Flight 447, the decision to follow a route through convective weather was interesting. It seems that at least some other flight crews chose to fly around it that night. Various factors may have influenced the captain. As discussed later, it is impossible to adequately assess a decision without knowing what was in the person's mind, but the question is worth asking—was this actually a good decision?

JUST CULTURE

Healthcare has traditionally had a culture in which the role and responsibility of individuals were emphasized and individuals were blamed when things went wrong. This phase was overtaken by a period in which there was strong advocacy for a *blame-free* response to failures in the safe delivery of healthcare. Not surprisingly, some hospital administrators and members of the public objected. At least some of the things that go wrong in healthcare reflect negligence or recklessness on the part of practitioners, making calls for greater accountability understandable. Gradually, the idea of a blame-free culture in healthcare is giving way to that of a *just culture*. The underlying notion is that it is possible, when harm occurs to a patient, to differentiate between actions for which an individual should be held blameless responsible and actions.[27] An important assumption is that the majority of things that go wrong reflect blameless errors. Few, if any, healthcare workers intentionally harm a patient. Indeed, they are typically very distressed when things go wrong, and may also become a *second victim* of an error that was not only unintentional but, in a statistical sense, unavoidable.

More on Deterrence

It is often said that an important difference between pilots and physicians is that pilots are at the front of the airplane and are therefore more safety conscious than doctors. In the early days of air mail, there was great pressure on pilots to fly even when the weather was bad, and accidents occurred frequently. Eventually, it was decided that the person making the call on whether to fly or not should go on the airplane, resulting in more conservative decisions and a sharp reduction in crashes. The pilots on Flight 447, however, were not deterred from error by being on the plane. In general, safety in the airline industry was not achieved by changing the position of the pilots. It was achieved by adopting a systems approach to safety, probably on account of the high cost of jet aircraft—crashes simply became too expensive to tolerate.

There is an important distinction between violations, which involve choice and can therefore be deterred, and errors, which are involuntary. This does not mean that errors should be tolerated. Patients who have been injured through error do have a right to expect that everything reasonable will be done to prevent a recurrence and to save other people from similar harm. Punishing a person who has made a genuine error is not an effective way of achieving that objective, however.

The Requirements of a Just Culture: Distinguishing Acceptable From Unacceptable Behavior

A just culture is, in effect, a social contract between an organization and its employees. In a just culture, the minimal requirement from the organization is a commitment to patient safety that is demonstrated by making every systems-level effort to facilitate doing the right things, combined with a commitment to those employees who are indeed trying to do the right thing that they will not be punished for genuine errors. The minimal requirement from individuals would seem to be a conscientious effort to comply with good practice and to support initiatives to improve safety and reduce avoidable harm to patients.

Where both sides have met this contract, the response to a failure in process (e.g., omitting to administer a required prophylactic antibiotic before the start of surgery) that contributes to a bad outcome should be an open report, a review, and an attempt to address contributory systems issues that are identified in the review. In the example in Box 3.4, such an omission arguably reflected errors on the part of both the individual and the organization, and the response was appropriate.

Not everyone agrees with every initiative intended to enhance safety. If one disagrees with rules or initiatives (such as the use of the SSC, for example), the solution is to articulate the reasons for the disagreement, and to work constructively with colleagues to address perceived shortcomings and improve the initiative, or to overturn it if that is justifiable. Conversely, repeatedly and deliberately flouting attempts to improve safety must be construed as violation. In a just culture, persistent violations of this type are not acceptable and should not be tolerated.

Deliberate recklessness, such as working under the influence of alcohol or drugs, is also unacceptable in a just culture. Intent to harm is obviously unacceptable, but is very unusual in the context of healthcare, notwithstanding some highly publicized exceptions.

Published algorithms can assist in differentiating between blameworthy and blameless acts (Figure 3.3). The problem is that applying these algorithms depends upon a sophisticated understanding of the way humans make decisions and act on them.[27] This task should not be delegated to mid-level administrators with

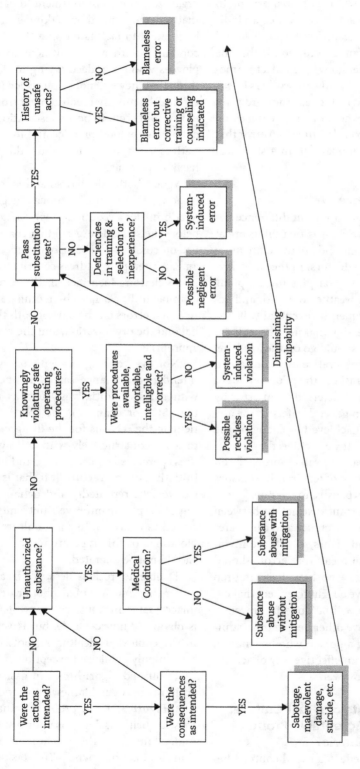

FIGURE 3.3: An algorithm to ascertain whether an act was blameworthy or blameless.

Reprinted with permission from A decision tree for determining the culpability of unsafe acts. In: Reason J, *Managing the Risks of Organizational Accidents*.Farnham, UK: Ashgate, 1997, p. 209.

little if any expertise in this field. It is critical to the success of a just culture in any institution that those who take on the responsibility of assessing and triaging events in this way are qualified to do so, and have high levels of trust from all concerned.

Reason has explained that "the boundaries between errors and violations are by no means hard and fast, either conceptually or within a particular accident sequence." Violations and errors in thinking from first principles (10 in Figure 3.1) can have much in common, but the difference lies in the intent. In the end, the only way to tell the difference between an error and a violation is through accessing the thought processes of the person concerned at the time of the action. This can only be done by asking the person. Ironically, honest people may be more likely than dishonest ones to incriminate themselves by telling the truth. There are, however, some features that can be helpful in assessing a situation. If a person has a track record of conscientiousness (in context), error is a more plausible explanation than if the person is known to disregard considerations of safety. This is not completely reliable, of course, but within a medical context, routine, typical, or usual behavior is probably what matters most.

REDUCING THE RISK OF FAILURE IN HEALTHCARE

Early in this chapter I noted the persistent nature of the problem of iatrogenic harm.[17] Safety in both healthcare and in anesthesia is, however, improving steadily and substantially, though the challenges in achieving and maintaining this progress are considerable. There is no quick fix or simple answer. Calls for top-down solutions, such as changing the culture, discount the diverse nature of failures in complex systems, and also the outstandingly well-motivated and committed culture that already exists in much of healthcare.

The foundation of safe care is, and always has been, the adequate training of healthcare professionals and the adequate resourcing of the facilities in which they work. Expertise in the form of subject-relevant knowledge and craft-relevant skills are absolutely fundamental to safe and effective care, as are the equipment and drugs needed to provide that care. Anesthesiologists can be proud of their achievements in this regard. Anesthesiologists have long concentrated on doing things right, but a focus on doing the right things is equally important. This implies making decisions about anesthesia for and with each patient that are evidence based and address the issues that matter to him or her as an individual. More generally, the "big picture" issues discussed earlier are an important part of the responsibility of anesthesiologists as perioperative physicians. Many aspects of the practice of anesthesia warrant collective review (within institutions at least, and at the level of national anesthesia organizations) to reduce variation and promote effective care. The development of standards[97] integral to anesthesia practice in most well-resourced countries makes an important contribution to reducing variation.

It is also part of anesthesiologists' collective responsibility to contribute to the debate on what surgical procedures are or are not appropriate in the context of their institutional, regional, or national circumstances. As physicians, we are as responsible for our patients as surgeons are, and we should not facilitate practices that are inadequately justified. Equally, we should support the provision of adequate access to procedures that are appropriate. Effective care should be the goal. The place and time for such debate is usually at the departmental level and within the ongoing work of committees and other organizational structures of the institutions and countries in which anesthesiologists work, rather than the OR and the heat of the moment, but contributing to the debate is part of promoting safety.

Unfortunately, standards do vary substantially around the world. Setting and maintaining appropriate standards are important, and supporting anesthesia professionals who have limited resources in improving their expertise and facilities is critically important in any genuine attempt to achieve the goals of the Anesthesia Patient Safety Foundation (APSF), globally.[98] The biggest potential gains lie in improving the care given to those in low-income regions of the world.

Even highly trained and adequately resourced anesthesiologists make errors from time to time. Violations, too, are not unknown, and often these reflect failures by organizations to support and insist on accepted practices. An understanding of the nature of error and violation provides a basis for reducing both, or for reducing harm arising from either. Hard engineering solutions, such as pin indexing, are highly effective in reducing error, but it is likely that most of the low hanging fruit has been picked in this regard. Mitigating the consequences of error may at times be more effective than trying to prevent error. For example, the road casualty toll has been reduced by a combination of prevention and mitigation: stricter enforcement of speed and alcohol limits to reduce the risk of accidents have gone hand in hand with safer designs of roads (e.g., median strips) and cars (e.g., air bags) to mitigate the consequences when accidents occur.

We are now in an era in which process tools used in other industries, such as briefings, checklists, and barcodes or radio frequency identification devices, are increasingly important. Unlike hard engineering solutions, these solutions require the engagement of practitioners to achieve their full potential. Part of that engagement lies in reading the literature on teamwork, communication, process engineering (e.g., checklists[99] and the new APSF's paradigm for drug safety in anesthesia[100]) and other major developments in improving patient safety, as well as the literature on the craft-specific aspects of our specialty.

It is important that all concerned feel safe to report failures or risks, and to comment critically on any processes and aspects of the infrastructure that appear to create risk, in order that the iterative process of ongoing review and improvement can continue to promote safety. Proactive efforts focused on optimizing success are also very important.

CONCLUSIONS

It is only reasonable for patients and those who lead organizations to expect that practitioners will engage in all reasonable attempts to enhance safety. This dual expectation is the basis of a just culture, and a just culture is a fundamental requirement for improving safety in healthcare. Establishing and maintaining a just culture depends on a sophisticated understanding of error and violations, and the difference between them, and also of systems, and the challenges imposed by complexity.

REFERENCES

1. *Medication Safety in the Operating Room: Time for a New Paradigm.* Indianapolis, IN: Anesthesia Patient Safety Foundation; 2010.
2. Pronovost P, Needham D, Berenholtz S, et al. An intervention to decrease catheter-related bloodstream infections in the ICU. *N Engl J Med.* 2006;355(26):2725–2732.
3. Seddon ME, Hocking CJ, Bryce EA, Hillman J, McCoubrie V. From ICU to hospital-wide: extending central line associated bacteraemia (CLAB) prevention. *N Z Med J.* 2014;127(1394):60–71.
4. Wikipedia contributors. Air France Flight 447. *Wikipedia, The Free Encyclopedia.* http://en.wikipedia.org/w/index.php?title=Air_France_Flight_447&oldid=651444057. Accessed March 17, 2015.
5. Perrow C. *Normal Accidents: Living With High Risk Technologies.* New York: Basic Books; 1984.
6. Perrow C. *Normal Accidents: Living With High Risk Technologies.* 2nd ed. Princeton, NJ: Princeton University Press; 1999.
7. Jarman B. Quality of care and patient safety in the UK: the way forward after Mid Staffordshire. *Lancet.* 2013;382(9892):573–575.
8. Institute of Medicine. *To Err Is Human: Building a Safer Health System.* Washington, DC: National Academies Press; 1999.
9. Leape LL. Error in medicine. *JAMA.* 1994; 272(23):1851–1857.
10. Runciman WB, Webb RK, Helps SC, et al. A comparison of iatrogenic injury studies in Australia and the USA. II: reviewer behaviour and quality of care. *Int J Qual Health Care.* 2000;12(5):379–388.
11. Hayward RA, Hofer TP. Estimating hospital deaths due to medical errors: preventability is in the eye of the reviewer. *JAMA.* 2001;286(4):415–420.
12. Runciman B, Merry A, Walton M. *Safety and Ethics in Healthcare: A Guide to Getting it Right.* Aldershot, UK: Ashgate; 2007.
13. Cook TM, Woodall N, Frerk C. Major complications of airway management in the UK: results of the Fourth National Audit Project of the Royal College of Anaesthetists and the Difficult

Airway Society. Part 1: anaesthesia. *Br J Anaesth.* 2011;106(5):617–631.

14. Merry AF, Peck DJ. Anaesthetists, errors in drug administration and the law. *N Z Med J.* 1995;108(1000):185–187.

15. Greenland KB, Acott C, Segal R, Goulding G, Riley RH, Merry AF. Emergency surgical airway in life-threatening acute airway emergencies: why are we so reluctant to do it? *Anaesth Intensive Care.* 2011;39(4):578–584.

16. Brennan TA, Leape LL, Laird NM, et al. Incidence of adverse events and negligence in hospitalized patients: results of the Harvard Medical Practice Study I. *N Engl J Med.* 1991;324(6):370–376.

17. Landrigan CP, Parry GJ, Bones CB, Hackbarth AD, Goldmann DA, Sharek PJ. Temporal trends in rates of patient harm resulting from medical care. *N Engl J Med.* 2010;363(22):2124–2134.

18. Cooper JB, Gaba D. No myth: anesthesia is a model for addressing patient safety. *Anesthesiology.* 2002;97(6):1335–1337.

19. Gaba DM, Maxwell M, DeAnda A. Anesthetic mishaps: breaking the chain of accident evolution. *Anesthesiology.* 1987;66(5):670–676.

20. Cooper JB, Long CD, Newbower RS, Philip JH. Critical incidents associated with intraoperative exchanges of anesthesia personnel. *Anesthesiology.* 1982;56(6):456–461.

21. Runciman WB, Sellen A, Webb RK, et al. The Australian Incident Monitoring Study: errors, incidents and accidents in anaesthetic practice. *Anaesth Intensive Care.* 1993;21(5):506–519.

22. Denson JS, Abrahamson S. A computer-controlled patient simulator. *JAMA.* 1969;208(3):504–508.

23. Gaba DM, DeAnda A. A comprehensive anesthesia simulation environment: re-creating the operating room for research and training. *Anesthesiology.* 1988;69:387–394.

24. Schwid HA. A flight simulator for general anesthesia training. *Comput Biomed. Res.* 1987;20(1):64–75.

25. Good ML, Gravenstein JS. Anesthesia simulators and training devices. *Int Anesthesiol Clin.* 1989;27(3):161–168.

26. Cooper J. Patient safety and biomedical engineering. In: Kitz R, ed. *This Is No Humbug: Reminiscences of the Department of Anesthesia at the Massachusetts General Hospital.* Boston: Department of Anesthesia and Critical Care, Massachusetts General Hospital; 2002:377–420.

27. Merry AF, McCall Smith A. *Errors, Medicine and the Law.* Cambridge: Cambridge University Press; 2001.

28. Merry A. How does the law recognize and deal with medical errors? In: Hurwitz B, Sheik A, eds. *Health Care Errors and Patient Safety.* Hoboken, NJ: Wiley Blackwell BMJ Books; 2009:75–88.

29. Reason J. *Human Error.* New York: Cambridge University Press; 1990.

30. Reason J. Human error: models and management. *Br Med J.* 2000;320:768–770.

31. Hollnagel E. *Safety-I and Safety-II: the past and future of safety management*: Aldershot, UK: Ashgate; 2014.

32. Merry AF, Weller J, Mitchell SJ. Improving the quality and safety of patient care in cardiac anesthesia. *J Cardiothorac Vasc Anesth.* 2014;28(5):1341–1351.

33. Gargiulo DA, Sheridan J, Webster CS, et al. Anaesthetic drug administration as a potential contributor to healthcare-associated infections: a prospective simulation-based evaluation of aseptic techniques in the administration of anaesthetic drugs. *BMJ Qual Saf.* 2012;21(10): 826–834.

34. Runciman B, Merry A, McCall Smith A. Improving patients' safety by gathering information: anonymous reporting has an important role. *Br Med J.* 2001;323(7308):298.

35. Merry AF. Safety in anaesthesia: reporting incidents and learning from them. *Anaesthesia.* 2008;63(4):337–339.

36. Kluger MT, Bullock MF. Recovery room incidents: a review of 419 reports from the Anaesthetic Incident Monitoring Study (AIMS). *Anaesthesia.* 2002;57(11):1060–1066.

37. Leape LL. Errors in medicine. *Clin Chim Acta.* 2009;404(1):2–5.

38. Swensen SJ, Kaplan GS, Meyer GS, et al. Controlling healthcare costs by removing waste: what American doctors can do now. *BMJ Qual Saf.* 2011;20(6):534–537.

39. Funk LM, Weiser TG, Berry WR, et al. Global operating theatre distribution and pulse oximetry supply: an estimation from reported data. *Lancet.* 2010;376(9746):1055–1061.

40. Walker IA, Wilson IH. Anaesthesia in developing countries-a risk for patients. *Lancet.* 2008;371(9617):968–969.

41. Merry AF, Eichhorn JH, Wilson IH. Extending the WHO "Safe Surgery Saves Lives" project through Global Oximetry. *Anaesthesia.* 2009; 64(10):1045–1048.

42. Gornall BF, Myles PS, Smith CL, et al. Measurement of quality of recovery using the QoR-40: a quantitative systematic review. *Br J Anaesth.* 2013;111(2):161–169.

43. Weiser TG, Makary MA, Haynes AB, et al. Standardised metrics for global surgical surveillance. *Lancet.* 2009;374(9695):1113–1117.

44. Catchpole KR, Giddings AEB, Wilkinson M, Hirst G, Dale T, de Leval MR. Improving patient safety by identifying latent failures in

successful operations. *Surgery.* 2007;142(1): 102–110.

45. Berwick DM, Nolan TW, Whittington J. The triple aim: care, health, and cost. *Health Aff (Millwood).* 2008;27(3):759–769.

46. Davies JI, Meara JG. Global surgery-going beyond the Lancet Commission. *Lancet.* 2015; 386: 507–509.

47. POISE Study Group, Devereaux PJ, Yang H, et al. Effects of extended-release metoprolol succinate in patients undergoing non-cardiac surgery (POISE trial): a randomised controlled trial. *Lancet.* 2008;371(9627):1839–1847.

48. Myles PS, Leslie K, Chan MT, et al. The safety of addition of nitrous oxide to general anaesthesia in at-risk patients having major non-cardiac surgery (ENIGMA-II): a randomised, single-blind trial. *Lancet.* 2014;384(9952):1446–1454.

49. Myles PS, Leslie K, McNeil J, Forbes A, Chan MT. Bispectral index monitoring to prevent awareness during anaesthesia: the B-Aware randomised controlled trial. *Lancet.* 2004;363(9423):1757–1763.

50. Institute of Medicine. *Crossing the Quality Chasm: A New Health System for the 21st Century.* Washington, DC: National Academy Press; 2001.

51. McGlynn E, Asch S, Adams J, et al. The quality of health care delivered to adults in the United States. *N Engl J Med.* 2003;348(26):2635–2645.

52. Wennberg JE, Peters PG, Jr. Unwarranted variations in the quality of health care: can the law help medicine provide a remedy/remedies? *Spec Law Dig Health Care Law.* 2004(305):9–25.

53. Fisher ES, Wennberg DE, Stukel TA, Gottlieb DJ, Lucas FL, Pinder EL. The implications of regional variations in Medicare spending. Part 2: health outcomes and satisfaction with care. *Ann Intern Med.* 2003;138(4):288–298.

54. Weiser TG, Regenbogen SE, Thompson KD, et al. An estimation of the global volume of surgery: a modelling strategy based on available data. *Lancet.* 2008;372(9633):139–144.

55. Fisher ES, Wennberg JE. Health care quality, geographic variations, and the challenge of supply-sensitive care. *Perspect Biol Med.* 2003;46(1):69–79.

56. Fisher ES. Medical care: is more always better? *N Engl J Med.* 2003;349(17):1665–1667.

57. Van Brabandt H, Neyt M, Hulstaert F. Transcatheter aortic valve implantation (TAVI): risky and costly. *BMJ.* 2012;345:e4710.

58. Glouberman S, Zimmerman B. *Complicated and Complex Systems: What Would Successful Reform of Medicare Look Like?* Saskatoon: Commission on the Future of Health Care in Canada; 2002.

59. Webster CS . *Implementing Safety in Medicine: The Problem, the Pitfalls and a Successful Safety Initiative in Anaesthesia.* Saarbrucken, Germany: VDM Verlag; 2008.

60. Webster CS, Merry AF, Larsson L, McGrath KA, Weller J. The frequency and nature of drug administration error during anaesthesia. *Anaesth Intensive Care.* 2001;29(5):494–500.

61. Skegg PDG. Criminal prosecutions of negligent health professionals: the New Zealand experience. *Med Law Rev.* 1998;6:220–246.

62. Cooper JB, Newbower RS, Kitz RJ. An analysis of major errors and equipment failures in anesthesia management: considerations for prevention and detection. *Anesthesiology.* 1984;60(1):34–42.

63. Runciman WB. Report from the Australian Patient Safety Foundation: Australasian Incident Monitoring Study. *Anaesth Intensive Care.* 1989;17(1):107–108.

64. Runciman WB, Merry AF, Tito F. Error, blame, and the law in health care: an antipodean perspective. *Ann Intern Med.* 2003;138(12):974–979.

65. Kahneman D. *Thinking, Fast and Slow.* London: Penguin Books; 2011.

66. Thaler R, Sunstein C. *Nudge: Improving Decisions About Health, Wealth and Happiness.* New Haven, CT: Yale University Press; 2008.

67. Stanovich KE, West RF. Individual differences in reasoning: implications for the rationality debate? *Behav Brain Sci.* 2000;23(5):645–665; discussion 665–726.

68. Klein G. *Sources of Power: How People Make Decisions.* Cambridge, MA: MIT Press; 1999.

69. Rudolph JW, Simon R, Rivard P, Dufresne RL, Raemer DB. Debriefing with good judgment: combining rigorous feedback with genuine inquiry. *Anesthesiol Clin.* 2007;25(2):361–376.

70. Wegner DM, Ansfiled M, Pilloff D. The putt and the pendulum: ironic effects of the mental control of action. *Psychol Sci.* 1998;9(3):196–199.

71. Rudolph JW, Repenning NP. Disaster dynamics: understanding the role of quantity in organizational collapse. *Adm Sci Q.* 2002;47:1–30.

72. Yerkes R, Dodson J. The relation of strength of stimulus to rapidity of habit formation. *J Comp Neurol Psychol.* 1908;18:459–482.

73. *Executive Summary of the 2002 "Sleep in America" Poll.* Washington DC: National Sleep Foundation; 2002.

74. Dawson D, Reid K. Fatigue, alcohol and performance impairment. *Nature.* 1997;388:235.

75. Greenberg SL, Vega MP, Bowder AN, Meara JG. The Lancet commission on global surgery makes progress in first year of work: an update. *Bull Am Coll Surg.* 2015;100(4):23–29.

76. Alkire BC, Raykar NP, Shrime MG, et al. Global access to surgical care: a modelling study. *The Lancet. Global Health.* 2015; e316–23.

77. Bonnet MH, Balkin TJ, Dinges DF, et al. The use of stimulants to modify performance during sleep loss: a review by the Sleep Deprivation and Stimulant Task Force of the American Academy of Sleep Medicine. *Sleep*. 2005;28(9): 1163–1187.

78. Howard SK, Gaba DM, Smith BE, et al. Simulation study of rested versus sleep-deprived anesthesiologists. *Anesthesiology*. 2003;98(6):1345–1355; discussion 1345A.

79. Moller HJ, Kayumov L, Bulmash EL, Nhan J, Shapiro CM. Simulator performance, microsleep episodes, and subjective sleepiness: normative data using convergent methodologies to assess driver drowsiness. *J Psychosom Res*. 2006;61(3):335–342.

80. Russo MB, Kendall AP, Johnson DE, et al. Visual perception, psychomotor performance, and complex motor performance during an overnight air refueling simulated flight. *Aviat Space Environ Med*. 2005;76(7 Suppl):C92–103.

81. Zohar D, Tzischinsky O, Epstein R, Lavie P. The effects of sleep loss on medical residents' emotional reactions to work events: a cognitive-energy model. *Sleep*. 2005;28(1):47–54.

82. Lockley SW, Cronin JW, Evans EE, et al. Effect of reducing interns' weekly work hours on sleep and attentional failures. *N Engl J Med*. 2004;351(18):1829–1837.

83. Landrigan CP, Rothschild JM, Cronin JW, et al. Effect of reducing interns' work hours on serious medical errors in intensive care units. *N Engl J Med*. 2004;351(18):1838–1848.

84. Griffiths JD, McCutcheon C, Silbert BS, Maruff P. A prospective observational study of the effect of night duty on the cognitive function of anaesthetic registrars. *Anaesth Intensive Care*. 2006;34: 621–628.

85. Barger LK, Cade BE, Ayas NT, et al. Extended work shifts and the risk of motor vehicle crashes among interns. *N Engl J Med*. 2005;352(2):125–134.

86. Morgan L, Hampton S, Gibbs M, Arendt J. Circadian aspects of postprandial metabolism. *Chronobiol Int*. 2003;20(5):795–808.

87. Lockley SW, Landrigan CP, Barger LK, Czeisler CA. When policy meets physiology: the challenge of reducing resident work hours. *Clin Orthop*. 2006(449):116–127.

88. Mathis BR, Diers T, Hornung R, Ho M, Rouan GW. Implementing duty-hour restrictions without diminishing patient care or education: can it be done? *Acad Med*. 2006;81(1):68–75.

89. Rosekind MR, Smith RM, Miller DL, et al. Alertness management: strategic naps in operational settings. *J Sleep Res*. 1995;4(S2):62–66.

90. Jewett ME, Wyatt JK, Ritz-De Cecco A, Khalsa SB, Dijk DJ, Czeisler CA. Time course of sleep inertia dissipation in human performance and alertness. *J Sleep Res*. 1999;8(1):1–8.

91. Meara JG, Leather AJ, Hagander L, et al. Global Surgery 2030: evidence and solutions for achieving health, welfare, and economic development. *Lancet*. 2015; 386 569–624.

92. Reason J. *Managing the Risks of Organizational Accidents*. Aldershot, UK: Ashgate; 1997.

93. Kristensen M, Teoh W, Baker P. Percutaneous emergency airway access; prevention, preparation, technique and training. *Br J Anaesth*. 2015;114(3).

94. Fletcher G, Flin R, McGeorge P, Glavin R, Maran N, Patey R. Anaesthetists' Non-Technical Skills (ANTS): evaluation of a behavioural marker system. *Br J Anaesth*. 2003;90(5):580–588.

95. Weller JM, Torrie J, Boyd M, et al. Improving team information sharing with a structured call-out in anaesthetic emergencies: a randomized controlled trial. *Br J Anaesth*. 2014;112(6):1042–1049.

96. Bolsin S, Colson MW. The use of the Cusum technique in the assessment of trainee competence in new procedures. *Int J Qual Health Care*. 2000;12(5):433–438.

97. Merry AF, Cooper JB, Soyannwo O, Wilson IH, Eichhorn JH. International standards for a safe practice of anesthesia 2010. *Can J Anaesth*. 2010;57(11):1027–1034.

98. Lifebox. http://www.lifebox.org/about-lifebox/the-pulse-oximetry-gap/. Accessed September 6, 2012.

99. Birkmeyer JD. Strategies for improving surgical quality: checklists and beyond. *N Engl J Med*. 2010;363(20):1963–1965.

100. Eichhorn J. APSF hosts medication safety conference: consensus group defines challenges and opportunities for improved practice. *APSF Newsletter* 2010;25(1):1–7.

4

The Human-Technology Interface

FRANK A. DREWS AND JONATHAN R. ZADRA

SOCIO-TECHNICAL SYSTEMS PERSPECTIVE

The introduction of computer technology into many non-healthcare environments is a story of successes, but also of problems and challenges.[1,2] Until very recently, the adoption of technology in healthcare, and more specifically in anesthesiology, was perceived to be overwhelmingly positive. Over the last decade, however, a number of studies indicate that the same problems have occurred in healthcare as have happened in other domains for some time: the introduction and adoption of technology come at a price.[3,4] The adoption of new technology is often perceived as a problem of development and implementation, ignoring the social dimension of its use. In the following sections, we describe a potentially more suitable approach toward the implementation of technology: the socio-technical design approach. This approach attempts to raise awareness of the complexity of technology adoption.

The initial work on a socio-technical perspective was done by Trist (1981) and Cherns (1976) to investigate the impact of technology on social processes at work.[5,6] A similar approach was introduced in healthcare in the form of the Systems Engineering Initiative for Patient Safety (SEIPS) model.[7] A socio-technical approach pursues the goal of developing a coherent human-technology interface (HTI). While the direct interface between a user and the technical system is important,[8] a socio-technical perspective also involves consideration of the entire network of users, system developers, potential technology limitations, and the use context. The underlying assumption is that a thorough understanding is required of the social system, the technical system, and the ways in which the two interact, in order to develop HTIs that present complex and integrated, but still usable, information without disrupting system functioning.[9] Clearly, this socio-technical perspective is significantly different from a more traditional user-centered approach that uses a task-level analysis.[10]

Until recently, it was assumed that complex technology could be designed and implemented all the way from the drawing board to a complete, correct, and consistent system without any substantial user feedback or involvement. It has become clear over the last decade, however, that the implementation of HTI can create unintended consequences (e.g., error and workarounds) if the socio-technical perspective is ignored.[11]

MONITORING NATURAL SYSTEMS IN A COMPLEX ENVIRONMENT

Several aspects of healthcare, especially anesthesia, present unique challenges to healthcare professionals. The human body is an extremely complex system with a high degree of inter- and intra-individual variability. Medical care requires monitoring a large number of parameters and making constant adjustments as the body adjusts to the physiologic stress of surgery. Furthermore, all of this must be accomplished in a complex working environment, with regular interruptions and many stimuli that simultaneously compete for practitioners' attention, requiring precise coordination among team members.

Natural Systems

Healthcare, in general, and anesthesia, in particular, deal with a natural system at the core: the patient. While this may sound trivial, monitoring a natural system as opposed to a technical system (e.g., an aircraft) involves a number of important implications.

One important aspect of natural systems is that they exist as a result of reorganization and evolution.[12-14] Changes in the environment force natural systems to respond to those changes by adapting.[13,15] For example, maintaining the proper depth of general anesthesia involves continuous adjustments that ideally anticipate the patient's physiological adaptations to surgery in order to maintain the desired level of unconsciousness. Another problem is that natural systems are opaque; the algorithms that describe the component interactions and the state variables must be deduced.[16,17] Prediction of the future state of a natural system requires constant monitoring. Although an anesthesiologist's mental model may closely approximate the functioning of a patient, such a model is merely an explanation of the system, which may be inaccurate and which therefore leaves space for surprises. Glass and Rampil support the idea that the monitoring of biological systems is more challenging because of the variance that can be found within a population.[18] They argue that designing a closed-loop patient monitoring system is difficult because the requirements are significantly higher than those in a technical system such as aviation.

Similarly, Drews and Doig argue that inter- and intra-individual variability causes potential problems for monitoring.[19] The authors found that nurses' diagnostic performance improved when they used a vital sign display that visualized parameter variability in patients, as compared to a control condition in which nurses used a conventional representation of patient vital signs.

Complex Environment

The overall number of tasks that are being performed by anesthesiologists has increased significantly over the last decades. Today, anesthesiologists work in a wide range of environments (e.g., the OR, the ICU, and the ED). Anesthesiologists provide a wide range of services: they provide intraoperative care, are involved in perioperative patient management, and participate in organizational and management activities in hospitals. Given the complexity of this work environment and the diverse tasks that are being performed, maintaining a high level of performance becomes an even greater challenge. Finally, due to the growth of medical and engineering knowledge, the complexity of the medical field and of the equipment and devices that are being used increases constantly. For example, equipment-related challenges emerge when problems with connectivity and inter-operability of devices cause unexpected behavior.

Anesthesiologists face additional challenges related to workflow: they perform in a context that is dominated by frequent task interruptions, requiring multitasking. Task interruptions have been shown to occur frequently in healthcare in areas ranging from the ED[20] to the ICU.[21] Grundgeiger et al.[22] found that anesthesiologists' performance in a simulator was negatively affected by interruptions.

Another aspect of anesthesia care is that it occurs in a dynamic environment that requires constant group coordination in order to collaborate effectively.[23] The effectiveness of responses to interruptions can be impaired by a lack of awareness of what is happening beyond an individual's specific workspace, a lack of information system integration, and the absence of information pooling and organizational learning.

HUMAN FACTORS TO GUIDE THE DEVELOPMENT OF THE HUMAN TECHNOLOGY INTERFACE

We now discuss some of the issues that contribute to performance breakdowns in anesthesia. Understanding these contributors can provide guidance for the development of an improved HTI that reduces the likelihood of performance breakdowns.

Situation Awareness

The ability to identify problems before patient injury occurs is a function of the anesthesiologist's mental representation of the patient in the context of the dynamically changing task environment (the "mental model").[24] Such cognitive representation of the patient's state includes at least the following elements: (a) detection of deviations from a monitored variable's expected value, (b) prediction of future values or trends in these variables, and (c) revision of the representation of the patient's state after an intervention or event. Current models of anesthesiologists' problem-solving processes include these elements.[25,26]

In her domain-independent approach to conceptualizing cognition in context, Endsley[27–29] (see also [30], a special issue of *Human Factors* on situation awareness) describes the concept of situation awareness. Situation awareness (SA) is the understanding of the state of a system and the relevant parameters of an environment. SA provides the primary basis for subsequent decision-making, with effective SA enhancing performance during the control and operation of complex, dynamic, and tightly coupled systems. Endsley[28] distinguished three levels of situation awareness:

- *Level 1 (detection)*: A person perceives relevant information and detects a change in the environment. The person discovers that an event has happened.
- *Level 2 (diagnosis)*: The user integrates various pieces of data, in conjunction with his or her present goals, and gains an understanding of the meaning of that information. At this level of SA, a number of variables often constitute a familiar pattern, which can then be used to make an almost effortless assessment.[31–33]
- *Level 3 (prediction)*: A user predicts future system states based on existing system knowledge and situation awareness. This involves formulating a plan and considering the effects of its implementation.

The enhancement of operators' situation awareness has become a major goal for HTI development in many non-medical domains, such as aviation, surface transportation, and power plant control.[34–38] In anesthesia, where a significant number of adverse events and close calls are related to breakdowns in situation awareness, an improved HTI could have a positive impact on patient safety.

Situation awareness was introduced to anesthesiology by Gaba, Howard, and Small (1995),[39] and a recent review surveys the small body of empirical work on SA in anesthesia.[40] The first SA study in anesthesiology evaluated a new graphical display by asking anesthesiologists to manage several clinical scenarios.[41] The authors found that a graphical display results in faster response times and higher SA in some, but not all, of the scenarios that were tested. Ford, Daniels, Lim, et al. evaluated vibrotactile displays in the context of a simulated anaphylaxis scenario.[42] While participants using the vibrotactile display delivered treatment more rapidly than the control group, they did not show a higher level of SA. This lack of improvement might also be related to the fact that the authors used a SA measurement in a different manner from its initial design. It is possible that the measure was not sensitive to potential changes in SA.

More recently, an approach that emphasizes the importance of the team component in situation awareness was proposed by Schulz, Endsley, Kochs, et al..[43] The authors define team SA as "the degree to which every team member possesses the SA required for his or her responsibilities." The authors argue that in an effective team, decisions are made based on information derived from all team members, rather than only from an individual or a small subgroup. The authors describe factors that influence team situation awareness; among them are team SA devices, which include communications (verbal and nonverbal), shared displays (visual, audio, and other), and the shared environment.

Information Integration

One of the main challenges for anesthesiologists, who must interact with complex environments, is the availability of large amounts of data that cannot be processed effectively.

Patient monitoring interfaces frequently follow the traditional *single sensor, single indicator* approach,[44] which displays a single variable for each sensor that is used. These designs are suboptimal from a cognitive perspective due to an increase in cognitive workload, as they require sequential, piecemeal data gathering. This makes it more difficult for an anesthesiologist to develop a coherent understanding of the relationships between monitored variables and their underlying mechanisms.[45]

A better approach is to design an interface that supports the anesthesiologist by providing integrated patient information, thus allowing rapid detection, diagnosis and treatment. For example, Drews, Agutter, Syroid, Albert, Westenskow, and Strayer[46] developed a cardiovascular display that incorporates anesthesiologists' mental model of the cardiovascular system (see also [47]). In this graphical display, symmetry shows normal values, and asymmetry shows deviations from normal. The authors incorporated emerging features and implemented patterns that matched particular diagnoses. (An analysis of the cognitive implications of patient monitoring in anesthesiology and the design requirements to support this task can be found in [48].)

Another challenge relates to the effective exchange of information. Making patient information accessible within a single hospital (i.e., scheduling, billing, pharmacy, material management, and patient administration) but also allowing information exchange with other hospitals is critical to effective care. The challenge is that many of the currently used systems are heterogeneous, incompatible, and designed to meet local needs only. Rarely, if ever, are these systems designed to support cognition and to improve performance.

HUMAN TECHNOLOGY INTERFACES IN ANESTHESIA

Types of Interfaces

Computers and software operate in a highly invisible way: often, the user receives only limited information about the operational or organizational state of the system.[49] The user interface provides the operating environment that allows interaction with the system and provides feedback about the system's status. Several types of interfaces can be found in the clinical environment.

Character-based user interfaces are still in common use throughout medicine. These systems were developed to meet the specific aims of particular organizations. One challenge of these interfaces to novice and intermediate users is the high cognitive load they impose. The user must remember the command syntax, the spelling, and the specific procedures required by the system. Having "knowledge in the head",[50] i.e., having learned the computer commands prior to using them, is the only way to interact with a computer that uses a character-based interface .

A more complex variant of character-based interfaces is the full screen interface in which the user switches between entry fields on the screen. Full-screen interfaces can be found, for example, in patient documentation systems where a form-filling dialogue is used to enter the patient information. The interaction with these displays uses a combination of menus and function keys. One problem associated with full-screen interfaces is that the menu structure must be optimized for the user's needs, but an analysis to identify those needs is often not performed. Another problem with these systems is that moving through entry boxes can be time-consuming; consequently, interacting with full-screen interfaces is suboptimal. In addition, functionality such as auto-completion of entries increases the probability of an error.

Graphical user interfaces (GUIs) consist of windows, icons, menus, and a direct (e.g., touchscreen) or indirect (e.g., mouse) control, and allow the user to directly manipulate visual representations of the dialogue objects on the screen. Using a GUI supports the user in multiple ways. The interface supports recognition, as opposed to character-based interfaces that require recall. Graphical user interfaces can also use metaphors (e.g., desktop metaphor or patient anatomy) that allow a user to apply knowledge about the real objects represented in the metaphor to directly and intuitively interact with the interface.

Finally, hypertext-based interfaces allow the user to assess information by clicking on hyperlinks, facilitating navigation through the information space. Internet browsers use this interface by allowing navigation by clicking on hyperlinks on web pages. In healthcare a growing number of applications use this approach.

Anesthesia Devices and Interfaces

There is a growing body of evidence that suggests that hazards resulting from medical device use might far exceed hazards caused by device failures. These problems can partly be attributed to professionals who must deal with these devices' interfaces, illustrating that effective human-computer interaction design needs to be part of the device development process. According to Leape, Woods, Hatlie, Kizer, Schroeder, and Lundberg,[51] many systems are not designed for safety, but rely on "error-free performance enforced by punishment." Sustained, error-free performance in a high-stress and high-stakes environment is impossible,[52] but human error can be reduced by good interface design. We now describe the functions of devices that pose different requirements for the interface designer.

Patient Monitoring

Devices designed to support patient monitoring use their interface to provide feedback about the status of the patient. Gardner and Shabot[53] defined *patient monitoring* as "repeated or continuous observations or measurement of the patient, his or her physiological function, and the function of life support equipment, for the purpose of guiding management decisions." Patient monitoring is of critical importance in the perioperative period, and it is also used in other contexts (e.g., intensive care, perinatal care, and coronary care). A broad variety of devices serve the monitoring function. For example, multiparameter physiological monitoring systems are used in the operating room while pulse oximeters might be used in perinatal care. Monitoring systems provide the anesthesiologist with critical, real-time information

about the patient's current status. In this function, devices support patient assessment, diagnosis, and monitoring of treatment.

One major limitation of these devices is that, with few exceptions, development of systems that facilitate information processing has been slow. Some progress has been made, however. For example, Cole and Stewart[54] developed an integrated graphical display that shows respiratory variables. This display then was developed further by Michels, Gravenstein and Westenskow[55] into a more comprehensive display that presented a total of 32 patient variables in an integrated fashion. Evaluation of this display demonstrated a significant improvement in the detection of adverse events. (A review of several graphical displays in anesthesia can be found in [48].)

Advanced Displays

Limitations in attention are common in the operating room, because an anesthesiologist must divide attention between the vital sign displays and the patient. During certain procedures such as intubation, it may be difficult to monitor vital signs as visual attention is required for the procedure, yet at the same time, vital signs can be of critical importance during this period. Newer technologies, such as head-mounted displays, have been developed in an attempt to resolve this issue by presenting vital signs within the anesthesiologists' field of view. Although experimental trials with these displays indicate that users are able to spend more time looking at the patient, there is no clear improvement in detection of adverse events or overall performance.[56–58]

Computer-Controlled Devices

Another type of interface is used to control computer-operated equipment (e.g., an infusion pump). An infusion pump interface provides information about the pump's current status (for example, its mode of operation) and the means of changing its status. Equipment device interfaces are ideally designed to make the interaction with the device simple and fast in order to minimize user error. They should therefore provide information or request input in a way that reflects the task structure, the workflow, or the procedure that is being performed. It is also critical to provide information about the current or last operational status of the device and the status of variables, because interruptions and multitasking make it impossible for the anesthesiologist to constantly monitor the device. Finally, equipment interfaces should facilitate easy and natural navigation for the user, provide information about actions that were performed previously, have an option to reverse and cancel actions to correct potential error, and facilitate correct operation while preventing or discouraging potentially hazardous actions.

Clinical Data Systems

Clinical data systems (e.g., electronic health records; EHR) are not considered safety critical; the main function of these systems is to maintain the patient record.

Anesthesia Information Management Systems

The adoption of anesthesia information management systems (AIMS) in the United States has been relatively slow as compared to the adoption of other health IT systems. A recent survey[59] indicates that 44% of 140 surveyed US academic anesthesia departments had either implemented, were planning to acquire, or were actively searching for AIMS. At a more detailed level, the study revealed a current AIMS implementation and usage rate of 23% in responding academic anesthesia departments; an additional 21% of the programs were in the process of identifying an AIMS. The expectations associated with AIMS implementation are that the system will improve clinical documentation and data collection for clinical research and will enhance quality improvement programs and regulatory compliance. Challenges related to the adoption include acquisition and maintenance costs, low return of investment for the hospital, complexity of implementation, lack of interoperability with other HIT systems, immaturity of the software, and lack of clear evidence of benefits.

All currently available AIMS use standard GUIs[60] and follow general design principles that make them relatively easy to use. Inconsistency of clinical definitions can create problems related to data capture and entry. Variation in those definitions with or between institutions can severely compromise the quality of the collected data, and both the Anesthesia Patient Safety Foundation and the Anesthesia Quality Institute have made it a priority to develop data dictionaries. These dictionaries serve to standardize data collection, and their development is guided by a yearly meeting and a task force, respectively. While not directly an HTI issue, the emphasis these organizations place on development of such a tool should underscore the importance of the institutional context of technology use.

Decision Support Systems

Anesthesiologists must monitor a large number of complex patient variables. Decision support systems (DSS) aim to aggregate these data into more meaningful units, providing suggestions for action or reminders based on models and algorithms throughout the perioperative period. Anesthetic risk assessments, potential airway management issues, and preoperative test selection can be aided by a DSS that uses patient history as input.[61] These systems can improve patient outcomes while reducing cost by reducing unnecessary use of drugs and issuing reminders about documenting billable activities.[62]

Some advantages of DSS may be offset over the long term by loss of knowledge or expertise and increasing dependence on the DSS.[63,64] Brody, Kowalczyk, and Coulter tested subjects who engaged in a hypothetical decision task with the aid of either a DSS system or standard text-based information materials.[65] Those who used the DSS had poorer memory encoding and did not develop the same level of knowledge. A number of other studies have similarly shown that allowing subjects to externalize information (e.g., take a picture, or save a list in a file) results in poorer recall of this information at a later time.[66]

Extended use of DSS can lead to system reliance. As users trust the system to do more of the information processing for them, their skills and expertise are degraded, causing a negative impact on performance. Users may therefore not be able to take over if the automation fails. They may also be unable to detect failure of the automation because they do not recognize that their decisions differ from those suggested by the automation. While DSS may ameliorate information overload, they may ultimately cause loss of decision-making skills, knowledge, and memory of the criteria upon which decisions were based.

Finally, real-time decision support can only be provided if the required data entry is correct and timely, because the quality of the support is a direct function of the comprehensiveness of the data that are included in the system's assessment and diagnosis. Consequentially, delayed data entry can have a negative impact on the utility of DSS[67] and negatively affect trust in the support.

ANESTHESIA AUTOMATION
Automation is often implemented to perform functions that are associated with significant operator error. The inherent assumption is that automation will remove the source of error by replacing the human. (This is also referred to as the orthodox engineering approach; see [52].)

Anesthetic complications are relatively rare, but are often attributable to human error.[68] One study found that 25% of equipment errors were due to human error.[69] Another determined that human error was one of three main causes of adverse incidents related to medical devices.[70] In the United States, an 18-month study in one hospital found that 411 of 549 reported problems in anesthesia were attributable to human error,[71] and a larger study covering the period 1962–1991 found that 75% of adverse outcomes related to gas delivery were related to human error.[72] Anesthesia is already a highly automated area of healthcare, and current developments suggest that automation is poised to increase significantly in the near future.

Closed-Loop Control Systems
Anesthesiologists must make adjustments to intravenous infusions, drug delivery rates, and other factors in response to changes in patient status that are indicated by proxy variables such as physiological indicators. This response inherently involves delays, because a process of recognition, diagnosis, and treatment must occur. The speed of each stage is limited by both cognitive factors and the interface design, which has an impact on the rate and accuracy of cognition. Errors can also be caused by physiological changes that are unnoticed because of failure to monitor or a lack of awareness. An alternative approach is to use closed-loop systems that are intended to reduce these delays by automatically adjusting dosages in response to physiological changes. These systems could also theoretically reduce error rates because critical variables are constantly monitored, and no change in a physiological parameter goes unnoticed. This approach permits finely grained adjustments in response to subtle physiological changes. Experimental closed-loop systems exist, but currently there is no evidence for a widespread adoption in clinical use.[73] Although there is a wealth of data about a patient's status that is available to an automated system, there are certain factors (such as visual observation of the patient) that only a human operator is currently capable of monitoring.

Target-Controlled Infusion
Target-controlled infusion (TCI) was originally developed in the 1990s[74] and is relatively popular in Europe, where it is used in 10%–25% of total intravenous anesthetics.[75] Unlike closed-loop systems, TCI functions as an open-loop system in which infusion rates are determined with pharmacokinetic algorithms without measuring the actual effect of the infused drug. Leslie, Clavisi, and Hargrove performed a systemic literature review comparing TCI with manually controlled infusion of propofol and found that using target-controlled infusion offered limited benefits.[76] The only benefit found associated with the use of TCI was a decrease in the requirement for manual intervention as compared to manually controlled infusion. Total propofol consumption was increased in patients who received TCI. Finally, there were

no differences in terms of quality of delivery of anesthesia or adverse events.

Automation: Problems and Challenges

Errors in the design of automated systems may be more difficult to recover from than operator errors. If the automation fails, the operator must suddenly take over control and may have lost the skills necessary to do so.[77] Complicating matters further, the failure of automated systems is less predictable and more difficult to diagnose for the operator. When a process is under operator control, the operator is aware of its state and is inherently able to complete the process manually. One implication is that failures shift from easily observable slips, occurring when the operator is performing the task, to difficult-to-detect mistakes when automation and designer error contribute to breakdowns.

Automated systems are introduced to increase system performance in addition to reducing human error. As the level of automation increases, so does the opacity of the system due to the larger complexity of the underlying algorithms. A high level of knowledge about the system is required in order for the operator to understand what the system is doing. Consequently and somewhat counterintuitively, the higher the level of automation, the more training is required for the operator of the system.[78]

Increasing levels of automation can yield better performance when all is well, but may become problematic since they contribute to degradation of performance when the system fails[79] (for an health care (HC) example, see [80]). Increasing the complexity and support provided by an automated system may significantly increase the impact of adverse effects on system performance. As operator involvement decreases, there is less opportunity to support system recovery in the face of an automation error.

Using automation to increase system performance should lower clinician workload and leave a healthcare worker with more time to focus on patients, thereby enhancing patient safety, but several factors work against this goal. Firstly, "clumsy automation" frequently increases the operator's workload[81,82] by forcing the clinician to monitor and second-guess the automated system while continuing to perform the task at hand. Improvement in the level of automation results in increased performance pressure: the system is stretched to again operate at capacity by requiring a greater level of activity on the part of the operator.

HUMAN-CENTERED AUTOMATION

Although traditional automation does not focus on socio-technical elements of the work and often requires the operator to accommodate the system, human-centered automation aims to design systems that work in conjunction with the human operator. It is possible to identify a number of principles that should be implemented to have "true" human-centered automation in anesthesiology (for application of this to aviation, see [83]). Criteria that should be included are subject to ongoing controversy; this section covers some of the least controversial criteria. Tasks should be allocated such that the human performs those for which he or she is best suited, while the automation is responsible for tasks that it can perform best. The human operator should be kept in the decision and control loop; the automation should not have complete control. The human operator should be the final authority over automation, and the job of the operator should be made easier and more satisfying through automation, not more difficult and less satisfying, and the automation should be engineered to reduce human error and minimize response variability.

Design Principles

The design of user interfaces is often described as a process that focuses on the user and the user's task. Taking a socio-technical perspective into account requires a broader perspective in healthcare in general and anesthesiology in particular. Several cognitive stages of information processing are involved when interacting with a computer interface. Following a standard information-processing framework, these stages are a *perceptual stage*, a *cognitive stage*, and a *response stage*. Each stage should be carefully considered in interface design. Common design elements often optimize the human-technology interface at more than one stage. The next sections describe general principles of interface design.

Perception

Interface design, especially for patient monitoring and device interfaces, offers an interesting challenge: the design must support rapid perception of information because rapid intervention may be needed, but the response to the information provided must be error-free while the operator is under stress or with concurrent cognitive demand from other tasks. The following principles of interface design support visual perception.

Interfaces should be transparent: it should be easy to identify how an interface works and how to interact with it simply by observing it.[50] A good GUI supports this by clearly showing the features that are available, rather than forcing a user to remember them (although alternatives such as keyboard shortcuts may not be immediately visible but can speed the interaction for expert users). The features should have clear affordances—that is, available actions that will accomplish the desired goal should be immediately obvious. Again, a good GUI will use graphical elements that have obvious activities associated with them (e.g., buttons, icons, folders, or sliders).

Information display should support rapid recognition and quick search. Important information can be made more salient by differentiating it from other information—for instance, by displaying it in a different color or a bolder or larger font, or by varying it on any other dimension. This can be done redundantly on more than one dimension to improve saliency. The greater the degree of difference in one or more dimensions, the more information will be obvious to a user who is searching for it, dramatically reducing the time required to find it. Information can also be grouped using gestalt principles to support faster perception and acquisition of information.[84]

Among those gestalt principles are that items that are located proximally, enclosed, move, or change together, or that look alike in size, shape, or color, are automatically perceived as a group. Grouping items that have something in common (e.g., variables related to the respiratory system) allows the user to quickly scan and focus on that group while ignoring others, thereby limiting the scope of a search for a specific piece of information such as respiratory rate.[85]

Cognition/Planning

Perceived information must be processed and integrated into existing knowledge, either following a fast and effortless pattern-matching process or a serial, slow, and cognitively demanding process.[48] A mental model is used to perform complex tasks by making predictions and inferences about future states of the controlled system. An interface designer must understand a user's mental model in order to understand the goals, actions, and information needs that are required when performing a task. When there is a match between an interface and a user's mental model, task performance increases because less time is required for interaction and learning. Interfaces in current use often reflect the mental model of the developer and not the user, imposing an unnecessary burden on cognition and thus reducing the possibility of successful and efficient interaction.

Using metaphors to exploit a user's existing mental models is a good approach for design—for example, using a patient's anatomy to structure information. Allowing such fit between a display and a user's conceptual knowledge facilitates interaction.[86,87]

Response Processes

After the information has been processed, a response must be generated and/or selected, to be executed. This response may require interaction with an HTI, and the goal is to facilitate the response so that is can be executed without delay.

Mapping

Controls should be related to their effects and should be consistent with the relationship between the object and the required action (e.g., knobs should be turned). This relationship can be representative, as is described by the principle of *pictorial realism*, in which the information on a display has the appearance of the variable it represents. It is also described by the principle of moving parts, in which there is a relationship between the movement of a control and its effects (for instance, increasing the value of a variable with a vertical slider should involve upward, rather than downward, movement.[88] Mapping should be logical, expected, and consistent. One example of consistent mapping is in older anesthesia machines where control was executed by turning mechanical knobs. These mechanical controls have been replaced with electronic "knobs," and most machines require two steps to modify the settings: first turning the knob, and then pushing the knob to actually apply the changes.[89]

Direct Manipulation

When at all possible, the user should be able to perform actions directly on the objects that are visible. Such actions are easier to learn and are consistent with the user's mental model of a task, thus reducing error and enhancing performance.

Providing a Natural Dialogue

Interfaces should present information in the natural language of the task. Task analysis that determines specific terminology that can simplify the labeling in an interface will minimize the effort required to navigate the system.

Error-Tolerant Systems and Ease of Error Recovery

Because human error is common, interfaces should be designed for rapid error recovery by minimizing the negative consequences of errors. This includes the prevention or mitigation of dangerous consequences when error occurs. One characteristic that predisposes a system to operator error is numerous modes within it. Ramundo and Larach report a case in which physicians noticed a mismatch between their patient observations and the variables on the patient monitor: the patient's blood pressure was constantly 120/70.[90] Wondering about the constant values, the physicians realized that the monitor was in demonstration mode and was not displaying patient data.

Individual User Characteristics

Individual user characteristics need to be considered in the context of the HTI. For example, designers must take into account the high percentage of color-blind users (8% of the male population) because anesthesiologists in the United States are predominantly male. Aging is another important consideration because it affects perceptual, cognitive, and response processes. Although these changes are gradual and begin in the late twenties, they become more serious with increasing age. User experience, level of education, work experience, and previous computer experience must also be considered.

Designing for Teams

The design principles outlined thus far focus mostly on the design for individual users, but a socio-technical perspective should include the design of the HTI. There is currently only limited work on how to facilitate team interaction by using specific design principles. Although some studies have evaluated shared information boards used to visualize the scheduling of operating rooms, not much is known about how to provide information that facilitates teamwork. Given the increasing amount of collaboration in anesthesia, there is a need for guiding principles that allow interdisciplinary and intradisciplinary sharing of information in surgical teams. Development of these technologies may be guided by studies of the effectiveness of electronic whiteboards in the OR to increase adherence to pre-incision safety practices.[91]

A Universal Interface Grammar

It is important to establish a grammar of information display so that devices that are designed by different people and produced by different manufacturers follow the same rules. The use of a new interface requires learning that will be accelerated by following familiar

GUI standards. For a unique GUI, however, maintaining a consistent interface can minimize the learning curve. That is, similar operations performed within the interface should use similar elements to achieve similar tasks, and coding, grouping, and action principles should be similar across interfaces. A consistent system enables faster learning, and it will have lower error rates and will be easier to use, especially when users must interact with multiple different systems simultaneously. These benefits will be realized to a greater degree if consistent design can be applied within a given interface and also between the interfaces of multiple devices in the healthcare setting.

TRAINING

Simulation is becoming an increasingly important component of training in healthcare. Aviation was one of the earliest disciplines to introduce simulation at the beginning of the twentieth century. Drews and Bakdash[92] identified some of the differences between the social, natural, and technical systems of simulation training in aviation and healthcare, and illustrated some of the limitations associated with simulation use.

The specialty of anesthesiology has been among the leaders in adapting new technologies and approaches within healthcare. Although increases in automation can enhance patient safety and reduce operator workload, a higher level of knowledge is needed to use systems safely and effectively as they become more complex, especially when automation fails. This implies that due to the increase in the complexity of the technological interfaces, the requirement for training increases significantly.[93] One method of providing the necessary training is the use of simulation-based training.

Full-body, mannequin simulators for anesthesiologists were developed for training and assessment in the mid-1980s by two groups: the Stanford CAE-Link simulator by Gaba and DeAnda[25] and the Gainesville Anesthesia Simulator by Good and Gravenstein at the University of Florida in Gainesville. Both groups focused on recognizing and managing critical events during anesthesia, but used different approaches. For example, Gaba and DeAnda were teaching Crew Resource Management, which originated in aviation to develop more effective teams and uses elements from a socio-technical systems perspective. Gaba's Simulation-Based Training in Anesthesia Crisis Resource Management (ACRM) consisted of highly realistic scenarios in which anesthesiologists had to manage emerging acute events. To improve the effectiveness of the simulation, a detailed debriefing was performed at the end of a scenario that focused on both technical and non-technical skills. Non-technical skills included principles of crisis management, which focused on leadership, teamwork, workload distribution, resource utilization, re-evaluation, and communication. Adoption of the approach was relatively fast in the United States and Canada, and non-technical skills training now represents the majority of all anesthesia simulation training.[94-96]

Recently developed simulation technology includes virtual reality, mannequins, and computer-based simulations.[97-99] Cook et al. performed a large meta-analysis of the effectiveness of technology-enhanced simulation training (609 studies) and found consistent large effects.[97] Virtual anesthesia machine simulators can be either photorealistic or diagrammatic. Fischler et al. suggested that a transparent simulator might lead to a deeper understanding of the structure and function of the machine. They found that users who were allowed to see and explore the entire system built a stronger mental model of how it worked, and they suggest that this will aid in managing adverse events.[100]

As simulators have become more realistic, a focus on training for technical skills has become increasingly possible. Simulators are now used to teach skills such as intubation and cricothyroidotomy,[101-103] identification of performance gaps,[104-108] and usability testing of new equipment.[109]

Non-Technical Skills Training

Simulation training can be used to develop non-technical skills such as interpersonal skills, including communication,[110] teamwork and leadership, and cognitive skills that include task management, situation awareness,[39] and decision-making.[111,112] There has recently been an emergence of non-technical skills training, especially in anesthesia and surgery,[25,113–115] and other medical specialties are following suit. Rall, Gaba, and Miller[116] point out the similarity of the non-technical skills required in anesthesia and those required in other areas of healthcare (e.g., the ICU). Fletcher et al.[113] provide an example of how to identify important non-technical skills for anesthesiologists. The Anesthetist's Non-Technical Skills (ANTS) behavioral marker system includes four core non-technical skills: task management, teamworking, situation awareness, and decision-making. Flin and Maran[117] describe a simulator-based course that targets these non-technical skills.

Simulator-Based Performance Assessment
Individual Performance

The assessment of individual performance in the context of medical training has been described in detail by Drews and Bakdash[92] with an emphasis on human factors. In one study[118] a human-factors-based program was used to train first-year anesthesiology residents in difficult airway management. The intervention group received *part task training* (PTT), which focuses on dividing complex tasks into components, followed by intensive concentrated training on individual components. They also received *variable priority training* (VPT), which focuses on the distribution of attention while performing multiple simultaneous tasks in order to facilitate flexible allocation of attention. The control group participated in a standard didactic program. While participants in both groups showed a significant improvement in all metrics after a year of training, the intervention group was able to complete more tasks and correctly answer more comprehension questions. This suggests that introducing human-factors approaches toward training can improve simulation-based training in anesthesiology.

Boulet and Murray[119] reviewed the literature regarding simulation-based performance assessment with a specific focus on anesthesia.

Relatively low inter-rater reliability when assessing performance is among the challenges of assessing individual performance, especially non-technical skill; inter-rater reliability is usually higher when focusing on technical skills and clinical management tasks. Overall, one current limitation is that simulation-based performance has yet to be proven to generalize to the clinical context or to be a valid predictor of performance.

Team Performance

An increasing level of attention is being directed toward the assessment of team performance because recent work establishes that gaps in team coordination and team communication are often a significant contributor to the genesis of adverse events. Among the challenges, despite some recent progress,[113,120–124] there is a lack of valid and reliable methods to assess team performance. As with individual performance assessment, there is no evidence of how team-based performance in the simulator generalizes into the clinical context.

CONCLUSIONS

Much of the recent progress in healthcare has trended toward more information, more complex working environments, and the adoption of new technologies. These developments have led to a variety of challenges that must be addressed: How can automation be made to function as part of the healthcare team? How can information from a growing number of sensors be displayed in a more effective manner to facilitate more effective patient management? How can the performance of the anesthesiologist be maintained or improved in an environment with increasing responsibilities and task complexity? Given that components of the socio-technical system in anesthesia are developed by different designers and manufacturers, how can a consistent user interface be maintained? How can training be improved and focused on individual and team performance? While automation provides some answers to these questions, it is human-centered automation that will have a significant impact on performance.

Future Outlook

As healthcare requires increasing levels of specialization, healthcareprofessionals will necessarily function as part of a team. Automation of some functions is changing the work that anesthesiologists do, and automation must be made to function as part of the team. Future efforts toward automation must be guided by a socio-technical perspective instead of an engineering perspective only.

Each specialty uses specific equipment, and each device has a unique interface that is determined by the tasks to be performed and the information that is relevant. Although the tasks and information will always be different, other unrelated design differences can somewhat arbitrarily and unnecessarily add to the complexity of a socio-technical system. Some information will inevitably be common to multiple specialties—basic vital signs, for instance—and this information should be presented similarly to both the surgeon and the anesthesiologist in such way that it is easily accessible for each of them.

Future systems should be designed for all practitioners who are part of a team. A common interface grammar could make a system immediately familiar to users from a range of backgrounds. Actions should be accomplished in the same manner, and information should be presented similarly (location, color, and iconography should all be standardized).

In addition, there is a need to develop integrative displays for the anesthesia team. Sensor data need to be integrated in such way that they provide information and tell the "story of the patient," with specific attention to patient idiosyncrasies. While some basic work has been done to develop such displays, more work is required to develop displays that are intuitive and that follow the design principles outlined. Similar to aviation, there is a move toward a glass cockpit for anesthesiologists. However, developers will have to be careful to not use the large available display space as an excuse for not integrating the information to support anesthesiologists' cognition. In addition, following Herbert Simon's quote of "a wealth of information leads to poverty of attention,"[125] it is critical to not provide all information that is available, but only that which is necessary.

Overall, in the future the use of advanced technology in healthcare and especially anesthesia will inevitably continue to grow. The changes associated with this development require a socio-technical systems approach, coupled with human factors, to guide HTI development in a way that avoids many of the potential drawbacks and realizes the full potential of advanced technology.

REFERENCES

1. Rochlin, GI. *Trapped in the Net: The Unanticipated Consequences of Computerization* Princeton: MA: Princeton University Press. 1997.
2. Tenner, E. *Why Things Bite Back: Technology and the Revenge of Unintended Consequences.* New York: Knopf; 1997.
3. Garg AX, Adhikari NK, McDonald H, Rosas-Arellano MP, Devereaux PJ, Beyene J, ... Haynes RB. Effects of computerized clinical decision support systems on practitioner performance and patient outcomes: a systematic review. *JAMA.* 2005;293(10):1223–1238.
4. Koppel R, Metlay JP, Cohen A, Abaluck B, Localio AR, Kimmel SE, Strom BL. Role of computerized physician order entry systems in facilitating medication errors. *JAMA.* 2005;293(10):1197–1203.
5. Trist E. The evolution of sociotechnical systems as a conceptual framework and as an action research program. In: Van de Ven A, Joyce W, eds. *Perspectives on Organization Design and Behavior.* New York: Wiley; 1981:19–75.
6. Cherns A. The principles of sociotechnical design. *Hum Relat.* 1976;29(8):783–792.
7. Carayon P, Hundt AS, Karsh BT, Gurses AP, Alvarado CJ, Smith M, Brennan PF. Work system design for patient safety: the SEIPS model. *Qual Saf Health Care.* 2006;15(Suppl 1):i50–i58.
8. Scacci W. Socio-technical design. In: Bainbridge WS, ed. *The Berkshire Encyclopedia of Human-Computer Interaction.* Great Barrington, MA: Berkshire Publishing; 2004:656–659.
9. Harrison MI, Koppel R, Bar-Lev S. Unintended consequences of information technologies in health care: an interactive sociotechnical analysis. *J Am Med Inform Assn.* 2007;14(5):542–549.
10. Dillon A. Group dynamics meet cognition: combining socio-technical concepts and usability engineering in the design of information systems. In: Coakes E, ed. *The New Socio Tech: Graffiti on the Long Wall.* London: Springer; 2000:119–126.

11. Han YY, Carcillo JA, Venkataraman ST, Clark RS, Watson RS, Nguyen TC, ... Orr RA. Unexpected increased mortality after implementation of a commercially sold computerized physician order entry system. *Pediatrics.* 2005;116(6):1506–1512.

12. Bar-Yam Y. *Dynamics of Complex Systems*, Vol. 213. Reading, MA: Addison-Wesley; 1997.

13. Raichman N, Gabay T, Katsir Y, Shapira Y, Ben-Jacob E. Engineered self-organization in natural and man-made systems. In: Bergman, David J and Inan, Esin (Eds.) *Continuum Models and Discrete Systems*. Dordrecht: Springer; 2004:187–205.

14. Tompkins G, Azadivar F. Genetic algorithms in optimizing simulated systems. In: *Proceedings of the 27th Conference on Winter Simulation*. IEEE Computer Society, December 1995:757–762.

15. Collier JD, Hooker CA. Complexly organised dynamical systems. *Open Syst Inform Dyn*, 1999;6(3):241–302.

16. Kelso JS, Ding M, Schoner G. Dynamic pattern formation: a primer. In *Santa Fe Institute Studies in the Sciences of Complexity Proceedings* (Vol. 13, p. 397). Addison-Wesley; 1992.

17. Sterman JD. Learning in and about complex systems. *Syst Dyn Rev.* 1994;10(2–3):291–330. doi:10.1002/sdr.4260100214

18. Glass PS, Rampil IJ. Automated anesthesia: fact or fantasy? *Anesthesiology.* 2001;95(1):1–2.

19. Drews FA, Doig A. Evaluation of a configural vital signs display for intensive care unit nurses. *Hum Factors.* 2014;56(3):596–580.

20. Chisholm CD, Dornfeld AM, Nelson DR, Cordell WH. Work interrupted: a comparison of workplace interruptions in emergency departments and primary care offices. *Ann Emerg Med.* 2001;38(2):146–151. doi: 10.1067/mem.2001.115440.

21. Drews FA. The frequency and impact of task interruptions in the ICU. *Proceedings of the Human Factors and Ergonomics Society Annual Meeting*, 2007;51(11):683–686.

22. Grundgeiger T, Liu D, Sanderson PM, Jenkins S, Leane T. Effects of interruptions on prospective memory performance in anesthesiology. *Proceedings of the Human Factors and Ergonomics Society Annual Meeting*, 2008;52(12):808–812. doi: 10.1177/154193120805201209

23. Ren, Kiesler, and Fussell, Cambridge: Cambridge University Press, UK; 2008.

24. Craik K. *The Nature of Explanation*. Cambridge: Cambridge University Press; 1943.

25. Gaba DM, DeAnda A. The response of anesthesia trainees to simulated critical incidents. *Anesth Analg.* 1989;68(4):444–451. doi: 10.1213/00000539-198904000-00004.

26. Gaba DM, Fish K, Howard S. *Crisis Management in Anesthesia*. New York: Churchill-Livingstone; 1994.

27. Endsley MR. Predictive utility of an objective measure of situation awareness. In: *Proceedings of the Human Factors Society 34th Annual Meeting*. Santa Monica, CA: Human Factors and Ergonomics Society; 1990:41–45.

28. Endsley MR. *Situation Awareness Global Assessment Technique (SAGAT): Air-to-Air Tactical Version User Guide*. Hawthorne, CA: Northrop; 1990.

29. Endsley MR. Toward a theory of situation awareness in dynamic systems. *Hum Factors.* 1995;37(1):32–64. doi: 10.1518/001872095779049543.

30. Gilson RD. Situation awareness [Special section]. *Hum Factors.* 1995;37:3–157.

31. Klein G. The recognition-primed decision (RPD) model: Looking back, looking forward. In: Zsambrock CE, Klein G, eds. *Naturalistic Decision-Making*. Mahwah, NJ: Lawrence Erlbaum; 1997:285–292.

32. Klein G. *Sources of Power*. Cambridge, MA: MIT Press; 1998.

33. Nyssen AS, De Keyser V. Improving training in problem solving skills: analysis of anesthetists' performance in simulated problem situations. *Le travail humain.* 1998; 2:387–401.

34. Dinadis N, Vicente KJ. Designing functional visualizations for aircraft system status displays. *Int J Aviat Psychol.* 1999;9:241–269.

35. Niessen C, Eyferth K, Bierwagen T. Modelling cognitive processes of experienced air traffic controllers. *Ergonomics*, 1998;42:1507–1520.

36. Itoh J, Sakuma A, Monta K. An ecological interface for supervisory control of BWR nuclear power plants. *Control Engin Practice.* 1995; 3:231–239.

37. Pawlak WS, Vicente KJ. Inducing effective operator control through ecological interface design. *Int J Human-Comp Studies.* 1996;44(5):653–688. doi: 10.1006/ijhc.1996.0028.

38. Vicente KJ, Rasmussen J. The ecology of human-machine systems II: mediating "Direct Perception" in complex work domains. *Ecol Psychology.* 1990;2(3):207–249. doi: 10.1207/s15326969eco0203_2.

39. Gaba DM, Howard SK, Small SD. Situation awareness in anesthesiology. *Hum Factors.* 1995;37(1):20–31. doi: 10.1518/001872095779049435.

40. Fioratou E, Flin R, Glavin R, Patey R. Beyond monitoring: distributed situation awareness in anaesthesia. *Br J Anaesth.* 2010;105(1):83–90.

41. Drews FA, Zhang Y, Westenskow DR, Foresti S, Agutter J, Bermudez JC, ... Loeb R. Effects of

integrated graphical displays on situation awareness in anaesthesiology. *Cognit Technol Work*, 2002;4(2):82–90. doi: 10.1007/s101110200007.

42. Ford S, Daniels J, Lim J, Koval V, Dumont G, Schwarz SKW, Ansermino JM. A novel vibrotactile display to improve the performance of anesthesiologists in a simulated critical incident. *Anesth Analg.* 2008;106(4):1182–1188, table of contents. doi: 10.1213/ane.0b013e318163f7c2.

43. Schulz CM, Endsley MR, Kochs EF, Gelb AW, Wagner KJ. Situation awareness in anesthesia: concept and research. *Anesthesiology.* 2013; 118(3):729–742. doi: 10.1097/ALN.0b013e318-280a40f.

44. Goodstein LP. Discriminative display support for process operators. In: Rasmussen J, Rouse WB, eds. *Human Detection and Diagnosis of System Failure.* New York: Plenum; 1981:433–449.

45. Vicente KJ, Christoffersen K, Pereklita A. Supporting operator problem solving through ecological interface design. *IEEE Trans Syst Man Cybernetics.* 1995;25(4):529–545. doi: 10.1109/21.370186

46. Drews FA, Agutter J, Syroid ND, Albert RW, Westenskow DR, Strayer DL. Evaluating a graphical cardiovascular display for anesthesia. *Proceedings of the Human Factors and Ergonomics Society Annual Meeting*, 2001;45(17): 1303–1307.

47. Albert RW, Agutter JA, Syroid ND, Johnson KB, Loeb RG, Westenskow DR. A simulation-based evaluation of a graphic cardiovascular display. *Anesth Analg.* 2007;105(5):1303–1311.

48. Drews FA, Westenskow DR. The right picture is worth a thousand numbers: data displays in anesthesia. *Hum Factors.* 2006;48(1):59–71.

49. Norman D. *Things That Make Us Smart: Defending Human Attributes in the Age of the Machine.* Reading, MA: Addison-Wesley; 1993.

50. Norman D. *The Design of Everyday Things.* New York: Currency and Doubleday; 1990.

51. Leape LL, Woods DD, Hatlie MJ, Kizer KW, Schroeder SA, Lundberg GD. Promoting patient safety by preventing medical error. *JAMA.* 1998;280(16):1444–1447.

52. Reason JT. *Managing the Risks of Organizational Accidents.* Aldershot, UK: Ashgate; 1997.

53. Gardner RM, Shabot M. Patient monitoring systems. In Shortliffe EH, Perrault LE, Wiederhold G, Fagan LM (Eds) *Medical Informatics: Computer Applications in Health Care and Biomedicine.* 2nd ed. New York: Springer; 2001:443–484.

54. Cole WG, Stewart JG. Metaphor graphics to support integrated decision-making with respiratory data. *Int J Clin Monitor Comput.* 1993;10(2):91–100.

55. Michels P, Gravenstein D, Westenskow DR. An integrated graphic data display improves detection and identification of critical events during anesthesia. *J Clin Monitor.* 1997;13(4):249–259.

56. Liu D, Jenkins S, Sanderson PM, Leane T, Watson MO, Russell W. Simulator evaluation of head-mounted displays for patient monitoring. *Anesth Analg.* 2008;106(S2):34.

57. Liu D, Jenkins SA, Sanderson PM, Fabian P, Russell WJ. Monitoring with head-mounted displays in general anesthesia: a clinical evaluation in the operating room. *Anesth Analg.* 2010;110(4):1032–1038. doi: 10.1213/ANE.0b013e3181d3e647.

58. Sanderson PM, Watson MO, Russell WJ. Advanced patient monitoring displays: tools for continuous informing. *Anesth Analg.* 2005; 101(1):161–168, table of contents. doi: 10.1213/01.ANE.0000154080.67496.AE

59. Halbeis CBE, Epstein RH, Macario A, Pearl RG, Grunwald Z. Adoption of anesthesia information management systems by academic departments in the United States. *Anesth Analg.* 2008;*107*(4), 1323–1329.

60. Ehrenfeld JM, Rehman MA. Anesthesia information management systems: a review of functionality and installation considerations. *J Clin Monitor Comput.* 2011;25(1):71–79.

61. Hemmerling TM, Cirillo F, Cyr S. *Decision Support Systems in Medicine-Anesthesia, Critical Care and Intensive Care Medicine.* INTECH Open Access Publisher, 2012.

62. Nair BG, Newman S, Peterson GN, Schwid HA. Smart Anesthesia Manager™ (SAM): a real-time decision support system for anesthesia care during surgery. *IEEE Trans Bio-Med Engineering.* 2013;60(1):207–210. doi: 10.1109/TBME.2012.2205384.

63. Van Nimwegen C. *The Paradox of the Guided User: Assistance Can Be Counter-Effective.* Utrecht: Utrecht University; 2008.

64. van Nimwegen C, van Oostendorp H. The questionable impact of an assisting interface on performance in transfer situations.*International Journal of Industrial Ergonomics* 2009;*39*(3), 501–508

65. Brody R, Kowalczyk T, Coulter J. The effect of a computerized decision aid on the development of knowledge. *J Business Psychol.* 2003;18(2): 157–174.

66. Sparrow B, Liu J, Wegner DM. Google effects on memory: cognitive consequences of having information at our fingertips. *Science (New York).* 2011;333(6043):776–778. doi: 10.1126/science.1207745.

67. Epstein RH, Dexter F, Ehrenfeld JM, Sandberg WS. Implications of event entry latency on anesthesia information management decision

support systems. *Anesth Analg.* 2009;108(3):941–947. doi: 10.1213/ane.0b013e3181949ae6.

68. Cassidy CJ, Smith A, Arnot-Smith J. Critical incident reports concerning anaesthetic equipment: analysis of the UK National Reporting and Learning System (NRLS) data from 2006–2008. *Anaesthesia.* 2011;66(10), 879–888. doi: 10.1111/j.1365-2044.2011.06826.x.

69. Fasting S, Gisvold S. Equipment problems during anaesthesia: are they a quality problem? *Br J Anaesth.* 2002;89(6):825–831.

70. Beydon L, Conreux F. Analysis of the French health ministry's national register of incidents involving medical devices in anaesthesia and intensive care. *British Journal of Anesthesia,* 2001;86(3):382–387.

71. Chopra V, Bovill JG, Spierdijk J, Koornneef F. Reported significant observations during anaesthesia: a prospective analysis over an 18-month period. *Br J Anaesth.* 1992;68(1):13–17. doi: 10.1093/bja/68.1.13.

72. Caplan RA, Vistica MF, Posner KL, Cheney FW. Adverse anesthetic outcomes arising from gas delivery equipment. *Anesthesiology.* 1997;87:741–748. doi: 10.1097/00000542-199710000-00006.

73. Dumont GA, Ansermino JM. Closed-loop control of anesthesia: a primer for anesthesiologists. *Anesth Analg.* 2013;117(5), 1130–1138. doi: 10.1213/ANE.0b013e3182973687.

74. Schwilden H, Schuttler J. The determination of an effective therapeutic infusion rate for intravenous anesthetics using feedback-controlled dosages. *Anaesthesist.* 1990;39:603–606.

75. Schwilden H, Schuttler J. Target controlled anaesthetic drug dosing. *Handb Exp Pharmacol.* 2008;182:425–450.

76. Leslie K, Clavisi O, Hargrove J. Target-controlled infusion versus manually-controlled infusion of propofol for general anaesthesia or sedation in adults. Anesthesia and Analgesia, 2008;107:2089.

77. Lee JD. Review of a pivotal human factors article: "Humans and Automation: Use, Misuse, Disuse, Abuse." *Hum Factors.* 2008;50(3):404–410. doi: 10.1518/001872008X288547.

78. Bainbridge L. Ironies of automation. *Automatica.* 1983;19(6):775–779.

79. Onnasch L, Wickens CD, Li H, Manzey D. Human performance consequences of stages and levels of automation: an integrated meta-analysis. *Hum Factors.* 2013;56(3):476–488. doi: 10.1177/0018720813501549.

80. Wears RL, Cook RI, Perry SJ. Automation, interaction, complexity, and failure: a case study. *Reliab Engin Syst Saf.* 2006;91(12):1494–1501. doi: 10.1016/j.ress.2006.01.009.

81. Wiener, Earl L. Cockpit automation. In: Wiener EL, Nagel DC, eds. *Human Factors in Aviation.* Academic Press series in cognition and perception. San Diego, CA: Academic Press; 1998:433–461.

82. Wiener EL. Reflections on human error: matters of life and death. In *Proceedings of the Human Factors and Ergonomics Society Annual Meeting,* October 1989 (Vol. 33, no. 1, pp. 1–7). SAGE Publications.

83. Billings C. *Aviation Automation: The Search for a Human-Centered Approach.* Mahwah, NJ: Lawrence Erlbaum; 1997.

84. Rock I, Palmer S. The legacy of Gestalt psychology. *Sci Am.* 1990;263(6):84–90. doi: 10.1038/scientificamerican1290-84.

85. Wickens CD, Carswell CM. The proximity compatibility principle: its psychological foundation and relevance to display design. *Hum Factors.* 1995;37(3):473–494. doi: 10.1518/001872095779049408.

86. Carroll JM, Mack RL, Kellogg WA. Interface metaphors and user interface design. In: Helander M, ed., *Handbook of Human-Computer Interface.* Cambridge: Cambridge University Press; 1988:74–102.

87. Wozny LA. The application of metaphor, analogy, and conceptual models in computer systems. *Interact Comput.* 1989;1(3):273–283. doi: 10.1016/0953-5438(89)90015-5.

88. Roscoe SN. Airborne displays for flight and navigation. *Hum Factors.* 1968;10(4), 321–332.

89. Patil VP, Shetmahajan MG, Divatia JV. The modern integrated anaesthesia workstation. *Indian J Anaesth.* 2013;57(5):446–454. doi: 10.4103/0019-5049.120139.

90. Ramundo GB, Larach DR. A monitor with a mind of its own. *Anesthesiology.* 1995;82(1):317. doi:10.1097/00000542-199501000-00049.

91. Mainthia R, Lockney T, Zotov A, France DJ, Bennett M, St Jacques PJ, . . . Anders S. Novel use of electronic whiteboard in the operating room increases surgical team compliance with pre-incision safety practices. *Surgery.* 2012;151(5):660–666. doi: 10.1016/j.surg.2011.12.005.

92. Drews FA, Bakdash JZ. Simulation training in health care. *Rev Hum Factors Ergonom.* 2013;8(1):191–234.

93. Bainbridge L. The change in concepts needed to account for human behavior in complex dynamic tasks. *Syst Man Cybernet A.* 1997;27(3):351–359.

94. Cooper JB, Taqueti VR. A brief history of the development of mannequin simulators for clinical education and training. *Postgrad Med J.* 2008;84:563–570.

95. Gaba DM, Howard SK, Fish KJ, Smith BE, Sowb YA. Simulation-based training in anesthesia

crisis resource management (ACRM): a decade of experience. *Simulat Gaming.* 2001;32: 175–193.

96. Glavin R, Flin R. Review article: the influence of psychology and human factors on education in anesthesiology. *Can J Anaesth.* 2012;59(2):151–158. doi: 10.1007/s12630-011-9634-z.

97. Cook DA, Hatala R, Brydges R, Zendejas B, Szostek JH, Wang AT, Erwin PJ, Hamstra SJ. Technology-enhanced simulation for health professions education: a systematic review and meta-analysis. *JAMA.* 2011;306(9):978–988. doi: 10.1001/jama.2011.1234.

98. Chu LF, Young C, Zamora A, Kurup V, Macario A. Anesthesia 2.0: internet-based information resources and Web 2.0 applications in anesthesia education. *Curr Opin Anaesth.* 2010;23(2):218–227. doi: 10.1097/ACO.0b013e328337339c.

99. Rosen KR. The history of medical simulation. *J Crit Care.* 2008;23(2):157–166. doi: 10.1016/j.jcrc.2007.12.004.

100. Fischler IS, Kaschub CE, Lizdas DE, Lampotang S. Understanding of anesthesia machine function is enhanced with a transparent reality simulation. *Simulat Healthcare.* 2008;3(1):26–32. doi: 10.1097/SIH.0b013e31816366d3.

101. Boet S, Bould M, Schaeffer R. Learning fibreoptic intubation with a virtual computer program transfers to "hands on" improvement. *Eur J Anesth.* 2010;27(1):31–35.

102. Chandra DB, Savoldelli GL, Joo HS, Weiss ID, Naik VN. Fiberoptic oral intubation: the effect of model fidelity on training for transfer to patient care. *Anesthesiology.* 2008;109:1007–1013.

103. Friedman Z, You-Ten KE, Bould MD, Naik V. Teaching lifesaving procedures: the impact of model fidelity on acquisition and transfer of cricothyrotomy skills to performance on cadavers. *Anesth Analg.* 2008;107:1663–1669.

104. Lorraway PG, Savoldelli GL, Joo HS, Chandra DB, Chow R, Naik VN. Management of simulated oxygen supply failure: is there a gap in the curriculum? *Anesth Analg.* 2006;102(3):865–867. doi: 10.1213/01.ane.0000195548.38669.6c.

105. Blike G, Christoffersen K. A method for measuring system safety and latent errors associated with pediatric procedural sedation. *Anesth Analg.* 2005;101(1):48–58.

106. Lighthall GK, Poon T, Harrison TK. Using in situ simulation to improve in-hospital cardiopulmonary resuscitation. *Jt Comm J Qual Patient Saf.* 2010;36(5):209–216.

107. Harrison TK, Manser T, Howard SK, Gaba DM. Use of cognitive aids in a simulated anesthetic crisis. *Anesth Analg.* 2006;103(3):551–556. doi: 10.1213/01.ane.0000229718.02478.c4.

108. Mudumbai SC, Fanning R, Howard SK, Davies MF, Gaba DM. Use of medical simulation to explore equipment failures and human-machine interactions in anesthesia machine pipeline supply crossover. *Anesth Analg.* 2010;110(5), 1292–1296. doi:10.1213/ANE.0b013e3181d7e097

109. Dalle, P, Robinson B, Weller J, Caldwell C. The use of high-fidelity human patient simulation and the introduction of new anesthesia delivery systems. *Anesth Analg.* 2004;99(6): 1737–1741.

110. Baker DP, Gustafson S, Beaubien JM, Salas E, Barach P. *Medical Team Training Programs in Health Care.* Rockville, MD: Agency for Healthcare Research and Quality; 2005.

111. Cosby KS, Croskerry P. Patient safety: a curriculum for teaching patient safety in emergency medicine. *Acad Emerg Med.* 2003;10(1): 69–78.

112. Gaba DM. Dynamic decision-making in anesthesiology: cognitive models and training approaches. In: David A. Evans, Vimla L. Patel (Eds) *Advanced Models of Cognition for Medical Training and Practice.* Berlin and Heidelberg: Springer; 1992:123–147.

113. Fletcher G, Flin R, McGeorge P, Glavin R, Maran N, Patey R. Anaesthetists' Non-Technical Skills (ANTS): evaluation of a behavioural marker system. *Br J Anaesth.* 2003;90(5):580–588.

114. Helmreich RL, Merritt AR. *Culture at Work in Aviation and Medicine: National, Organizational and Professional Influences.* Ashgate Publishing: Surrey, United Kingdom;2001.

115. Yee B, Naik VN, Joo HS, Savoldelli GL, Chung DY, Houston PL, ... Hamstra SJ. Nontechnical skills in anesthesia crisis management with repeated exposure to simulation-based education. *Anesthesiology.* 2005;103(2), 241–248. doi: 10.1097/00000542-200508000-00006.

116. Rall M, Gaba D. Patient simulators. In: Miller R, ed. *Miller's Anesthesia,* 6th ed. Oxford: Elsevier, 2005, 3073–103.

117. Flin R, Maran N. Identifying and training non-technical skills for teams in acute medicine. *Qual Saf Health Care.* 2004;13(Suppl 1):i80–i84.

118. Johnson KB, Syroid ND, Drews FA, Ogden LL, Strayer DL, Pace NL, ... Westenskow DR. Part task and variable priority training in first-year anesthesia resident education: a combined didactic and simulation-based approach to improve management of adverse airway and respiratory events. *Anesthesiology.* 2008;108(5):831–840. doi: 10.1097/ALN.0b013e31816bbd54.

119. Boulet JR, Murray DJ. Simulation-based assessment in anesthesiology: requirements for practical implementation. *Anesthesiology.* 2010;112:1041–1052.

120. Cooper S, Cant R, Porter J, Sellick K, Somers G, Kinsman L, Nestel D. Rating medical emergency teamwork performance: development of the Team Emergency Assessment Measure (TEAM). *Resuscitation,* 2010;81(4):446–452.

121. Malec JF, Torsher LC, Dunn WF, Wiegmann DA, Arnold JJ, Brown DA, Phatak V. The Mayo high performance teamwork scale: reliability and validity for evaluating key crew resource management skills. *Simulat Healthcare.* 2007;2(1):4–10. doi: 10.1097/SIH.0b013e31802b68ee.

122. Morgan PJ, Pittini R, Regehr G, Marrs C, Haley MF. Evaluating teamwork in a simulated obstetric environment. *Anesthesiology.* 2007;106(5):907–915. doi: 10.1097/01.anes.0000265149.94190.04.

123. Thomas EJ, Sexton JB, Helmreich RL. Translating teamwork behaviours from aviation to healthcare: development of behavioural markers for neonatal resuscitation. *Qual Saf Health Care.* 2004;13(Suppl 1):i57–i64.

124. Wright MC, Phillips-Bute BG, Petrusa ER, Griffin KL, Hobbs GW, Taekman JM. Assessing teamwork in medical education and practice: relating behavioural teamwork ratings and clinical performance. *Med Teach.* 2009;31:30–38.

125. Simon HA. Designing organizations for an information-rich world. In: Martin Greenberger, Computers, *Communication, and the Public Interest, Baltimore.* MD: The Johns Hopkins Press; 1971:40–41

5

Deliberate Practice and the Acquisition of Expertise

KEITH BAKER

OVERVIEW

Modern medical reforms have focused mainly on system-level changes to drive improvement in the quality and safety of medical care, but reforms are infrequently focused on strategies for improving individual-level medical care. In this chapter we assert that the quality of medical care has significant room for improvement at the individual level. We describe the expert performance framework, and show that this approach is rarely used in the domain of medicine, including in anesthesiology. This current limitation stems from a lack of reliable measures to determine which individuals render superior performance. A distinction will be made between the processes used to attain expert performance and those used for general performance improvement. While the expert-performance approach is being developed in the coming years, physicians can begin to use more effective methods of practice to improve the quality of the care that they provide today. Overall improvement in the quality of medical care will require system-level changes, as well as improvements in individual performance that are based on the theoretical framework of *deliberate practice*.

THE QUALITY OF CURRENT MEDICAL CARE HAS ROOM FOR IMPROVEMENT

The United States spends nearly $3 trillion a year on healthcare.[1] Despite this massive expenditure, outcomes and other measures of quality are relatively poor compared to other developed nations.[2,3] For example, when Americans go to the doctor for illnesses for which there is a broad consensus on treatment strategy, appropriate care is given only about half of the time.[4] A recent study on the control of hypertension showed that patients have better control of their hypertension if they self-monitor their blood pressure, enter their blood pressure readings into a website, and then call a pharmacist for medication adjustments, instead of allowing a physician to manage their medications.[5] Patients can even get better control of their hypertension if they self-monitor their blood pressure and adjust their own medications using an algorithm, as compared to allowing their physician to manage their hypertension.[6] These findings show that a performance gap exists; it can be closed, but modern physicians have yet to close that gap themselves. Although the cause of this gap is multifactorial, physician performance is an important part of the problem. This begs the question of how to improve individual physician performance so that patients can have better outcomes.

MANY MEDICAL REFORMS ARE FOCUSED ON SYSTEM-LEVEL CHANGES TO ENHANCE THE QUALITY OF MEDICAL CARE

Current efforts to improve medical care in the United States are heavily focused on using system-level approaches. Examples of system-level approaches include pay-for-performance (P4P) systems,[7] installation of electronic health records (EHRs),[8,9] adoption of physician order entry (POE) systems,[10-12] creation of accountable care organizations (ACOs),[13] checklist initiatives,[14,15] and quality measurement and reporting programs.[16,17] These system-level approaches are well intended and have brought about some improvements in patient care,[16,17] but improvements have been more the exception than the rule. For example, recent large-scale efforts failed to show benefits of P4P systems,[16,17] checklists,[18] and quality measures.[16,17] Even if all of these system-level approaches eventually are shown to have benefit, they still do not address performance improvement at the level of the individual physician.

THE EXPERT-PERFORMANCE FRAMEWORK EXPLAINS THE DEVELOPMENT OF SUPERIOR PERFORMANCE

In this chapter an *expert* is defined as an individual who can reliably outperform his or her peers when performance is measured using an agreed-upon, objective, and representative measure in the domain of interest. For example, an expert laparoscopic bariatric surgeon has the best outcomes given that all else was equal (e.g., comparable patient populations, hospital infrastructure, etc). This definition can be applied to any area of medical practice in which reliable, objective measurements of meaningful outcomes are available. Based on this definition, there are very few identified experts in the field of medicine since there are very few available objective measures that can reliably distinguish average from superior care. Instead, most medical experts are identified though peer-nomination.[19]

In order to learn about the processes required for attaining expert performance in the domain of medicine, one must therefore look to other domains in which performance is measured and where these measures reliably distinguish average from superior performance. The process of studying and developing expert performance began in 1980 with a proof of concept experiment that involved SF, a college student with average memory. He was able to develop world-class memory for rapidly presented random

digits (1s/digit).[20] In this seminal study SF spent about an hour per day, 3–5 times per week, for one and a half years using trial and error to develop, by himself, an encoding method that allowed him to increase his memory of random digits from average to exceptional. He always worked at the edge of what he could successfully recall. For example, if he was able to recite back 21 random digits then he would subsequently be asked by the experimenter to recite back 22 digits. If he failed, he would reduce the next attempted digit span by 1. During the development of his exceptional memory for random digits, his memory for random letters did not change. Instead, his elite performance was confined to the area he was working on, namely, recall of random digits. The strategy of always working at the limits of his memory caused him, over time, to develop cognitive processes that allowed him to bypass the normal limits imposed by the severely constrained capacity of short-term or working memory.[21] SF bypassed the limits of short-term memory by learning how to interpret random digits as meaningful numbers based on his extensive experience and knowledge of running times for races. For example, 3584 might be encoded as three minutes and 58.4 seconds or almost a 4-minute mile. This approach was based on an acquired skill that he used to store and later retrieve sequences of digit groups using long-term memory. The essential feature of this feat is that SF developed the ability to recall random digits at an elite level despite starting with average abilities. In fact, his I.Q. and digit span were well within the normal range for college students at the outset of the experiment.

The study of expert performance was again advanced in 1993 when Ericsson and colleagues investigated the effects of teacher-guided training on the attained level of musical performance among elite-level musicians. They hypothesized that the amount of a particular form of practice (deliberate practice) would be related to attained level of performance.[22] *Deliberate practice* is "the individualized training activities specially designed by a coach or teacher to improve specific aspects of an individual's performance through repetition and successive refinement."[23] This type of practice involves one-on-one supervised training during which the teacher assesses the music student's performance and then assigns practice activities designed to improve a specific aspect of performance. During subsequent individualized training sessions, the teacher then provides immediate feedback to help the student monitor and adjust his or her actions in order to ensure gradual improvement. The student returns to the teacher on a regular basis for evaluation of his or her training and is eventually assigned new goals and training activities. They found that superior performance was attained after years of deliberate practice, and that the best performers had engaged in the most deliberate practice. Deliberate practice is thus designed to improve performance beyond its current level, is difficult, requires full attention, and is not inherently enjoyable.[22,24] In contrast to SF, who had to self-discover his encoding method, the music students received help from the teacher to identify areas in need of improvement. Specific training tasks, which had been developed over centuries, were then assigned by the teacher. Although deliberate practice requires many preconditions, it is possible to find training that relies on some of these conditions or features.[22] For example, a concert pianist may choose to work on the timing of a short, difficult musical passage involving only the left hand and repeatedly address how to improve that specific challenging aspect of the piece. This approach contrasts sharply with the idea of "practice," which can be thought of as playing a musical piece from start to finish, with no active plan for improving any particular aspect of the performance.

The expert-performance framework examines superior performance and the associated development of new cognitive processes that result from effective practice. During a typical professional career, repeated professional activities become less effortful and eventually become habitual. Improving one's performance, however, requires that the individual actively seek professional development by engaging in practice activities with features of deliberate practice. Continuous evaluation of performance by teachers and the performers themselves makes it possible to repeatedly identify areas for improvement, and to adapt training activities that help to improve performance. This process is repeated over and over again to reach ever-increasing and, finally, superior levels of performance.[25] A key axiom of performance improvement is that once automaticity occurs, growth in performance slows or stops. Automaticity is a double-edged sword that allows for relatively effortless performance yet causes performance stagnation. The comfort afforded by automaticity causes most individuals to remain on performance plateaus for long periods of time, eventually becoming an experienced non-expert.[26,27]

There is no evidence that the expert-performance framework requires innate talent or general ability to reach superior performance as long as the individual can engage in focused practice. Instead, it is the long-term and repeated application of conscious control and deliberate practice that eventually results in superior performance.[25] There are some genetic limitations to performance, and they relate to things like height and size. Ability and talent (IQ, for example) play a role in the initial rate of learning and in the rate of initial performance improvement in many domains, especially ones that have a significant cognitive component. Individuals who have higher ability and talent initially improve at a faster rate than less-able individuals. Irrespective of ability or talent, however, once an individual learns a new task and has used it repeatedly, automaticity ensues, and once automaticity is attained, performance improvement ceases. Thus, ability and talent play an important role in the rate at which automaticity is attained, and it may take less talented individuals longer to reach automaticity. This may explain why academically gifted medical students initially outperform their peers in medical school, but by the end of medical school they have indistinguishable test scores.[28] A key ingredient needed to reach superior levels of performance, according to the expert-performance framework, is the incessant reinvestment in performance improvement each time automaticity occurs. Although ability and talent may play a role in the acquisition of superior performance, to date, they have not been experimentally demonstrated.[25]

Some of the general features of deliberate practice are involved in the development of expert-level performance in a variety of domains. In each domain, the process involves finding an area that can be improved by repeated effortful practice, combined with checking for measurable improvement. There are now a variety of well-studied domains that have shown dose-response relationships between deliberate practice and measured performance. They include music,[22] sports,[29,30] chess,[31,32] typing,[33] spelling,[34] crisis decision-making in US Air Force fighter pilots,[35] and the game of Scrabble.[36]

The expert-performance framework proposes that long-term development in a domain causes the development of new cognitive processes that allow the individual to perform at superior levels. These processes are acquired and do not require underlying talent or ability. The domain of chess provides an example of the changes that occur with long-term focused practice. Initially, at the novice level of chess play, talent or IQ correlates with chess performance.[37] As the level of performance increases over time, IQ becomes less important as new cognitive processes are developed through long-term practice.[38] In chess, effective practice (entailing many features of deliberate practice) has been operationalized as "serious study alone," in which the player studies the moves of chess grandmasters.[32] For example, the player studies the board as the grandmaster experienced it (from real games with other elite chess players) and decides on a move, then checks to see if his or her move was the same as the grandmaster's move. These cognitive processes ultimately allow the developing player to manipulate vast amounts of information in long-term memory instead of relying upon limited working memory capacity.[39] This in turn allows more accomplished players to use their working memory to make decisions about the best next move. Early studies of expert chess players showed that they had near perfect memory for chess piece positions in mid-game positions. All of the pieces could be removed from the chessboard and expert chess players could replace each piece in its original position on the board.[39] When these same players were asked to replace chess pieces that were randomly placed on the chess board (pieces not placed in real game positions), the elite chess players' superior memory essentially vanished and their memory for chess piece positions returned to the levels of less skilled chess players. This showed that their superior memory performance was not talent-based, but rather had developed through years of chess study. The long-term pursuit of performance improvement that results in expert performance likely produces structural changes in the brain. Recent studies have shown changes in brain structure associated with long-term piano playing,[40] opera singing,[41] and expertise in the game "Baduk" (GO).[42]

The willingness to engage in long-term skill acquisition despite setbacks and difficulties is related to the concept of *grit*. Grit is defined as "perseverance and passion for long-term goals."[43] Grit involves working strenuously to overcome challenges, maintaining effort and interest over years despite failure, adversity, and intermittent plateaus in progress. "The gritty individual approaches achievement as a marathon; his or her advantage is stamina. Whereas disappointment or boredom signals to others that it is time to change trajectory and cut losses, the gritty individual stays the course."[43] Of note, grit appears to be unrelated to, or is even inversely related to, IQ.[43] In a recent analysis of spelling bee champions, success in spelling bees was related to cumulative amounts of deliberate practice, but the willingness to engage in deliberate practice was mediated by grit.[34] Grit appears to increase with age.[43,44]

Can Individual Differences in Physician Performance Affect Outcomes in Measurable and Meaningful Ways?

It is commonly assumed that some physicians are better than others, but demonstrating this, in a reliable and measurable fashion, has been difficult. Part of the difficulty stems from a lack of agreed-upon measures for what constitutes expert, or even just better, performance in medicine. In addition, there are many factors that go into determining patient outcomes, only one of which is physician performance.

The quantitative measurement of physician performance was recently advanced when a group of surgeons specializing in laparoscopic bariatric surgery agreed to have their operations videotaped and to have the videotapes blindly analyzed for technical performance.[45] The blindly assessed ratings of the surgeons' operative performance were strongly related to both operative and non-operative outcomes. This study effectively related measured physician performance to patient outcomes.

THE EXPERT-PERFORMANCE APPROACH TO INCREASING THE QUALITY OF MEDICAL CARE

The expert-performance approach identifies individuals who reliably outperform others in a measurable and reliable fashion in the domain of interest and then seeks to understand what they have done to achieve that level of performance. This has proven to be an effective approach in a number of domains, including chess, piano, spelling, and Scrabble. In order to apply the expert-performance approach to the practice of medicine, one must first find an area of medical practice that is measurable, valid, and important. This is currently a significant barrier to the application of the expert-performance approach to the domain of medicine because of the lack of agreement as to what constitutes superior performance. This is also manifested by the difficulty that many medical specialties have encountered when trying to identify meaningful and measureable clinical performance metrics. Even when measurable features of physician performance are found, there remains a complex interplay between the physician "performer," the unique aspects of the patient, and the many other individuals involved in the care of the patient. The modern "team approach" to patient care makes it increasingly difficult to attribute outcomes to a specific individual. The development of measures for various areas of medicine, including anesthesiology, will therefore require significant investment in research in the coming years. The recent example using bariatric surgery[45]

provides hope that this approach will find application in other areas of medicine.

The Expert-Performance Framework Differs from General Performance Improvement

The expert-performance framework incorporates the long-term use of processes that result in new cognitive support structures that ultimately allow an individual to reach superior performance. This level of performance is not attainable through talent alone, no matter how gifted the individual. Expert performance requires years of study and practice to develop the underlying cognitive changes that support this level of performance. Expert typists, for example, develop the skill of reading ahead of the actual material that they are typing.[46,47] This allows them to activate motor patterns that control their finger sequences so that they can execute these patterns very efficiently. If expert typists are not permitted to read ahead of the text that they are transcribing, their typing speed falls and approaches that of experienced non-experts.[33,46] Thus, their superior performance is not the result of an innate speed advantage,[33] but rather to highly developed processes that develop with extended practice.

General improvement can occur by using a variety of different strategies to enhance performance. The resulting improvement will be immediately available to anyone who uses the strategies. The initial rate of performance improvement will vary by the amount of effort expended, the ability of the individual, and a number of other factors. General performance improvement, though important, does not invariably result in expert performance. General improvement strategies will, however, likely lead to some enhancement in performance.

Physicians Are Required to Be Competent, Not Expert: Expert Performance Is a Choice

Today's physicians are required to be "competent," as determined by the residency programs that graduate them, the state medical boards that license them, the specialty boards that certify them, and the hospitals that credential them. There is currently no requirement for physicians to attain expert levels of performance, so the pursuit of expertise currently remains a personal choice.

Experience Is Not Enough

Physicians often assume that the "practice of medicine" will, in time, generate expertise. It has, however, been amply demonstrated that experience is not enough to ensure expert performance.[48-53] More commonly, experience or "practice" leads to the individual becoming an experienced non-expert.[26] For a variety of reasons, the use of deliberate practice has not been adopted to any significant extent by physicians in practice.[54] This may partly stem from the culture of medicine, which has trusted physicians to engage in self-assessment to identify areas for improvement. Unfortunately, self-assessment is often misleading, particularly for the poorest-performing physicians.[55] Because self-assessment is frequently inaccurate, physicians need external and valid feedback to identify areas for improvement.[56]

A GENERAL APPROACH TO IMPROVING PERFORMANCE IN MEDICINE: APPLICATION OF STRATEGIES

It is necessary to identify a specific goal before embarking on a targeted performance-improvement program. In the case where an "expert level" of performance has been reliably determined, then this level of performance can serve as the goal. In many areas of medicine there is no agreement about who renders expert performance (reliable, measurable performance that is "best in class"). The individual is therefore typically left to seek an area of practice that he or she personally wishes to improve. This approach entails the risk of using flawed self-assessment[55,56] to determine areas to focus on for improvement. External input should therefore be sought in choosing an area for improvement.

Goal Orientation

Deliberate practice requires the individual to work on areas that can be improved beyond his or her current highest levels of performance. This leads, by definition, to performance difficulties and results in frequent challenges, setbacks, and failure. People vary in how they construe or react to failure or challenging circumstances. Achievement goal orientation is a framework that addresses this response.[57,58] Individuals whose goal is to demonstrate their abilities to others and who interpret setbacks and challenges as diagnostic of low ability are said to have a *performance orientation*. An individual with a performance orientation is concerned that his or her performance will be judged as diagnostic of his or her inherent abilities and therefore prefers tasks that are easy and that can be readily accomplished. In contrast, an individual with a *learning orientation* wishes to increase his or her competence and master any challenges that may be encountered. The primary goal of a person with a learning orientation is to improve his or her performance; failure or setbacks are viewed as indicators that additional information, training, or coaching is needed for improvement. Learning-oriented individuals enjoy tasks that are challenging and that can be learned from and result in improvement. The most efficacious and functional approach to coping with setbacks and challenges is the adoption of a strong learning orientation. A learning orientation is also ideal when practice focuses on aspects of performance that are challenging and that result in failure before improved performance emerges. Numerous studies have demonstrated that a person's learning orientation can be increased by various interventions.[59,60] For example, when college students were randomized to a learning-oriented prime and then encountered a setback in their performance they accepted a tutorial designed to improve their performance, whereas students randomized to a performance-oriented prime did not accept the tutorial.[59] Recent evidence has shown that these two achievement goal orientations (learning and performance) are independent of each other, and thus features of each construct can be found, to varying degrees, in a single person.[58]

Mastery Learning

Mastery learning sets the target performance and the learner continues to improve, taking more or less time to do so, until performance goals are reliably attained. Mastery learning is suited for general performance improvement, particularly for basic skill development, because it ensures that all learners will eventually reach learning targets.[61] Conventional time-based learning curricula (e.g., lectures or courses) ensure that the learner receives training for a set period of time, but does not ensure mastery over the material. In fact, there is usually a wide variation in individual performance at the end of the course. Mastery learning typically incorporates features of deliberate practice (immediate feedback, repetition until mastery, focus on challenging aspects of the task) to achieve its results. Although mastery learning incorporates these features and is designed to ensure that all individuals attain "mastery," it does not ensure the attainment of expert performance. Indeed, mastery learning is often used to attain adherence to a checklist or algorithm that is limited in scope. Some recent mastery learning studies have found that individuals who take more time to attain performance targets also attain lower levels of final performance, even though they have attained "mastery."[62]

Deliberate Practice Can Be Used to Improve the Performance of Technical Procedures

The theoretical framework of deliberate practice has been applied to a variety of highly focused areas in medicine. The most commonly used performance standard is adherence to a checklist or an algorithm, but these studies have not used experts as the reference standard for achievement. They therefore fall short of the expert-performance approach because the level of performance is set well below the expert level; instead, performance goals are determined so that most individuals can attain "mastery" with a modicum of deliberate practice. Remarkably, even with this limitation, the use of mastery learning, with features of deliberate practice to achieve checklist

adherence, has been shown to significantly improve performance of advanced cardiac life support (ACLS),[63] central line placement,[64,65] thoracentesis,[62] lumbar puncture,[66] and laparoscopic surgery.[67] A number of studies have now shown benefits of this practice extending directly to patient outcomes.[64,68]

Deliberate Practice Can Be Used to Improve Medical Decision-Making

The theoretical framework of deliberate practice has been used to improve the accuracy of medical diagnosis when the *availability bias* acted as a barrier to performance.[69] This work incorporates several features of deliberate practice in that the resident physicians in the study were required to make a diagnosis, list aspects of that diagnosis that did not fit the clinical scenario, then list another diagnosis and the features that did not fit that diagnosis, until all possible diagnoses were considered. The final diagnosis was then chosen. This process improved performance, focused on an area of performance that was difficult (diagnosis in the presence of the availability bias), and was effortful and not inherently enjoyable. It did not, however, incorporate feedback or repeated practice to achieve its effects; nevertheless, it did improve performance.

Grit

Grit appears to mediate one's willingness to engage in significant amounts of deliberate practice.[34] This appears to be plausible because grit allows or enables the individual to endure setbacks and challenges while focusing on, and staying committed to the long-term goal of excellent performance. Grit is therefore essential for sustaining engagement in deliberate practice to develop superior performance. The degree to which grit can be externally altered is unknown.

Accurate Performance Assessment

Improving performance to very high levels requires knowing one's current level of performance and knowing how to reach the next level. Self-assessment in the domain of medicine is notoriously flawed[55,56] and thus external measures are needed.[56] In contrast to most elite-level performers in other domains, such as sports or music, very few physicians currently work with a coach. If a coach is not available, some other trusted, external measure of performance must be used to determine whether adequate improvement is being made. One area that holds promise is recording procedures or events for later review. This allows performance to be studied while looking for ways to improve.[70,71] This type of review is common during the debriefing that follows simulated events.

Feedback

Feedback can take many forms and is essential to performance improvement.[72-76] Video recording offers direct audio and visual feedback. Coaching will bring an external person's perspective. Measured outcomes can be compared to performance goals, and peer feedback can offer the collective wisdom of experienced others. Feedback's primary limitation is the learner's acceptance.[77] Studies have shown that physicians find many barriers to both giving and receiving feedback.[78,79] Feedback is often threatening to an individual but can be made more acceptable if a person holds a strong learning orientation.[80] Willingness to accept feedback also can be increased by interventions that increase an individual's learning orientation.[59,60]

Automaticity, Chunking, and Elaboration

Newly learned tasks, or difficult aspects of a task, must be practiced until automaticity develops. As automaticity develops, the new level of performance will be achieved with less and less attention and effort. This relieves the individual from thinking about each aspect of performance and allows cognitive resources to be focused on further enhancement of performance.[81] As automaticity develops, the cognitive, behavioral, and mechanical aspects of a task are incorporated into routines and habit.[82] In medicine, the learning of new diseases and their management results in the development of illness scripts.[27] With repeated application of new knowledge, the information also becomes "elaborated," meaning that it becomes connected to other knowledge in a meaningful way.[83] "Chunking" information refers to the encapsulation of large amounts of information into a single construct that represents all of the relevant information.[39] Chunking results from the repeated use of, and elaboration on, knowledge. For example, with extended study and practice, a hyperkalemic cardiac arrest caused by releasing the clamps on a recently implanted cold and ischemic liver will trigger a well-orchestrated response that addresses all of the maneuvers and decisions associated with understanding and managing that event. The encapsulation and chunking of information allows the individual to effectively bypass the severe limits imposed by normal working memory capacity,[39,84-87] which subsequently permits the active use of cognitive resources during such an event.

A Culture of Continuous Quality Improvement

Performance improvement requires a culture of continuous quality improvement. This is particularly true for residency and fellowship training programs in the United States. The Next Accreditation System (NAS) was launched by the Accreditation Council for Graduate Medical Education (ACGME) beginning in 2013.[88] The NAS includes frequent institutional site visits known as Clinical Learning Environment Review (CLER) visits.[89] These visits look for evidence that ACGME accredited residencies and fellowships promote a culture of continuous quality improvement. Maintenance of Certification (MOC) is now required by most member Boards of the American Board of Medical Specialties and includes a component that allows individuals to demonstrate continuous quality improvement.[90] Engaging in continuous quality improvement is increasingly considered as normal. This reflects a change in the culture of medicine from a view that a physician is completely trained at the end of his or her formal medical training to a view in which performance is continuously scrutinized for improvement.

Simulation

Simulation has unique features that make it especially valuable as part of a training program, and is a key adjunct in performance improvement. Simulation allows novices to practice in a safe environment that will not jeopardize patient safety and allows repeated trial and error, coupled with formative feedback, during the learning of a new skill. It is most commonly used to train for rare or high-stakes events such as malignant hyperthermia or local anesthetic toxicity. Simulation allows for repeated practice until mastery is achieved, without the risk of patient harm. A large body of evidence shows that simulation-based training is at least as effective as conventional clinical training for certain scenarios.[75,76,91,92] The major barrier to widespread adoption of simulator training programs is cost, which includes infrastructure, equipment, personnel, and coverage for clinicians who would otherwise be generating income.

Checklists and Protocols

Most clinical performance measures depend on following protocols or adhering to checklists, which serve as highly reliable measures but focus on process, and not patient outcomes. Moreover, they aspire to a level of performance that almost any practitioner can achieve with a modicum of time and effort. Thus the protocol and checklist approach to ensuring performance will not, by definition, result in expert performance. Checklists can also reduce cognitive investment in certain processes, which can foster a form of mindlessness[93] that will act to forestall performance improvement. The balance between ensuring basic performance using protocols and checklists and ensuring the development of advanced forms of performance has not been determined and requires further investigation.

The Reinvestment Model of Performance Improvement

The reinvestment model of performance improvement contains fundamental and essential features for attaining expert performance (Figure 5.1). In this model, a novice individual requires significant amounts of time and effort to learn a new skill. Learning the new

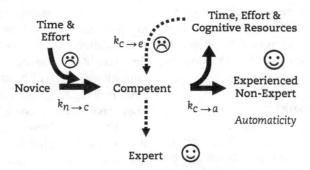

FIGURE 5.1: Reinvestment model of performance improvement. The novice learner requires significant time and effort to learn a new skill. This process is challenging, and setbacks are frequent as novices learn to become competent. The rate of transition from novice to competent ($k_{n \to c}$) is affected by ability, effort, and other factors. As the new skill is successfully repeated, automaticity develops, and the skill no longer requires conscious control. The transition rate from being competent to acting via automaticity and becoming an experienced non-expert ($k_{c \to a}$) is affected by repetition, time, and other factors. The transition from competent to expert is made when the individual chooses to reinvest time, effort, and cognitive resources or cognitive control (made available because of available working memory capacity) back into performance improvement through deliberate practice. The rate of transition from competent to expert ($k_{c \to e}$) depends on the extent to which time, effort, and cognitive resources are reinvested into the design and execution of deliberate practice for performance improvement. The use of deliberate practice is at least partly mediated by grit. The conversion of automaticity back into cognitive control (for use in deliberate practice) represents a latent opportunity for improvement which is available to almost all individuals.

skill consumes most of that person's working memory capacity (WMC), which is needed to process new information. WMC is the bottle-neck in cognitive processing.[94] The rate at which the novice acquires the new skill and approaches competence ($k_n \rightarrow_c$) is dependent on his or her ability or talent (in the case of cogni-tive skills, this is typically IQ[25]), the amount of effort exerted, and other factors. Once he or she can reliably carry out the skill at a basic level, then competency is attained. Automaticity is reached when the new skill has been used re-peatedly. Automaticity allows the skill to be executed with little need for cognitive control and without the need to significantly engage working memory capacity. The rate at which basic competence transitions to automatic-ity ($k_c \rightarrow_a$) depends upon repetition and time. When automaticity emerges, the task becomes relatively easy for the individual to complete, and he or she regains working memory capac-ity for processing new or more complex items. The key to performance improvement hinges on whether the individual chooses to reinvest their free working memory capacity back into performance improvement. Most individuals choose to simply enjoy the easy or effortless conduct of the skill once they have reached au-tomaticity, in which case skills will be arrested at this level of performance and the individual can be called an experienced non-expert. The reinvestment model of performance improve-ment requires reinvestment of time, effort, and cognitive resources such as working memory capacity into skill improvement through de-liberate practice. This "reinvestment of auto-maticity" into deliberate practice represents a latent improvement opportunity available to almost all individuals. The rate at which individuals move from competent toward becoming true experts ($k_c \rightarrow_e$) is related to the frequency with which they invest time, effort, and cognitive resources into the design and ex-ecution of deliberate practice for performance improvement. The use of deliberate practice is mediated by grit to at least some extent, since grit is required in order to remain dedicated to a long-term goal (becoming an expert), even when the task is arduous.

Deliberate Practice Can Be Used to Increase Performance of Some "Everyday Skills"

The theoretical framework of deliberate practice can be applied to many skill areas. We will use airway management as an example. Cormack and Lehane are best known for developing the grading system used to communicate the extent of glottic exposure during laryngoscopy.[95] They were aware of the difficulty and morbidity asso-ciated with intubating patients having a grade 3 glottic exposure at laryngoscopy. They realized that they would need to practice intubating pa-tients with these poor glottic exposures to im-prove their performance with these challenging airways. They also realized that very few such patients were available for practice, as these are infrequent occurrences.[95] To overcome the limitation of too few grade 3 views, they de-signed a technique to convert the common and easy grade 1 view to the more challenging and infrequent grade 3 view by relaxing the force on the laryngoscope handle to degrade the la-ryngoscopic view of the larynx. They could then practice intubating patients having an iat-rogenically created grade 3 view. This training incorporates most of the features of deliberate practice because it requires that the operator perform at the upper limit of his or her skill set, it improves performance with airway manage-ment, it is challenging, it takes time and effort, and it is not immediately needed at the time of practice. As skill develops, new and more ad-vanced methods can be introduced. Ironically, Cormack and Lehane did not address the grade 4 view because it required advanced airways skills with fiberoptics that few people possessed at the time. These skills are now commonly learned by resident physicians.

The theoretical framework of deliberate practice can be applied to many other aspects of medical care. For example, practice can be designed to enhance cognitive skills that re-quire knowledge and decision-making. Areas for development might include "what if" sce-narios for rare or life-threatening events such as cardiac arrest, difficult airway management, or life-threatening hemorrhage. Other forms of practice can also enhance behavioral skills that might be required for high-stress circumstances. The generic approach is the same for each: identify an area for improvement, determine a measure of performance, create a plan to accomplish the goal, obtain feedback on performance or seek coaching to help guide performance, attempt the new skill, evaluate the parts that did not work well and reflect on how to improve the most difficult aspects, seek advanced coaching if needed, practice repeatedly until full control develops, and then consider which aspect of performance to improve next.

LIMITATIONS

The primary limitation with applying the expert-performance framework to medicine, including anesthesiology, is the lack of measures that define superior performance. Without the ability to reliably measure superior performance, it becomes impossible to identify individuals who exemplify expert performance. Instead, we are often limited to using peer nominations to identify "expert" performance; unfortunately, these do not enjoy a strong track record.[96] Given that we are infrequently able to identify reliable and measurable examples of superior performance, we are limited to using general methods for performance improvement. Many of these methods are known to produce skill improvement. Because there are so few measures of superior performance, this implies that an individual may, or may not, be focusing on the correct strategies for improvement. The development of reliable measures so that superior performance can be identified is critical to this effort. Finally, since organized medicine requires only competence (a minimum standard), the development of expertise is wholly dependent on individual choice. The time, effort, and reinvestment of cognitive resources, all of which are needed for performance improvement, coupled with the absence of a requirement for expertise, will ensure that expert performance remains a high achievement.

REFERENCES

1. Asch DA, Weinstein DF. Innovation in medical education. *N Engl J Med.* 2014;371(9):794–795.
2. Banks J, Marmot M, Oldfield Z, Smith JP. Disease and disadvantage in the United States and in England. *JAMA.* 2006;295(17):2037–2045.
3. Davis K, Stremikis K, Schoen C, Squires D. Mirror, mirror on the wall, 2014 update: how the U.S. health care system compares internationally. *The Commonwealth Fund.* 2014: 1–32.
4. McGlynn EA, Asch SM, Adams J, et al. The quality of health care delivered to adults in the United States. *N Engl J Med.* 2003;348(26):2635–2645.
5. Green BB, Cook AJ, Ralston JD, et al. Effectiveness of home blood pressure monitoring, Web communication, and pharmacist care on hypertension control: a randomized controlled trial. *JAMA.* 2008;299(24):2857–2867.
6. McManus RJ, Mant J, Haque MS, et al. Effect of self-monitoring and medication self-titration on systolic blood pressure in hypertensive patients at high risk of cardiovascular disease: the TASMIN-SR randomized clinical trial. *JAMA.* 2014;312(8):799–808.
7. Jha AK, Joynt KE, Orav EJ, Epstein AM. The long-term effect of premier pay for performance on patient outcomes. *N Engl J Med.* 2012;366(17):1606–1615.
8. Menachemi N, Collum TH. Benefits and drawbacks of electronic health record systems. *Risk Manag Healthc Policy.* 2011;4:47–55.
9. Ludwick DA, Doucette J. Adopting electronic medical records in primary care: lessons learned from health information systems implementation experience in seven countries. *Int J Med Inform.* 2009;78(1):22–31.
10. Koppel R, Metlay JP, Cohen A, et al. Role of computerized physician order entry systems in facilitating medication errors. *JAMA.* 2005;293(10): 1197–1203.
11. Longo DR, Hewett JE, Ge B, Schubert S. The long road to patient safety: a status report on patient safety systems. *JAMA.* 2005;294(22):2858–2865.
12. Slight SP, Seger DL, Nanji KC, et al. Are we heeding the warning signs? Examining providers' overrides of computerized drug-drug interaction alerts in primary care. *PLoS One.* 2013;8(12):e85071.
13. Pham HH, Cohen M, Conway PH. The Pioneer accountable care organization model: improving quality and lowering costs. *JAMA.* 2014;312(16):1635–1636.
14. Haynes AB, Weiser TG, Berry WR, et al. A surgical safety checklist to reduce morbidity and mortality in a global population. *N Engl J Med.* 2009;360(5):491–499.
15. Pronovost P, Needham D, Berenholtz S, et al. An intervention to decrease catheter-related bloodstream infections in the ICU. *N Engl J Med.* 2006;355(26):2725–2732.

16. Howell EA, Zeitlin J, Hebert PL, Balbierz A, Egorova N. Association between hospital-level obstetric quality indicators and maternal and neonatal morbidity. *JAMA*. 2014;312(15):1531–1541.

17. Neuman MD, Wirtalla C, Werner RM. Association between skilled nursing facility quality indicators and hospital readmissions. *JAMA*. 2014;312(15):1542–1551.

18. Urbach DR, Govindarajan A, Saskin R, Wilton AS, Baxter NN. Introduction of surgical safety checklists in Ontario, Canada. *N Engl J Med*. 2014;370(11):1029–1038.

19. Ericsson KA. An expert-performance perspective of research on medical expertise: the study of clinical performance. *Med Educ*. 2007;41(12):1124–1130.

20. Ericcson KA, Chase WG, Faloon S. Acquisition of a memory skill. *Science*. 1980;208(4448):1181–1182.

21. Miller GA. The magical number seven, plus or minus two: some limits on our capacity for processing information. *Psychol Rev*. 1956;63(2):81–97.

22. Ericsson KA, Krampe RT, Tesch-Römer C. The role of deliberate practice in the acquisition of expert performance. *Psychol Rev*. 1993;100(3):363–406.

23. Ericsson KA, Lehmann AC. Expert and exceptional performance: evidence of maximal adaptation to task constraints. *Annu Rev Psychol*. 1996;47:273–305.

24. Coughlan EK, Williams AM, McRobert AP, Ford PR. How experts practice: a novel test of deliberate practice theory. *J Exp Psychol Learn Mem Cogn*. 2014;40(2):449–458.

25. Ericsson KA. Why expert performance is special and cannot be extrapolated from studies of performance in the general population: a response to criticisms. *Intelligence*. 2014;45:81–103.

26. Guest CB, Regehr G, Tiberius RG. The life long challenge of expertise. *Med Educ*. 2001;35(1):78–81.

27. Mylopoulos M, Regehr G. Cognitive metaphors of expertise and knowledge: prospects and limitations for medical education. *Med Educ*. 2007;41(12):1159–1165.

28. Kim KJ, Kee C. Gifted students' academic performance in medical school: a study of Olympiad winners. *Teach Learn Med*. 2012;24(2):128–132.

29. Greco P, Memmert D, Morales JCP. The effect of deliberate play on tactical performance in basketball. *Percept Mot Skills*. 2010;110(3, Pt1):849–856.

30. Ericsson KA, Nandagopal K, Roring RW. Toward a science of exceptional achievement: attaining superior performance through deliberate practice. *Ann N Y Acad Sci*. 2009;1172:199–217.

31. de Bruin ABH, Smits N, Rikers RMJP, Schmidt HG. Deliberate practice predicts performance over time in adolescent chess players and drop-outs: a linear mixed models analysis. *Br J Psychol*. 2008;99(4):473–497.

32. Charness N, Tuffiash M, Krampe R, Reingold E, Vasyukova E. The role of deliberate practice in chess expertise. *Appl Cogn Psychol*. 2005;19(2):151–165.

33. Keith N, Ericsson KA. A deliberate practice account of typing proficiency in everyday typists. *J Exp Psychol Appl*. 2007;13(3):135–145.

34. Duckworth AL, Kirby TA, Tsukayama E, Berstein H, Ericsson KA. Deliberate practice spells success: why grittier competitors triumph at the National Spelling Bee. *Soc Psychol Personal Sci*. 2011;2(2):174–181.

35. McKinney EH, Jr., Davis KJ. Effects of deliberate practice on crisis decision performance. *Hum Factors*. 2003;45(3):436–444.

36. Tuffiash M, Roring RW, Ericsson KA. Expert performance in SCRABBLE: Implications for the study of the structure and acquisition of complex skills. *J Exp Psychol Appl*. 2007;13(3):124–134.

37. de Bruin ABH, Kok EM, Leppink J, Camp G. Practice, intelligence, and enjoyment in novice chess players: a prospective study at the earliest stage of a chess career. *Intelligence*. 2014;45:18–25.

38. Grabner RH, Stern E, Neubauer AC. Individual differences in chess expertise: a psychometric investigation. *Acta Psychol (Amst.)*. 2007;124(3):398–420.

39. Gobet F, Charness N. Expertise in chess. In: Ericsson KA, Charness N, Feltovich PJ, Hoffman RR, eds. *The Cambridge Handbook of Expertise and Expert Performance*. New York: Cambridge University Press; 2006:523–538.

40. Bengtsson SL, Nagy Z, Skare S, Forsman L, Forssberg H, Ullen F. Extensive piano practicing has regionally specific effects on white matter development. *Nat Neurosci*. 2005;8(9):1148–1150.

41. Kleber B, Veit R, Birbaumer N, Gruzelier J, Lotze M. The brain of opera singers: experience-dependent changes in functional activation. *Cereb Cortex*. 2010;20(5):1144–1152.

42. Lee B, Park J-Y, Jung WH, et al. White matter neuroplastic changes in long-term trained players of the game of "Baduk" (GO): a voxel-based diffusion-tensor imaging study. *Neuroimage*. 2010;52(1):9–19.

43. Duckworth AL, Peterson C, Matthews MD, Kelly DR. Grit: P perseverance and passion for long-term goals. *J Pers Soc Psychol*. 2007;92(6):1087–1101.

44. Duckworth AL, Quinn PD. Development and validation of the Short Grit Scale (GRIT-S). *J Pers Assess*. 2009;91(2):166–174.

45. Birkmeyer JD, Finks JF, O'Reilly A, et al. Surgical skill and complication rates after bariatric surgery. *N Engl J Med.* 2013;369(15):1434–1442.

46. Salthouse TA. Perceptual, cognitive, and motoric aspects of transcription typing. *Psychol Bull.* 1986;99(3):303–319.

47. Legrand-Lestremau S, Postal V, Charles A. La vitesse de frappe est-elle liée au processus d'anticipation? [Does typing speed depend on the process of anticipation?]. *Le Travail Humain.* 2006;69(1):67–92.

48. Choudhry NK, Fletcher RH, Soumerai SB. Systematic review: the relationship between clinical experience and quality of health care. *Ann Intern Med.* 2005;142(4):260–273.

49. Friedman Z, Siddiqui N, Katznelson R, Devito I, Davies S. Experience is not enough: repeated breaches in epidural anesthesia aseptic technique by novice operators despite improved skill. *Anesthesiology.* 2008;108(5):914–920.

50. Weinger MB. Experience does not equal expertise: can simulation be used to tell the difference? *Anesthesiology.* 2007;107(5):691–694.

51. Eva KW. The aging physician: changes in cognitive processing and their impact on medical practice. *Acad Med.* 2002;77(10 Suppl):S1–6.

52. Hamers JP, van den Hout MA, Halfens RJ, Abu-Saad HH, Heijltjes AE. Differences in pain assessment and decisions regarding the administration of analgesics between novices, intermediates and experts in pediatric nursing. *Int J Nurs Stud.* 1997;34(5):325–334.

53. Ericsson KA, Whyte Jt, Ward P. Expert performance in nursing: reviewing research on expertise in nursing within the framework of the expert-performance approach. *ANS Adv Nurs Sci.* 2007;30(1):E58–71.

54. van de Wiel MWJ, Van den Bossche P, Janssen S, Jossberger H. Exploring deliberate practice in medicine: how do physicians learn in the workplace? *Adv Health Sci Educ.* 2011;16(1):81–95.

55. Davis DA, Mazmanian PE, Fordis M, Van Harrison R, Thorpe KE, Perrier L. Accuracy of physician self-assessment compared with observed measures of competence: a systematic review. *JAMA.* 2006;296(9):1094–1102.

56. Eva KW, Regehr G. Self-assessment in the health professions: a reformulation and research agenda. *Acad Med.* 2005;80(10 Suppl):S46–54.

57. Dweck CS. Motivational processes affecting learning. *Am Psychol.* 1986;41(10):1040–1048.

58. Attenweiler WJ, Moore D. Goal orientations: two, three, or more factors? *Educ Psychol Meas.* 2006;66(2):342–352.

59. Hong Y-y, Chiu C-y, Dweck CS, Lin DMS, Wan W. Implicit theories, attributions, and coping: a meaning system approach. *J Pers Soc Psychol.* 1999;77(3):588–599.

60. Nussbaum AD, Dweck CS. Defensiveness versus remediation: Self-theories and modes of self-esteem maintenance. *Pers Social Psychol Bull.* 2008;34(5):599–612.

61. Cook DA, Brydges R, Zendejas B, Hamstra SJ, Hatala R. Mastery learning for health professionals using technology-enhanced simulation: a systematic review and meta-analysis. *Acad Med.* 2013;88(8):1178–1186.

62. Wayne DB, Barsuk JH, O'Leary KJ, Fudala MJ, McGaghie WC. Mastery learning of thoracentesis skills by internal medicine residents using simulation technology and deliberate practice. *J Hosp Med.* 2008;3(1):48–54.

63. Wayne DB, Butter J, Siddall VJ, et al. Simulation-based training of internal medicine residents in advanced cardiac life support protocols: a randomized trial. *Teach Learn Med.* 2005;17(3):202–208.

64. Khouli H, Jahnes K, Shapiro J, et al. Performance of medical residents in sterile techniques during central vein catheterization: randomized trial of efficacy of simulation-based training. *Chest.* 2011;139(1):80–87.

65. Barsuk JH, Cohen ER, McGaghie WC, Wayne DB. Long-term retention of central venous catheter insertion skills after simulation-based mastery learning. *Acad Med.* 2010;85(10 Suppl):S9–12.

66. Barsuk JH, Cohen ER, Caprio T, McGaghie WC, Simuni T, Wayne DB. Simulation-based education with mastery learning improves residents' lumbar puncture skills. *Neurology.* 2012;79(2):132–137.

67. Zendejas B, Cook DA, Hernandez-Irizarry R, Huebner M, Farley DR. Mastery learning simulation-based curriculum for laparoscopic TEP inguinal hernia repair. *J Surg Educ.* 2012;69(2):208–214.

68. Zendejas B, Cook DA, Bingener J, et al. Simulation-based mastery learning improves patient outcomes in laparoscopic inguinal hernia repair: a randomized controlled trial. *Ann Surg.* 2011;254(3):502–509; discussion 509–511.

69. Mamede S, van Gog T, van den Berge K, et al. Effect of availability bias and reflective reasoning on diagnostic accuracy among internal medicine residents. *JAMA.* 2010; 304(11):1198–1203.

70. Hu YY, Peyre SE, Arriaga AF, et al. Postgame analysis: using video-based coaching for continuous professional development. *J Am Coll Surg.* 2012;214(1):115–124.

71. Ericsson KA. Necessity is the mother of invention: video recording firsthand perspectives of critical medical procedures to make simulated training more effective. *Acad Med.* 2014;89(1):17–20.

72. Archer JC. State of the science in health professional education: effective feedback. *Med Educ.* 2010;44(1):101–108.

73. Shute VJ. Focus on formative feedback. *Rev Educ Res.* 2008;78(1):153–189.

74. Boehler ML, Rogers DA, Schwind CJ, et al. An investigation of medical student reactions to feedback: a randomised controlled trial. *Med Educ.* 2006;40(8):746–749.

75. Cook DA. How much evidence does it take? A cumulative meta-analysis of outcomes of simulation-based education. *Med Educ.* 2014;48(8):750–760.

76. Issenberg SB, McGaghie WC, Petrusa ER, Lee Gordon D, Scalese RJ. Features and uses of high-fidelity medical simulations that lead to effective learning: a BEME systematic review. *Med Teach.* 2005;27(1):10–28.

77. Yaniv I. Receiving other people's advice: influence and benefit. *Organ Behav Hum Decis Process.* 2004;93(1):1–13.

78. Mann K, van der Vleuten C, Eva K, et al. Tensions in informed self-assessment: how the desire for feedback and reticence to collect and use it can conflict. *Acad Med.* 2011;86(9):1120–1127.

79. Delva D, Sargeant J, Miller S, et al. Encouraging residents to seek feedback. *Med Teach.* 2013;35(12):e1625–1631.

80. Teunissen PW, Stapel DA, van der Vleuten C, Scherpbier A, Boor K, Scheele F. Who wants feedback? an investigation of the variables influencing residents' feedback-seeking behavior in relation to night shifts. *Acad Med.* 2009; 84(7):910–917.

81. Kurahashi AM, Harvey A, MacRae H, Moulton CA, Dubrowski A. Technical skill training improves the ability to learn. *Surgery.* 2011; 149(1):1–6.

82. Bargh JA, Chartrand TL. The unbearable automaticity of being. *Am Psychol.* 1999;54(7):462.

83. Bordage G. Elaborated knowledge: a key to successful diagnostic thinking. *Acad Med.* 1994;69(11):883–885.

84. Young JQ, Van Merrienboer J, Durning S, Ten Cate O. Cognitive Load Theory: implications for medical education: AMEE Guide No. 86. *Med Teach.* 2014;36(5):371–384.

85. van Merrienboer JJ, Sweller J. Cognitive load theory in health professional education: design principles and strategies. *Med Educ.* 2010; 44(1):85–93.

86. Engle RW. Working memory capacity as executive attention. *Curr Dir Psychol Sci.* 2002;11(1):19–23.

87. Ericsson KA. Exceptional memorizers: made, not born. *Trends Cogn Sci.* 2003;7(6):233–235.

88. Nasca TJ, Philibert I, Brigham T, Flynn TC. The next GME accreditation system: rationale and benefits. *N Engl J Med.* 2012;366(11):1051–1056.

89. Weiss KB, Wagner R, Nasca TJ. Development, testing, and implementation of the ACGME Clinical Learning Environment Review (CLER) Program. *J Grad Med. Educ.* 2012;4(3):396–398.

90. Cook DA, Holmboe ES, Sorensen KJ, Berger RA, Wilkinson JM. Getting maintenance of certification to work: a grounded theory study of physicians' perceptions. *JAMA Intern Med.* 2015;175(1): 35–42.

91. Cook DA, Hatala R, Brydges R, et al. Technology-enhanced simulation for health professions education: a systematic review and meta-analysis. *JAMA.* 2011;306(9):978–988.

92. McGaghie WC, Issenberg SB, Cohen ER, Barsuk JH, Wayne DB. Does simulation-based medical education with deliberate practice yield better results than traditional clinical education? A meta-analytic comparative review of the evidence. *Acad Med.* 2011;86(6):706–711.

93. Barshi I, Healy AF. Checklist procedures and the cost of automaticity. *M & C.* 1993;21(4): 496–505.

94. Mayer RE. Applying the science of learning to medical education. *Med Educ.* 2010;44(6):543–549.

95. Cormack RS, Lehane J. Difficult tracheal intubation in obstetrics. *Anaesthesia.* 1984;39(11):1105–1111.

96. Ericsson KA. An expert-performance perspective of research on medical expertise: the study of clinical performance. *Med Educ.* 2007;41(12): 1124–1130.

6

Fatigue

MICHAEL KEANE

INTRODUCTION

Fatigue impairs human performance, making fatigue management an essential component of professional practice. In order to best design fatigue mitigation strategies, it is necessary to understand the causes and effects of fatigue. The study of fatigue incorporates concepts from neuroscience, dynamic systems, human factors, and risk management, and relates these elements to circumstances faced by all healthcare professionals. In addition to surveying those professional elements, this chapter will also consider how patients can experience fatigue and how it may affect their postoperative course.

Unfortunately, fatigue management is too complex to offer a single prescription. Although there is a growing body of data that can guide decisions, rational judgment, appropriate feedback, and adaptation will ultimately be required. It is also essential to consider the legitimate concerns of all stakeholders before imposing any changes in perioperative processes. For example, the US Federal Aviation Administration's (FAA) document outlining changes to flight-crew duty hours and rest requirements[1] openly discusses different stakeholders' legitimate concerns.

PHYSIOLOGY

Fatigue is a complex physiologic phenomenon that has a variety of effects on human performance, including cognitive and psychomotor performance as well as emotional states.[2] Fatigue can potentially also adversely affect nonneurologic systems such as the cardiovascular,[3] immune,[4,5] and metabolic systems.[6,7,8]

There are three types of sleep-related fatigue: *transient, cumulative,* and *circadian.* From the Federal Aviation Administration:[1]

1. *Transient fatigue* is acute fatigue brought on by extreme sleep restriction or extended hours awake within 1 or 2 days.
2. *Cumulative fatigue* is chronic fatigue brought on by repeated mild sleep restriction or extended hours awake across a series of days.
3. *Circadian fatigue* refers to the reduced performance during nighttime hours, particularly during an individual's window of circadian low (WOCL) (typically between 0200 and 0600.)

Mental fatigue is a phenomenon that is caused by repeated, demanding mental tasks. Mental fatigue can affect neurological processes that include attention, working memory, and action control, and can occur even in the setting of adequate sleep.[9] Thus, although fatigue is often caused by lack of sleep, it is not synonymous with sleep deprivation.

Sleep

In order to develop shift strategies within institutions, an appreciation of circadian biology is important. The circadian system synchronizes biological processes to a 24-hour cycle.[10] The innate circadian rhythm of humans is approximately 24.18 hours with a tight distribution[11] and is synchronized by environmental cues called *zeitgebers.*[10] The most import *zeitgeber* is light.[12] Different chronotypes are believed to have different underlying circadian physiology: night "owls" versus early morning "larks."[13]

Sleep is generally divided into two categories: non–rapid eye movement (non-REM) and rapid eye movement (REM) sleep.[14] Non-REM sleep is further subdivided into stages 1–4, identified by characteristic electroencephalography (EEG) patterns. Stages 3 and 4 are sometimes referred to as *slow wave sleep* because they are associated with high-amplitude, low-frequency waves on EEG. During REM sleep, the EEG appears erratic, with small amplitude waves that are similar to that of an awake encephalogram. The eyes demonstrate characteristic movements during REM sleep. Motor output also helps to characterize the stages of sleep. Non-REM sleep is associated with a reduction in muscle tone and movement. REM sleep is associated with characteristic ocular movements but otherwise a profound reduction of muscle tone and movement, with the exception of the diaphragm. Decreased tone to the upper airway dilator muscles, especially during REM sleep, is the cause of obstructive sleep apnea (OSA). In patients with OSA, the obstruction to breathing caused by loss of dilator tone during sleep causes hypoxia, which leads to arousal from sleep. This cycle of sleep-induced hypoxia followed by arousal can repeat many times per hour, precluding a restful and restorative sleep. OSA is now recognized as a significant cause of sleep deprivation and consequent fatigue.[15]

Two main drives promote sleep:[16] the circadian drive and a use-driven metabolic process that promotes sleep after a given period of wakefulness. These two drives are often conceptualized as a circadian clock (or "circadian rhythm") and a homeostatic fatigue clock. The circadian rhythm is an innate cycle, but it can be altered by environmental influences,[14] making it possible, for example, to adjust to a new time zone. The neurophysiological substrate for the circadian sleep cycle resides in the suprachiasmatic nucleus (SCN).[17] The most important of these environmental influences is light. Darkness in the evening contributes to increased secretion of melatonin by the pineal gland, which helps to initiate sleep. This response is known as the dim light melatonin onset (DLMO).[18] Blue light of approximately

460–480 nm wavelength is the strongest inhibitor of melatonin secretion.[17] Morning light therefore reduces the circadian drive to sleep. The *window of circadian low* (WOCL) describes the period in which sleep propensity is highest, from approximately 2 a.m. until 6 a.m.[1] A second less intense circadian low occurs in the afternoon from approximately 1 p.m. until 3 p.m.[19] These intervals represent the periods of greatest vulnerability to fatigue-related performance impairment.

The neurophysiology of sleep is complex and is still being elucidated. A variety of ascending pathways using a complex series of neurotransmitters underpins both wakefulness and sleep. Wakefulness-promoting neurotransmitters include acetylcholine, serotonin, norepinephrine, histamine, dopamine, glutamate and orexin.[8] Different systems are also thought to be responsible for different phases of sleep. Gamma-aminobutyric acid (GABA) is considered crucial in promoting slow-wave sleep.[14] REM sleep involves certain cholinergic, glutamatergic, and GABA-containing neurons and the inhibition of monoaminergic and orexin-secreting neurons.[20] The purine neurotransmitter adenosine is involved in sleep onset and is antagonized by caffeine, which explains its promotion of wakefulness.[21] Serotonin acts on many receptors and is involved in both the promotion of wakefulness and sleep.[22]

TIME ON TASK AS A CAUSE OF FATIGUE

As has been stated, even with adequate sleep, prolonged concentration on cognitive tasks can cause *mental fatigue*.[9] The longer a person has been continuously attending to work without a break, the more likely he or she is to be fatigued.[1] Prolonged cognitive demands can cause a decay in performance over time (the *time-on-task effect*).[23] Mental fatigue is a function of both the absolute length of a shift and the amount of concentration that is required during the shift. In the aviation industry, the maximum length of pilots' duty hours varies with the amount of time that they are required to attend to peak cognitive activity.[1] In a study of airline pilots, both the number of sectors flown (increasing the number of takeoffs and landings) and duty length were linearly associated with fatigue.[24] This might apply, for example, to anesthesiologists who are scheduled to care for a large number of pediatric patients who are undergoing short procedures.

Time on task outside of the peak cognitive tasks also causes mental fatigue.[1] While induction and emergence might be times of peak cognitive activity for an anesthesiologist, monitoring the patient while maintaining physiologic stability during a lengthy procedure is also mentally fatiguing. A review has concluded that "converging evidence using behavioral, neural, and subjective measures shows that vigilance requires hard mental work and is stressful."[25]

Some evidence suggests that the time on task effect is not solely a function of mental fatigue and might involve motivational circuits.[9] Moreover, mental fatigue is probably not a unitary phenomenon; different types of fatigue might affect different neurological circuitry.[26,27] Mental fatigue affects cognitive functions in different ways[28] and appears to exhibit genetic susceptibility.[23] Mental fatigue caused by both duration and intensity of time on task, including vigilance, induces cognitive dysfunction and may be one of the most significant causes of accidents in modern society.[29] This suggests that reducing the amount of extraneous and irrelevant tasks from front-line clinicians' workloads might improve safety.

EFFECTS ON HUMAN PERFORMANCE

Exactly how fatigue affects human performance in the clinical setting remains a topic of debate, with considerable variability among institutional and departmental regulations. In contrast, the aviation industry has a long-standing interest in fatigue risk management and has adopted policies and regulations designed to prevent errors caused by fatigue. The aviation industry endorses the following specific effects of fatigue:[30]

- Measurable reduction in speed and accuracy of performance;
- Lapses of attention and vigilance;
- Delayed reactions;
- Impaired logical reasoning and decision-making, including a reduced ability to assess risk or appreciate consequences of actions;
- Reduced situational awareness;
- Low motivation to perform optional activities.

In laboratory studies, fatigue caused by acute and chronic sleep loss causes significant deterioration on a number of indices of neurobehavioral function.[31]

Effects of Fatigue on Healthcare Professionals

An increasing body of laboratory and real-world studies suggests that fatigue-induced impairment decreases patient safety. Importantly, Zhou and colleagues have shown that "sleep-restricted individuals are likely to underestimate neurobehavioral impairment, particularly during the biological night."[32] Fatigue negatively affects all cognitive performance measures, including attention, reaction time, judgment, and accuracy. Sleep loss decreases vigilance and causes cognitive slowing, short-term memory failures, deficits in frontal lobe function, and rapid, involuntary "microsleep" episodes.[15] Interestingly, the detrimental effects caused by fatigue may demonstrate genetically determined variability between individuals.[33]

There is, however, some debate as to whether a reduction in psychomotor and cognitive performance actually translates into a decrease in safety, or whether healthcare professionals can compensate for some fatigue-related impairment with skills and knowledge.[34] Overall, the Harvard Work Hours, Health and Safety Group suggest that the evidence strongly suggests that sleep loss and mental fatigue from extended duration of work shifts significantly impair performance. In particular, they state that "[r]esidents' traditional work shifts of 24–30 consecutive hours unquestionably increase the risk of serious medical errors and diagnostic mistakes."[35]

McCormick et al. found that orthopedic residents were averaging 5.3 hours of sleep a night. With such a reduction in average sleep per night, the residents in the study reported that they were fatigued 48% of the time and at an impaired level of fatigue 27% of the time.[36] The authors calculated that the level of sleep deprivation experienced by the residents would be *predicted* to increase medical errors by 22% as compared to historical, well-rested controls.

Research on the effects of fatigue caused by sleep deprivation or circadian misalignment generally consists of either laboratory studies of individuals who have been deprived of sleep or epidemiological studies and case reports of accidents and errors committed at different times of the day by people who had various amounts of sleep deprivation. Mental fatigue in well-rested individuals also can be studied in the laboratory or by epidemiological studies, although epidemiological studies on the effects of shift length that may induce mental fatigue may also be associated with acute or chronic sleep deprivation.

Although it is unethical to randomly assign physicians to a fatigued state while performing their clinical duties, a degree of fatigue has historically been accepted in some clinical situations. These situations may allow for a study to legitimately randomize a group of physicians to interventions that reduce sleep deprivation and assess the effect on clinical outcome. A landmark ICU study investigated the effects of duty hours and the subsequent effects of fatigue on intern physician performance.[37,38] Interns were allocated to an intervention group (maximum of 16 hours per shift and an average of 65 hours per week) or to a control group whose duty hours were unchanged (shifts of up to 30 hours in duration and an average of 85 duty hours per week). The study found that those in the control group had more than twice the number of attention failures while working at night, and overall made 36% more serious medical errors, which included over five times as many serious diagnostic errors.

Epidemiological data demonstrating an increase in patient morbidity and mortality due to fatigued practitioners has been more ambiguous. In a survey of physician anesthesiologists from New Zealand, 86% percent reported fatigue-related errors, including 32% in the last 6 months.[39] In another study, the incidence of unintended dural puncture during obstetric epidural was increased during the night hours, although the overall incidence was low.[40] Two epidemiological studies that examine the relationships between experienced physicians' work hours, sleep, and patient safety have been widely cited.[41,42] Both studies examined complication rates among patients whose surgeons were on call the night before. Rothschild et al. reported an increased complication rate among surgeons who had less than 6 hours of sleep opportunity the previous night due to work. Conversely, Govindarajan and colleagues found no increase in complication rate. In this study by Govindarajan et al., surgeons were classified as working overnight if they had "treated patients in the preceding overnight hours (midnight to 7 a.m)," but without determining what sleep opportunities the surgeon had actually had. Draining an abscess at 6:30 a.m. before the start of a scheduled operating list would have potentially classified the surgeon as having worked overnight in this study. However, when the study examined patients "whose treating physician had performed two or more procedures at night" there was a statistically significant increase in risk of complications of 1.14 (95% CI, 1.00–1.29; $P = 0.05$).

Philibert performed a meta-analysis of 60 laboratory studies examining the effects of fatigue on both physicians (typically residents) and non-medical volunteers.[43] The meta-analysis found that sleep deprivation of 24–30 hours decreased performance by 1 to 1.5 standard deviations. The author of this paper commented that the effects of acute sleep loss may actually be larger than demonstrated, because the supposed "rested controls" in many of the physician studies were themselves in a state of chronic sleep deprivation. Howard et al. demonstrated that anesthesiology residents exhibited levels of sleepiness similar to those of patients with narcolepsy and obstructive sleep apnea during their normal work schedule.[44] The sleepiness was reversed with four nights of extended sleep opportunities.

In a simulated operating room environment, resident anesthesiology physicians were tested after both a period with at least 25 hours of wakefulness and after a period of extended sleep opportunities for four consecutive nights.[45] The residents who were sleep deprived performed worse on laboratory tests of cognitive performance, and approximately one-third fell asleep during simulated laparoscopic cases. One meta-analysis found that partial sleep deprivation can have as profound an effect on functioning as acute total sleep loss.[2] Awareness of the detrimental effect of chronic partial sleep deprivation should therefore be considered for professional standards of practice.

Because of the large number of factors affecting safety and the complexity of sleep neurobiology, it may be difficult to isolate specific effects caused by solely by fatigue. For example, the natural, circadian rhythm promotes alertness in the mid- to late morning hours, even after a lack of sleep the previous night. This effect may reduce the ability to detect decrements of performance during research studies, and might itself be an intrinsic safety factor.[45]

Sleep deprivation can negatively affect mood,[2] teamwork, and cooperation—all important components of safety in the perioperative environment. In general, sleep-deprived individuals demonstrate a number of behaviors that exacerbate conflict situations, including increased aggression and a propensity to blame others.[46] Interns showed an association between chronic sleep deprivation and depression.[47]

The fatigued practitioner is also at increased risk of personal harm. In one study, interns sustained more sharps injuries (e.g., needle sticks) during extended work shifts and at night.[48] Extended-duration work shifts were associated with over twice the risk of a motor vehicle crash and over 5 times the rate of a near-crash.[49] Because fatigue is widely recognized as a road safety issue, non-professional drivers can be found guilty of negligent homicide if involved in a fatal accident after being awake for more than 24 hours.[50]

Increasing awareness of the effects of fatigue is influencing a change within medical culture; simply trying to "fight through fatigue" is seen less as heroic dedication and may be considered reckless. The legal system may consider fatigued practitioners to be impaired; one anesthesiologist was convicted of criminal medical negligence in the death of a pediatric patient after anesthetizing the child while fatigued.[16]

REDUCING FATIGUE
Duty Hour Limits

After a report by the Institute of Medicine,[51] new duty hour requirements[52] were introduced in 2011 by the Accreditation Council for Graduate Medical Education (ACGME) in order to decrease the possibility that trainees would be performing clinical duties while fatigued from both acute and chronic sleep deprivation. However, these regulations did not specifically address circadian-related times of fatigue. There were, however, legitimate concerns from a variety of stakeholders about the unintended consequences of rapid and dramatic systems changes. Many medical educators were concerned that duty-hour reductions would degrade trainees' educational experience.[53] Systematic reviews have examined the growing literature on effects of duty-hour limitations, and reported mixed findings on both resident well-being and patient outcomes.[54,55,56]

Overall, the ACGME concedes that

> [t]he preponderance of this new published research suggests that the additional 2011 duty hour requirements may not have had an incremental benefit in patient safety, and that there might be significant negative impacts to the quality of physician education, professional development, and socialization to the practice of medicine.[57]

Although some authors claim that a reduction in duty hours reduces clinical experience,[58] some programs have responded by logistical restructuring to maintain clinical experience.[59] One internal medicine program, after restructuring to accommodate the 16-hour duty limit for interns, noted that the interns saw more patients and "produced more detailed notes, and attended more conferences."[60] Although duty-hour restrictions may reduce clinical experience, the Institute of Medicine report highlights the fact that performing clinical tasks while fatigued impairs the higher-order cognitive functions needed for learning.[51] Similarly, an adequate amount of sleep is required for memory consolidation.[61] However, reducing duty hours may actually impose a higher workload if trainees are expected to do the same amount of work in a reduced number of hours. This time pressure and stress also impair higher order cognitive learning.[51]

Even in the presence of predictable fatigue, many advocate preventing unnecessary handoffs of patient care. Ineffective handoffs have been identified as the cause of adverse patient outcomes, and the importance of clinical handoffs was highlighted in the Institute of Medicine duty-hour recommendations.[51] This implies that ineffective handoffs might be a confounding factor in studies that failed to find an overall patient benefit from reduced resident duty hours. Three recent studies [62,63,64] have shown that increased intraoperative handoffs among anesthesia professionals resulted in increased adverse outcomes for patients.[65] These studies use data collected over several years (starting in 2006, 2005, 1999) and might have been initiated before the importance of handoffs was fully understood. In contrast, high-quality, efficient clinical handoffs might actually be a positive moment for both the patient and the practitioner.[65]

Trainees in some programs might be pressured not to comply with duty-hour regulations[66] or may even falsify their hours.[67] In one survey, 60% of neurosurgical residents admitted underreporting their duty hours, with nearly 25% doing so at least weekly.[68] When surveyed, residency program directors were in favor of the 2011 duty-hour regulations, except for duty-period limits, with 71% opposed to the 16-hour limit for interns.[69]

In order to gain more data regarding the effects on patients and trainees of mandating rigid duty-hour limits, two prospective randomized trials were established. The Flexibility in Duty Hour Requirements for Surgical Trainees (FIRST) Trial was a national, cluster-randomized, non-inferiority trial in which General surgery programs were randomly assigned to either a standard group which adhered to all current ACGME duty-hour regulations or a flexible group where ACGME regulations for maximum shift lengths and time off between shifts were waived.[70]

Those programs that were allowed flexibility in duty hour limits were associated with "non-inferior patient outcomes and no significant difference in residents' satisfaction with overall well-being and education quality".[70] However, there have been very different interpretations of what this study means to the future of duty-hours regulation.[71,72,73]

A similar study of internal medicine programs the (iCOMPARE trial) is due for completion in 2017

Sleep Within Duty Period

Promoting fatigue awareness as part of a safety culture, rather than adhering to rigid shift lengths, may be a more effective way to mitigate fatigue-related impairment. Duty-hour limits are usually designed to protect against the worst-case scenario in which there was no sleep opportunity during the shift. Commercial aviation, for example, places the onus on pilots to make a "fatigue call" if they reasonably believe that they are too fatigued to safely carry out their duties. If, however, there is an opportunity to sleep during a duty period, offering the discretion to continue clinical care might help to ensure continuity of care without affecting safety. The Institute of Medicine report on resident fatigue recognizes this possibility, stating that "[i]f 4–5 hours of sleep are obtained in the protected nocturnal period, improved alertness and performance generally will remain for the final 9–10 hours of a 30-hour extended duty period"[51]

Naps also reduce the effects of sleep deprivation in the perioperative environment.[16] An often quoted study by NASA showed that a planned 40-minute nap significantly improved crew performance during long-haul flight operations.[74] Scheduling naps at a set time minimizes fatigue, while "emergency" naps may ameliorate the effects of already established fatigue.[75] *Sleep inertia* (see the next section) reduces performance immediately after an extended nap lasting 60 minutes or longer.[76]

A recent review of studies of scheduled naps taken during night shift found that although naps were followed by a brief period of sleep inertia, overall performance was improved.[77]

Sleep Inertia

A residual reduction in neurocognitive ability occurs immediately after awakening from sleep.[78] This phenomenon, which used to be called *sleep drunkenness*,[78] is now referred to as *sleep inertia*. The maximal decrement in performance lasts for 15 to 30 minutes after awakening[35] but can have subtle residual effects for hours.[79] Sleep inertia is increased in personnel with sleep deprivation, and is especially pronounced if someone is awoken from slow wave sleep.[78]

Sleep inertia has been listed as potentially contributing to a "very high risk of fatigue-related error."[35] However, studies of sleep inertia typically involve administering batteries of tests to volunteers in a non-stressful environment after they are awakened. Endogenous adrenaline[80] and other environmental stressors[81] may, however, reduce the effect of sleep inertia. Moreover, different cognitive domains are differentially affected by sleep inertia.

The American College of Occupational and Environmental Medicine has issued a Guidance Statement entitled "Fatigue Risk Management in the Workplace"[82] for organizations to consider when developing fatigue risk management systems (FRMS), and should be reviewed by anyone who is creating a fatigue mitigation program. This report is especially relevant to industries that run 24-hour operations. The Guidance Statement outlines four principles that organizations should follow in developing an FRMS.

- An FRMS is analogous to (or a subset of) a safety management system (SMS).
- An FRMS is science based, data driven, and subject to continuous improvement; in short, it is a system to manage risk associated with fatigue.
- Fatigue risk management systems are designed to improve outcomes and are more flexible than duty-rest and hours-of-service regulations.

- All stakeholders share responsibility for complying with and improving an FRMS.

In the United States, federal legislation requires all commercial passenger airlines to run fatigue risk management programs (FRMPs), and all levels of management are required to participate in these programs in order to understand the implications of fatigue among aircrew.[1]

Implementing fatigue reduction strategies potentially carries significant upfront costs.[51] Some programs may require large-scale restructuring in order to mitigate fatigue, and will entail significant financial challenges. In the short run at least, the benefits might not outweigh the costs. In one study, however, 57% of patients indicated a preference for a "fresh physician who had received a sign out" than a familiar physician who "may be tired from a long shift."[83] Perhaps even more instructive was that the patients in this study wanted to be notified if a resident looking after them had been working longer than 12 hours. Whether adverse outcome risk is actually increased or not, these preferences are important in the modern context of patient-centered care and patient satisfaction.

MITIGATING FATIGUE

Although it is not currently possible to completely eliminate fatigue, its harmful effects can be mitigated. A comprehensive strategy should maximize the opportunity to achieve adequate sleep and to increase awareness of the personal responsibility to sleep when able to do so. Most adults need between 7 and 9 hours of sleep per night,[84] depending upon age. Sleep requirements are higher for adolescents.[85] The American Academy of Pediatrics recommends that high school students start school no earlier than 8:30 a.m. to reduce the detrimental effects of chronic sleep deprivation.[85] In many countries, studies for a basic medical degree might begin at age 19 years or younger, so this recommendation might also have practical implications for medical educators. As people age, they tend to go to bed earlier and wake up earlier.[86] Practically, early morning ward rounds might work well for senior clinicians, but may be cognitively more difficult for students and younger trainees.

Shift Strategies

In an ideal world, physicians would avoid tasks related to patient care during the periods of high sleep propensity, especially the WOCL. However, this is not possible; patients routinely require care at night. There is no single shift strategy to eliminate the effects of fatigue. Ideal shift schedules remain the topic of debate, and the concept is considered industry specific and highly complex[12] Anyone who works overnight and especially during the WOCL during the early morning hours will be fatigued. Even if a person has rested during the day, he or she will still be affected by the nighttime circadian drive for sleep.[12] This effect occurs in other domains: the odds ratio of road accidents at 4 a.m. was 5.7 compared to the daytime reference hour, even after removing other potential confounding factors.[87] Both the circadian clock and the metabolic drive for sleep (the fatigue clock) must therefore be aligned in order to prevent fatigue.

Fatigue caused by shift work (shift lag) produces disruptions to the circadian clock, similar to those of jet lag. Traveling east to west implies a later bedtime and is called a *phase delay*. Traveling west to east produces an earlier bedtime (and earlier awakening) and is called a *phase advance*. Although the circadian clock cannot be adjusted immediately, people tend to adjust more rapidly to a phase delay rather than to a phase advance.[88] For this reason, some advocate that rotational shift schedules should start progressively later and lead into a night shift. However, the American College of Occupational and Environmental Medicine states, "There is no strong evidence that sleep or accident risk differs based on direction of rotation (of shifts)."[82] In order to adjust to a new time zone, both the circadian clock and the fatigue clock must align. This adds complexity to shift work scheduling because environmental cues are not consistent with the shift times.

Physiological cues for sleep, such as light and melatonin activity, as well as social cues, are affected by night shifts. Although shift times that progressively "travel" from east to west may permit some level of adaptation, a massive "west to east" change is then required to reacclimate to the day shift. Shift strategies should therefore include the direction and rate of shift changes as well as the shift length. Perhaps the lack of success of different shift strategies, including progressively later start times, is due to the fact that it is difficult to adapt the circadian rhythm to night shift.[89] It is difficult to attain quality sleep out of the circadian phase, and as Sack and colleagues point out, this leads to increased homeostatic sleep drive during the shift.[12] Furthermore, it does not seem to be the case that people can truly adapt to chronic shift work.[82]

The propensity for fatigue to accumulate during consecutive night shifts was acknowledged by the FAA when designing duty-hour regulations. They found that performance could substantially deteriorate after the third consecutive night when crew worked through the WOCL and slept during the day. They ruled that pilots could work 5 consecutive nights if they had a 2-hour sleep opportunity per night.[1] Interestingly, Leff et al. found that simulated laparoscopic skills exhibited the greatest level of deterioration in junior surgeons after the first night, but then improved over the remaining 6 nights of their night rotation.[90] However, many of the physicians in this study had sleep opportunities during their night shifts. A position paper adopted by the Aerospace Medical Association makes the following recommendations:[88]

Recommendations for Rotating to Different Shift Schedules

- When remaining within the same time zone but rotating to night duty, avoid morning sunlight by wearing dark glasses and by staying indoors as much as possible prior to sleeping.
- For daytime sleep, make sure the sleep environment is dark and cool.
- For daytime sleep, use eye masks and earplugs (or a masking noise like a

box fan) to minimize light and noise interference.

- When on duty at night, try to take a short nap before reporting for duty.
- After waking from daytime sleep, get at least 2 hours of sunlight (or artificial bright light) in the late afternoon or early evening if possible.

An alternative strategy to working a series of night shifts is to have a different person work a shift each night without attempting to readjust the circadian clock, possibly performing regular duties during the day and then being on call during the evening. Alternately, the person performing the night duties might have the day off to obtain adequate sleep. It is often difficult for a well-rested person to obtain sleep during the day[1] when preparing for night shift, but it may be easier to fall asleep out of circadian phase if one is chronically sleep deprived. If the first night is potentially the night when fatigue causes the most impairment to physician trainees' skills,[90] then this strategy also increases risk.

Sleep During the Shift

Scheduling shifts that allow healthcare professionals to be rested, with both circadian and fatigue clock alignment, is difficult and frequently impractical. An alternative strategy is to consider opportunities for sleep *during* the shift. More extensive sleep opportunities during a night duty period have been incorporated into both the ACGME duty-hour regulations and FAA regulations. These opportunities include the requirement to provide dedicated sleep facilities. Sleep during shift work does, however, predispose to sleep inertia. Although ACGME regulations promote opportunities for trainees to sleep during the shift, similar protections are not likely to be feasible for the supervising attending physicians.

PHARMACOLOGICAL AGENTS AND FATIGUE RISK MITIGATION

Although not widely used in clinical medicine (with the exception of caffeine), pharmacological agents are used in other industries, especially the military, to mitigate the effects of fatigue. This section provides an overview of pharmacological fatigue mitigation strategies.

Pharmacological Aids to Promote Sleep

Although sleep is important, the drive to sleep is not always aligned with the times that shift-working health professionals are able to sleep. Hypnotic agents are therefore sometimes used to induce or maintain sleep when a person is unable to sleep at the allocated time. Restorative sleep is not the same as central nervous system depression or a decreased level of consciousness. The restorative value of sleep is derived from a complex array of neural systems that cannot be replicated by a single pharmacological agent. In order to be effective, therefore, pharmacological sleeping aids must facilitate the initiation and/or maintenance of the endogenous sleep apparatus, while not affecting the function of the sleep centers once sleep has been initiated.

Caldwell et al. review benzodiazepine and non-benzodiazepine drugs and their strategic use to reduce fatigue from sleep deprivation in aviation medicine.[88] Overall, they recommend the strategic use of hypnotic drugs to induce sleep "where natural sleep is difficult or impossible due to circadian or other reasons," and advocate that "facilitating quality sleep with the use of a well-tested, safe pharmacological compound is far better than having pilots return to duty when sleep deprived."

Part of the endogenous sleep apparatus is thought to be mediated by the neurotransmitter gamma-aminobutyric acid (GABA). Benzodiazepines, which facilitate GABA transmission, promote the onset of sleep.[14] Zolpidem (Ambien®, Stilnox®), although not chemically a benzodiazepine, also acts at the benzodiazepine receptor.[91] Because of its favorable pharmacodynamics and pharmacokinetics, zolpidem has been used by shift-working residents.[92,93] Despite reports that zolpidem can be associated with sleep walking and other parasomnias,[94] it has become the sleeping tablet of choice for astronauts; 78% of space shuttle crew members reported using hypnotic drugs, a sleeping tablet was used on over half the in-flight nights, and zolpidem was by far the most common drug used.[95] Although Zolpidem's relatively short half-life helps to prevent a hangover effect, drug levels that impair driving ability have been observed in some people more than 8 hours after a 10-mg dose.[96] If an emergency situation arose during the allocated sleep time, the presence of a hypnotic agent might impair one's ability to respond.

Antihistamines are common over-the-counter sleeping aids and were reportedly used by 31% of shift-working emergency medicine residents.[92] Although alcohol is often used to relax and promote sleep, the effect of alcohol on sleep architecture means that it often reduces the quality and quantity of sleep.[16]

Melatonin and Light

Pharmacologic interventions other than hypnotic agents have been investigated as a means to alter the body's circadian physiology to promote sleep in the context of jet lag and shift work. Melatonin facilitates the initiation of the endogenous sleep mechanisms, and series of studies have demonstrated the beneficial effects of melatonin and light to both advance and delay the circadian phase.[97] Melatonin is also helpful to facilitate sleep during times when the circadian rhythm would not otherwise be promoting sleep.[98,99,100] Taking melatonin early can advance the onset of sleep (phase advance), while taking it in the morning hours can delay the time at which the individual would naturally awaken (phase delay). Similarly, light can be used in the early morning to advance the sleep phase and at night to delay the sleep phase.

Wakefulness-Promoting Drugs

Caffeine is the most widely used pharmacologic agent to promote wakefulness. It is rapidly absorbed after oral ingestion and its peak plasma concentration occurs in approximately 30–90 minutes, although absorption is slower in some individuals, taking several hours.[101] Caffeine absorption is more rapid through the oral mucosa.[102] In doses of 100 mg to 600 mg,

caffeine promotes wakefulness, increases vigilance, and reduces cognitive deficits caused by sleep deprivation.[102] A review by Vanderveen and colleagues also found that "[n]o differential dosing is recommended for habitual and first-time caffeine users, since there is no general agreement regarding the extent to which tolerance develops to caffeine's cognitive effects in habitual users."[102] Caffeine is a methylxanthine that causes a mild increase in norepinephrine and dopamine,[103] but its behavioral effects are mainly caused by its action as an adenosine antagonist and inhibitor of cyclic nucleotide phosphodiesterases.[102]

The half-life of caffeine varies significantly between individuals, between 1.5 to over 10 hours.[101,102] CYP450 1A2 is the main enzyme responsible for the metabolism of caffeine;[104] its activity varies among individuals due to genetic and environmental influences. Smoking increases clearance and reduces the half-life of caffeine,[102,104,105,106] while pregnancy and the oral contraceptive pill decrease clearance.[106] As a result, using caffeine for short-term fatigue mitigation might come at the cost of a long period of insomnia for certain individuals. As well, because adenosine promotes sleep,[21] the antagonizing effect of caffeine on adenosine may interfere with an unscheduled sleep opportunity.

Although caffeine is generally recognized as safe (GRAS) by the FDA,[107] it may rarely induce adverse effects, including severe anxiety, panic attacks, and psychosis.[106] Given this range in metabolism and effects, healthcare professionals must understand their individual response to caffeine before using it as an antifatigue measure. In military operations it has been suggested that caffeine be used in 100-mg increments, with a total dose not exceeding approximately 600 mg.[102]

Amphetamines have historically been employed to combat fatigue in the military. Dexamphetamine in doses of 10–20 mg (not exceeding 60 mg) is recommended for severely sleep-deprived military personnel who must complete a mission.[88] However, amphetamine's abuse potential and harmful side effects[97] render it unsuitable for civilian use.

Modafinil promotes wakefulness by mechanisms that have not yet been completely elucidated, and is currently used in the military. It has been demonstrated to improve cognitive function and alertness in sleep-deprived individuals.[88] Modafinil acts upon central norephiniphrine and dopamine transporters and has secondary effects upon glutamate, serotonin, histamine, GABA transmission,[108] and orexin.[109] It is approved by the FDA for sleepiness associated with (1) narcolepsy, (2) obstructive sleep apnea, and (3) shift-work sleep disorder.[110] Modafinil is also used off-label for jet lag and it has become popular on college campuses and among individuals in a variety of professions who seek not only wakefulness but cognitive enhancement.[111] Evidence for cognitive enhancement in non-sleep-deprived healthy individuals is inconclusive, and varies between individuals,[112] however it may improve performance in more complex tasks.[109] Modafinil's ability as a cognitive enhancer may be inversely related to underlying cognitive ability.[108]

In one study, modafinil improved "cognitive processes critical for efficient information processing, flexible thinking, and decision making under time pressure [in sleep-deprived physicians] but was not effective in improving clinical psychomotor performance."[113] In sleep-deprived emergency physicians, modafinil "increased certain aspects of cognitive function and subjectively improved participants' ability to attend post-night-shift didactic sessions but made it more difficult for participants to fall asleep when opportunities for sleep arose."[114] Insomnia during sleep opportunities is consistent with modafinil's half-life of 12–15 hours.[115]

Although modafinil seems to increase cognitive performance in fatigued individuals, its effect on cognitive performance and especially its effect on reasoning in fatigued physicians who are providing clinical care have not been fully established. Aggression has been reported with modafinil.[110] There is also debate as to whether modafinil induces overconfidence,[97] which might increase the possibility of risky behavior by physicians using the drug.

HEALTHCARE AND SOCIETAL CHANGES IN RELATION TO FATIGUE MANAGEMENT

Fatigue management strategies must also take into account primary sleep disorders and sleep pathology caused by medical and psychiatric conditions. For example, a healthcare professional might function adequately on a stable, fixed dose of a psychiatric medicine that may be taken at night and have sedating effects.[116] Legitimate medications for chronic and stable medical conditions may be acceptable, despite their potential to affect sleep and wakefulness.

From a societal perspective, the recognition of fatigue from both lack of sleep and heavy mental activity raises some difficult questions. If we accept the ACGME rule that moonlighting in a second job must be counted toward the fatigue load for the primary training position, society may need to develop strategies to help healthcare professionals with other sources of fatigue. Raising young children, for example, can contribute an intense mental load as well as fatigue from sleepless nights with ill or poorly sleeping children. Similarly, there are many primary sleep disorders and those secondary to medical and neuropsychiatric disorders. This raises a question of how to facilitate the needs of these individuals to optimize their ability to perform their professional roles as healthcare providers.

Fatigue in the Patient

This chapter has been focusing on the effects of fatigue on healthcare professionals. However, there is growing concern about, and investigations into, the effects of sleep deprivation on patients. Patients have reduced total sleep time, reduced REM, and reduced slow-wave sleep (SWS) for several days after a surgical procedure. Thereafter, they are subject to a rebound phenomenon in which total REM sleep is increased.[117] The initial lack of sleep is consistent with known disruptors of sleep, for example, pain, unfamiliar and stressful environments, noise, surgical drains or catheters, frequent observations and monitor alarms that activate at night. There also seem to be more fundamental effects on the sleep apparatus from surgery, including neurohumoral stress and inflammatory responses. Although the contributing factors to this lack of sleep are multifactorial, anesthesia does not seem to contribute significantly to this effect. In one study, healthy volunteers who were anesthetized for 3 hours without undergoing surgery had only minor changes to sleep.[118]

Major surgery causes more disruption to sleep than minor surgery.[117] Minimally invasive surgery results in lower surgical stress response[119] and might be predicted to result in less disruption to sleep. However, patients undergoing laparoscopic colon resection had worse subjective sleep quality than those undergoing open resection on the first postoperative night,[120] possibly because the laparoscopic patients had slightly higher pain scores. Even in a fast-track program for major joint replacement, patients still demonstrated a 93% decrease in REM sleep on the first postoperative night, which normalized by the fourth night, when they were at home.[121] Similarly, the use of a hypnotic, zolpidem (10 mg), did not improve objective measures of sleep as recorded by EEG, but did decrease the number of arousals and improve subjective reports of fatigue.[122]

If restorative sleep is important for immune function and healing, then sleep deprivation might affect recovery, including infection rates. Sleep disruption is a hallmark of obstructive sleep apnea (OSA). Although OSA is associated with a number of postoperative complications, [123,124] it is not well recognized as a significant risk factor for surgical site infection.[125] However, a recent study of colectomy patients found that the risk of surgical site infection was nearly triple in OSA patients.[125]

Delirium is a major postoperative complication. It has been found that melatonin secretion is reduced after surgery.[126] Studies have investigated whether exogenous melatonin to reverse sleep disruption after surgery reduces delirium; some have not demonstrated a significant effect.[127,128,129] However, some investigators have reported improvements,[130,131,132] and the strategic use of melatonin might become a clinical option. Interestingly, melatonin appears to consistently reduce preoperative anxiety.[133,134]

There has been significant interest in reducing sleep deprivation in sedated and intubated patients in the intensive care unit (ICU). Although sedated, with a reduced level of consciousness, intubated patients have very poor sleep. This lack of physiological sleep is thought to contribute to delirium, which is common in the ICU, as well as potentially inhibiting normal system homeostasis, including immune function.

Dexmedetomidine is an α-2 agonist that is indicated for the sedation of intubated patients. Dexmedetomidine sedation produces an EEG pattern that is characteristic of non-REM sleep, particularly stage 2,[135] and its mechanism of action involves the activation of endogenous sleep pathways, including the ventrolateral preoptic nucleus (VLPO).[136] This is believed to produce better restorative sleep than modulation of the system by GABAergic agents.[136] In one study, compared to a standard regimen of benzodiazepine, dexmedetomidine was associated with a decrease in delirium.[137] In another study, patients intubated long term for respiratory failure and sedated with dexmedetomidine during the evenings had increased sleep and a more normal circadian rhythm compared to those patients who did not receive sedation.[138]

SUMMARY

A variety of factors contribute to whether an individual experiences fatigue as well as the severity of that fatigue. The FAA summarizes the major factors affecting fatigue:[30]

1. *Time of day.* Fatigue is, in part, a function of circadian rhythms. All other factors being equal, fatigue is most likely and, when present, most severe between the hours of 0200 and 0600.
2. *Amount of recent sleep.* If a person has had significantly less than 8 hours of sleep in the past 24 hours, he or she is more likely to be fatigued.
3. *Time awake.* A person who has been continually awake for a long period of time since his or her last major sleep period is more likely to be fatigued.

4. *Cumulative sleep debt.* For the average person, cumulative sleep debt is the difference between the amount of sleep a person has received over the past several days, and the amount of sleep he or she would have received with 8 hours of sleep a night.

5. *Time on task.* The longer a person has continuously been doing a job without a break, the more likely he or she is to be fatigued.

6. *Individual variation.* Individuals respond to fatigue factors differently and may become fatigued at different times, and to different degrees of severity under the same circumstances.

Because of circadian factors, most people find it hard to sleep during the day and do not get good quality sleep even if they have been working overnight and their level of fatigue is high.[1] Awareness of fatigue is increasing in society at large and within the health professions. Considering that people can be charged with manslaughter if involved in an automobile accident after being awake for more than 24 hours, it should only be under the most exceptional circumstances that a licensed healthcare professional should be treating patients after a similar period without sleep.

REFERENCES

1. Federal Aviation Administration; 14 CFR Parts 117, 119, and 121; Docket No.: FAA-2009-1093; Amdt. Nos. 117-1, 119-16, 121-357; RIN 2120–AJ58; Flightcrew Member Duty and Rest Requirements. https://www.faa.gov/regulations_policies/rulemaking/recently_published/media/2120-AJ58-FinalRule.pdf, accessed January 2016.
2. Pilcher JJ, Huffcutt A. Effects of sleep deprivation on performance: a meta-analysis. *Sleep.* 1996;19(4):318–326.
3. Cappuccio FP, Cooper D, D'Elia L, Strazzullo P, Miller MA. Sleep duration predicts cardiovascular outcomes: a systematic review and meta-analysis of prospective studies. *Eur Heart J.* 2011;32(12):1484–1492.
4. Cohen S, Doyle WJ, Alper CM, Janicki-Deverts D, Turner RB. Sleep habits and susceptibility to the common cold. *Arch Intern Med.* 2009;169(1):62–67.
5. Thompson CL, Larkin EK, Patel S, Berger NA, Redline S, Li L. Short duration of sleep increases risk of colorectal adenoma. *Cancer.* 2011 Feb 15;117(4): 841–847.
6. Hart CN, Carskadon MA, Considine RV, et al. Changes in children's sleep duration on food intake, weight, and leptin. *Pediatrics.* 2013;132(6): e1473–1480.
7. Capers PL, Fobian AD, Kaiser KA, Borah R, Allison DB. A systemic review and meta-analysis of randomized controlled trials of the impact of sleep duration on adiposity and components of energy balance. *Obes Rev.* 2015;16(9):771–782
8. Zaremba S, Chamberlin NL, Eikermann M. Sleep Medicine. In: Miller RD, Lars I, Eriksson LI, Fleisher LA, Wiener-Kronish JP, Cohen NH, Young WL, eds. *Miller's Anesthesia.* 8th ed. Philadelphia: Elsevier Saunders; 2015.
9. Möckel T, Beste C, Wascher E. The effects of time on task in response selection: an ERP study of mental fatigue. *Scientific Reports.* 2015;5:10113. doi:10.1038/srep10113.
10. Bordyugov G, Abraham U, Granada A, et al. Tuning the phase of circadian entrainment. *J R Soc Interface.* 2015;12:20150282; DOI: 10.1098/rsif.2015.0282.
11. Czeisler CA, Duffy JF, Shanahan TL. Stability, precision, and near-24-hour period of the human circadian pacemaker. *Science.* 1999;284(5423): 2177–2181.
12. Sack RL, Auckley D, Auger RR, et al. Circadian rhythm sleep disorders: Part I, basic principles, shift work and jet lag disorders: an American Academy of Sleep Medicine review. *Sleep.* 2007;30(11): 1460–1483.
13. Dijk D, Lockley SW. Invited review: Integration of human sleep-wake regulation and circadian rhythmicity. *J Appl Physiol.* 2002;92(2):852–862.
14. Schupp M, Hanning CD. Physiology of sleep. *BJA CEPD Rev.* 2003;3:69–74.
15. Ruskin KJ, Caldwell JA, Caldwell JL, Boudreau EA. Screening for sleep apnea in morbidly obese pilots. *Aerosp Med Hum Perform.* 2015 Sep;86(9): 835–841.
16. Howard SK, Rosekind MR, Katz JD, Berry AJ; Fatigue in anesthesia implications and strategies for patient and provider safety. *Anesthesiology.* 2002;97:1281–1294.
17. Bonmati-Carrion MA, Arguelles-Prieto R, Martinez-Madrid MJ, et al. Protecting the melatonin rhythm through circadian healthy light exposure. *Int J Mol Sci.* 2014 Dec 17;15(12): 23448–23500.
18. Keijzer H, Smits MG, Duffy JF, Curfs LM. Why the dim light melatonin onset (DLMO) should be measured before treatment of patients with circadian rhythm sleep disorders. *Sleep Med Rev.* 2014 Aug;18(4):333–339.
19. Sinha A, Singh A, Tewari A. The fatigued anesthesiologist: a threat to patient safety? *J Anaesthesiol*

Clin Pharmacol. 2013;29(2):151–159. doi:10.4103/0970-9185.111657.

20. Lu J, Sherman D, Marshall Devor M, Saper CB. A putative flip–flop switch for control of REM sleep. *Nature.* 2006 June;441:589–594.

21. Huang ZL, Zhang Z, Qu WM. Roles of adenosine and its receptors in sleep-wake regulation. *Int Rev Neurobiol.* 2014;119:349–371.

22. Monti JM. Serotonin control of sleep-wake behavior. *Sleep Med Rev.* 2011;15(4):269–281.

23. Lim J, Ebstein R, Tse C-Y, et al. Dopaminergic polymorphisms associated with time-on-task declines and fatigue in the psychomotor vigilance test. *PLoS ONE.* 2012;7(3):e33767. doi:10.1371/journal.pone.0033767.

24. Powell DMC, Spencer MB, Holland D, Broadbent E, Petrie KJ. Pilot fatigue in short-haul operations: effects of number of sectors, duty length, and time of day. *Aviat Space Environ Med.* 2007;78:698–701.

25. Warm JS, Parasuraman R, Matthews G. Vigilance requires hard mental work and is stressful. *Human Factors.* 2008;50:433–441.

26. Tanaka M, Shigihara Y, Ishii A, Funakura M, Kanai E, Watanabe Y. Effect of mental fatigue on the central nervous system: an electroencephalography study. *Behav Brain Functions.* 2012;8:48. doi:10.1186/1744-9081-8-48.

27. Shigihara Y, Tanaka M, Ishii A, Kanai E, Funakura M, Watanabe Y. Two types of mental fatigue affect spontaneous oscillatory brain activities in different ways. *Behav Brain Functions.* 2013;9:2. doi:10.1186/1744-9081-9-2.

28. van der Linden D, Frese M, Meijman TF. Mental fatigue and the control of cognitive processes: effects on perseveration and planning;. *Acta Psychol (Amst).* 2003;113(1):45–65.

29. Ishii A, Tanaka M, Watanabe Y. Neural mechanisms of mental fatigue. *Rev Neurosci.* 2014;25(4):469–479.

30. FAA Flight Standards Information Management System; Volume 3, General Technical Information; Chapter 58, Management of aviation fatigue; Section 2, Understanding and applying Part 117. http://fsims.faa.gov/PICDetail.aspx?docId=8900.1,Vol.3,Ch58,Sec2. Accessed January 2016.

31. Van Dongen HPA, Maislin G, Mullington JM, Dinges DF. The cumulative cost of additional wakefulness: dose-response effects on neurobehavioral functions and sleep physiology from chronic sleep restriction and total sleep deprivation. *Sleep.* 2003;26(2);117–126.

32. Zhou X, Ferguson SA, Matthews RW, et al. Mismatch between subjective alertness and objective performance under sleep restriction is greatest during the biological night. *J Sleep Res.* 2012;21:40–49.

33. Groeger JA, Viola AU, Lo JCY, von Schantz M, Archer SN, Dijk D-J. Early Morning executive functioning during sleep deprivation is compromised by a *PERIOD3* polymorphism. *Sleep.* 2008;31(8):1159–1167.

34. Sugden C, Athanasiou T, Darzi A. What are the effects of sleep deprivation and fatigue in surgical practice? *Semin Thorac Cardiovasc Surg.* 2012;24(3); 166–175.

35. Lockley SW, Barger LK, Ayas NT, et al., for the Harvard Work Hours, Health and Safety Group. Effects of health care provider work hours and sleep deprivation on safety and performance. *Joint Comm J Qual Patient Safety.* 2007;33(11)(Suppl):7–18.

36. McCormick F, Kadzielski J, Landrigan CP, Evans B, Herndon JH, Rubash HE. Surgeon Fatigue: A prospective analysis of the incidence, risk, and intervals of predicted fatigue-related impairment in residents. *Arch Surg.* 2012;147(5): 430–435.

37. Lockley SW, Cronin JW, Evans EE, Cade BE, Lee CJ, Landrigan CP, et al. Effect of reducing interns' weekly work hours on sleep and attentional failures. *N Engl J Med.* 2004;351: 1829–1837

38. Landrigan CP, Rothschild JM, Cronin JW, Kaushal R, Burdick E, Katz JT, et al. Effect of reducing interns' work hours on serious medical errors in intensive care units. *N Engl J Med.* 2004;351:1838–1848.

39. Gander PH, Merry A, Millar MM, Weller J. Hours of work and fatigue-related error: a survey of New Zealand anaesthetists. *Anaesth Intensive Care.* 2000 Apr;28(2):178–183.

40. Aya AG, Mangin R, Robert C, Ferrer JM, Eledjam JJ. Increased risk of unintentional dural puncture in night-time obstetric epidural anesthesia. *Can J Anaesth.* 1999;46(7):665–669.

41. Rothschild JM, Keohane CA, Rogers S,et al. Risks of complications by attending physicians after performing nighttime procedures. *JAMA.* 2009;302(14):1565–1572.

42. Govindarajan A, Urbach DR, Kumar M, et al. Outcomes of daytime procedures performed by attending surgeons after night work. *N Engl J Med.* 373;9: 845–853.

43. Philibert I. Sleep loss and performance in residents and nonphysicians: a meta-analytic examination. *Sleep.* 2005;28(11):1392–1402.

44. Howard SK, Gaba DM, Rosekind MR, Zarcone VP. The risks and implications of excessive daytime sleepiness in resident physicians. *Acad Med.* 2002;77(10):1019–1025.

45. Howard SK, Gaba DM, Smith BE, et al. Simulation study of rested versus sleep-deprived anesthesiologist. *Anesthesiology.* 2003;98:1345–1355.

46. Kahn-Greene ET, Lipizzi EL, Conrad AK, Kamimori GH, Killgor WDS. Sleep deprivation adversely affects interpersonal responses to frustration. *Pers Indiv Differ*. 2006;41:1433–1443.

47. Rosen IM, Gimotty PA, Shea JA, Bellini LM. Evolution of sleep quantity, sleep deprivation, mood disturbances, empathy, and burnout among interns. *Acad Med*. 2006;81(1):82–85.

48. Ayas NT, Barger LK, Cade BE, et al. Extended work duration and the risk of self-reported percutaneous injuries in interns. *JAMA*. 2006;296(9):1055–1062.

49. Barger LK, Cade BE, Ayas NT, et al for the Harvard Work Hours, Health, and Safety Group. Extended work shifts and the risk of motor vehicle crashes among interns. *N Engl J Med*. 2005;352(2):125–134.

50. National Conference of State Legislatures. http://www.ncsl.org/research/transportation/summaries-of-current-drowsy-driving-laws.aspx. Accessed December 2015.

51. Ulmer C, Wolman DM, John MME, Committee on Optimizing Graduate Medical Trainee (Resident) Hours and Work Schedules to Improve Patient Safety. Resident duty hours: enhancing sleep, supervision, and safety. Washington, DC: Institute of Medicine of the National Academies; National Academies Press; 2009.

52. Accreditation Council For General Medical Education. Duty hours, common program requirements. https://www.acgme.org/acgmeweb/Portals/0/PDFs/Common_Program_Requirements_07012011[2].pdf. Accessed December 2015.

53. Dacey RG. Editorial: Our continuing experience with duty-hours regulation and its effect on quality of care and education. *J Neurosurg Spine*. 2014;21(4):499–501.

54. Ahmed N, Devitt KS, Keshet I, et al. A systematic review of the effects of resident duty hour restrictions in surgery: impact on resident wellness, training, and patient outcomes. *Ann Surg*. 2014;259(6):1041–1053.

55. Jamal MH, Doi SA, Rousseau M, et al. Systematic review and meta-analysis of the effect of North American working hours restrictions on mortality and morbidity in surgical patients. *Br J Surg*. 2012 Mar;99(3):336–344.

56. Harris JD, LT, Staheli G, LeClere L, Andersone D, McCormick F. What effects have resident work-hour changes had on education, quality of life, and safety? A systematic review. *Clin Orthop Relat Res*. 2015;473:1600–1608.

57. ACGME. News and update: update on two multicenter trials, December 7, 2015. https://www.acgme.org/acgmeweb/Portals/0/PDFs/NascaLetterCommunityDutyHoursMulticenter-TrialsUpdateDec2015.pdf.

58. Schwartz SI, Galante J, Kaji A, et al. Effect of the 16-hour work limit on general surgery intern operative case volume. *JAMA Surg*. 2013;148(9):829–833.

59. Freischlag JA. There are just not enough hours in the day. *JAMA Surg*. 2013;148(9):833.

60. Theobald CN, Stover DG, Choma NN, et al. The effect of reducing maximum shift lengths to 16 hours on internal medicine interns' educational opportunities. *Acad Med*. 2013; 88(4):512–518

61. Stickgold R. Sleep-dependent memory consolidation. *Nature*. 2005; 437(7063):1272–1278.

62. Hyder JA, Bohman JK, Kor DJ, et al. Anesthesia care transitions and risk of postoperative complications. *Anesth Analg*. 2016;122:134–144.

63. Saager L, Hesler BD, You J, et al. Intraoperative transitions of anesthesia care and postoperative adverse outcomes. *Anesthesiology*. 2014;121:695–706.

64. Hudson CC, McDonald B, Hudson JK, Tran D, Boodhwani M. Impact of anesthetic handover on mortality and morbidity in cardiac surgery: a cohort study. *J Cardiothorac Vasc Anesth*. 2015;29:11–16.

65. Lane-Fall MB. No matter the perspective, anesthesia handoffs are problematic. *Anesth Analg*. 2016;122(1):7–9.

66. Drolet BC, Schwede M, Bishop KD, Fischer SA. Compliance and falsification of duty hours: reports from residents and program directors. *J Grad Med Educ*. 2013;5(3):368–373.

67. Byrne JM, Loo LK, Giang DW. Duty hour reporting: conflicting values in professionalism. *J Grad Med Educ*. 2015;7(3):395–400.

68. Fargen KM, Dow J, Tomei KL, Friedman WA. Follow-up on a national survey: American neurosurgery resident opinions on the 2011 Accreditation Council for Graduate Medical Education-implemented duty hours. *World Neurosurg*. 2014;81(1): 15–21.

69. Drolet BC, Khokhar MT, Fischer SA. Perspective: The 2011 duty-hour requirements—a survey of residency program directors. *N Engl J Med*. 2013;368:694–697.

70. Bilimoria KY, Chung JW, Hedges LV, et al. National cluster-randomized trial of duty-hour flexibility in surgical training. *N Engl J Med* 2016;374:713–727.

71. Birkmeyer JD. Surgical Resident Duty-Hour Rules — Weighing the New Evidence. *N Engl J Med* 2016;374:783–784

72. Rosenbaum, Lisa. Leaping without Looking—Duty Hours, Autonomy, and the Risks of Research and Practice. *N Engl J Med* 2016;374:8, 701–703

73. American College of Surgheons. Extending the Length of Surgical Trainees' Shifts Does Not Affect Surgical Patients' Safety. https://www.facs.org/media/press-releases/2016/first0216 Accessed April 2016

74. Rosekind MR, Graeber RC, Dinges DF, Connell LJ, Rountree MS, Spinweber CL, Gillin KA. Crew factors in flight operations IX: effects of planned cockpit rest on crew performance and alertness in long-haul operations. NASA Technical Memorandum #108839. Moffett Field, CA: NASA Ames Research Center, 1994.

75. National Sleep Foundation. https://sleepfoundation.org/sleep-topics/napping. Accessed December 2015.

76. Kubo T, Takahashi M, Takeyama H, et al. How do the timing and length of a night-shift nap affect sleep inertia? *Chronobiol Int.* 2010;27(5):1031–1044.

77. Ruggiero JS, Redeker NS. Effects of napping on sleepiness and sleep-related performance deficits in night-shift workers: a systematic review. *Biol Res Nurs.* 2014;16(2):134–142.

78. Tassi P, Muze A. Sleep inertia. *Sleep Med Rev.* 2000;4(4):341–353.

79. Jewett ME, Wyatt JK, Ritz-De Cecco A, Khalsa SB, Dijk DJ, Czeisler CA. Time course of sleep inertia dissipation in human performance and alertness. *J Sleep Res.* 1999;8(1):1–8.

80. St. Pierre M, Hofinger G, Buerschaper C, Simon R. Attention: the focus of consciousness. In: *Crisis Management in Acute Care Settings: Human Factors, Team Psychology, and Patient Safety in a High Stakes Environment.* Berlin and Heidelberg: Springer-Verlag; 2011:Chapter 8.

81. Tassi P, Nicolas A, Dewasmes G, et al. Effects of noise on sleep inertia as a function of circadian placement of a one hour nap. *Percep Motor Skills.* 1992;75(1):291–302.

82. American College of Occupational and Environmental Medicine. ACOEM guidance statement: fatigue risk management in the workplace; ACOEM Presidential Task Force on Fatigue Risk Management. http://www.acoem.org/uploadedFiles/Public_Affairs/Policies_And_Position_Statements/Fatigue%20Risk%20Management%20in%20the%20Workplace.pdf. Accessed December 2015

83. Drolet BC, Hyman CH, Ghaderi KF, Rodriguez-Srednicki J, Thompson JM, Fischer SA. Hospitalized patients' perceptions of resident fatigue, duty hours, and continuity of care. *J Grad Med Educ.* 2014;6(4):658–663.

84. Gregory P, Edsell M. Fatigue and the anaesthetist. *Contin Educ Anaesth Crit Care Pain.* 2014;14(1):18–22.

85. American Academy of Pediatrics. http://pediatrics.aappublications.org/content/early/2014/08/19/peds.2014-1697. Accessed January 2016.

86. Duffy JF, Czeisler CA. Age-related change in the relationship between circadian period, circadian phase, and diurnal preference in humans. *Neurosci Lett.* 2002;318(3):117–120.

87. Akerstedt TL, Kecklund G, Hörte LG. Night driving, season, and the risk of highway accidents. *Sleep.* 2001;24(4):401–406.

88. Caldwell JA, Mallis MM, Caldwell JL, Paul MA, Miller JC, Neri DF, Aerospace Medical Association Aerospace Fatigue Countermeasures Subcommittee of the Human Factors Committee. Fatigue countermeasures in aviation. *Aviat Space Environ Med.* 2009;80:29–59.

89. Gallo LC, Eastman CI. Circadian rhythms during gradually delaying and advancing sleep and light schedules. *Physiol Behav.* 1993;53(1):119–126.

90. Leff, DR, Aggarwal R, Rana M, et al. Laparoscopic skills suffer on the first shift of sequential night shifts: program directors beware and residents prepare. *Ann Surg.* 2008;247(3):530–539.

91. Trevor, Anthony J. Sedative-hypnotic drugs. In: Katzung BG, Trevor AJ, eds. *Basic and Clinical Pharmacology.* 13th ed. New York: McGraw-Hill; 2015.

92. Shy BD, Portelli I, Nelson LS. Emergency medicine residents' use of psychostimulants and sedatives to aid in shift work. *Am J Emerg Med.* 2011;29(9):1034–1036.

93. McBeth BD, McNamara RM, Ankel FK, Mason EJ, Ling LJ, Flottemesch TJ, Asplin BR. Modafinil and zolpidem use by emergency medicine residents. *Acad Emerg Med.* 2009;16(12): 1311–1317.

94. Food and Drug Administration. Ambien CR product information. http://www.fda.gov/downloads/Drugs/DrugSafety/ucm085908.pdf. Accessed December 2015.

95. Barger LK, Flynn-Evans EE, Kubey A, et al. Prevalence of sleep deficiency and use of hypnotic drugs in astronauts before, during, and after spaceflight: an observational study. *Lancet Neurology.* 2014;13(9):904–912.

96. Farkas RH, Unger EF, Temple R. Zolpidem and driving impairment: identifying persons at risk. *N Engl J Med.* 2013;369:689–691.

97. Paul MA, Gray GW, Lieberman HR, Love RJ, Miller JC, Arendt J. Management of circadian desynchrony (jetlag and shiftlag) in CF Air Operations. Defence R&D Canada—Toronto Technical Report. DRDC Toronto TR 2010-002. December 2010.

98. Paul MA, Gray G, Sardana TM, Pigeau RA. Melatonin and zopiclone as facilitators of early circadian sleep in operational air transport crews. *Aviat Space Environ Med.* 2004;75(5):439–443.

99. Paul MA, Brown G, Buguet A, Gray G, Pigeau RA, Weinberg H, Radomski M. Melatonin and zopiclone as pharmacologic aids to facilitate crew rest. *Aviat Space Environ Med*. 2001;72(11):974–984.

100. Arendt J. Melatonin: characteristics, concerns, and prospects. *J Biol Rhythms*. 2005;20:291–303.

101. Newton R, Broughton LJ, Lind MJ, Morrison PJ, Rogers HJ, Bradbrook ID. Plasma and salivary pharmacokinetics of caffeine in man. *Eur J Clin Pharmacol*. 1981;21(1):45–52.

102. Vanderveen JE (Chair), Committee on Military Nutrition Research. Caffeine for the sustainment of mental task performance: formulations for military operations. Washington, DC: Food and Nutrition Board; Institute of Medicine; 2001.

103. O'Brien CP. Drug addiction. In: Brunton LL, Chabner BA, Knollmann BC. eds. *Goodman and Gilman's: The Pharmacological Basis of Therapeutics*. 12th ed. New York: McGraw-Hill; 2011: 649–668.

104. Almira Correia M. Drug biotransformation. In: Katzung BG, Trevor AJ, eds. *Basic and Clinical Pharmacology*. 13th ed. New York: McGraw-Hill; 2015.

105. Arnaud MJ. Pharmacokinetics and metabolism of caffeine. In: Lorist M, Snel J eds. *Nicotine, Caffeine and Social Drinking: Behaviour and Brain Function*. Amsterdam: Harwood Academic Publishers; 1998: Chapter 6, 153–166.

106. Winston AP, Hardwick E, Jaberi N. Neuropsychiatric effects of caffeine. *Adv Psychiat Treat*. 2005;11(6):432–439.

107. FDA Code of Federal Regulations, title 21. http://www.accessdata.fda.gov/scripts/cdrh/cfdocs/cfcfr/CFRSearch.cfm?fr=182.1180. Accessed January 2016.

108. Minzenberg MJ, Cameron S Carter CS. Modafinil: a review of neurochemical actions and effects on cognition. *Neuropsychopharmacology*. 2008;33:1477–1502. doi:10.1038/sj.npp.1301534.

109. Battleday RM, Brem AK. Modafinil for cognitive neuroenhancement in healthy non-sleep-deprived subjects: a systematic review. *Eur Neuropsychopharmacol*. 2015;25(11):1865–1881.

110. Medication Guide Provigil. http://www.fda.gov/downloads/Drugs/DrugSafety/UCM231722.pdf. Accessed December 2015.

111. Kim D. Practical use and risk of modafinil, a novel waking drug. *Environmental Health Toxicol*. 2012;27:e2012007.

112. Ragan CI, Bard I, Singh I. What should we do about student use of cognitive enhancers? An analysis of current evidence. *Neuropharmacology*. 2013;64:588–595.

113. Sugden C, Housden C, Aggarwal R, Sahakian B, Darzi A. Effect of pharmacological enhancement on the cognitive and clinical psychomotor performance of sleep-deprived doctors: a randomized controlled trial. *Ann Surg*. 2012;255(2):222–227.

114. Gill M, Haerich P, Westcott K, Godenick KL, Tucker JA. Cognitive performance following modafinil versus placebo in sleep-deprived emergency physicians: a double-blind randomized crossover study. *Acad Emerg Med*. 2006;13(2):158–165.

115. Robertson PJr, Hellriegel ET. Clinical pharmacokinetic profile of modafinil; *Clin Pharmacokinet*. 2003;42(2):123–137.

116. Levine M, Quan D. Levine M, Quan D Levine, Michael, and Dan Quan. Nonbenzodiazepine Sedatives. Chapter 184 In: Tintinalli JE, Stapczynski J, Ma O, Yealy DM, Meckler GD, Cline DM. eds. *Tintinalli's Emergency Medicine: A Comprehensive Study Guide, 8e*. New York, NY: McGraw-Hill; 2016: 1240–1243

117. Rosenberg-Adamsen S, Kehlet H, Dodds C et al. Postoperative sleep disturbances: mechanisms and clinical implications. *Br J Anaesth*. 1996;76:552–559.

118. Moote CA, Knill RL. Isoflurane anesthesia causes a transient alteration in nocturnal sleep. *Anesthesiology*. 1988;69(3):327–331.

119. Klemann N, Hansen MV, Gögenur I. Factors affecting post-operative sleep in patients undergoing colorectal surgery: a systematic review. *Dan Med J*. 2015;62(4):A5053.

120. Basse L, Jakobsen DH, Bardram L, et al. Functional recovery after open versus laparoscopic colonic resection: a randomized, blinded study. *Ann Surg*. 2005;241(3):416–423.

121. Krenk L, Jennum P, Kehlet H. Sleep disturbances after fast-track hip and knee arthroplasty *Br J Anaesth*. 2012;109(5):769–775.

122. Krenk L, Jennum P, Kehlet H. Postoperative sleep disturbances after zolpidem treatment in fast-track hip and knee replacement. *J Clin Sleep Med*. 2014;10(3):321–326. doi:10.5664/jcsm.3540.

123. Kaw R, Chung F, Pasupuleti V, Mehta J, Gay PC, Hernandez AV. Meta-analysis of the association between obstructive sleep apnoea and postoperative outcome. *Br J Anaesth*. 2012;109(6): 897–906.

124. Gaddam S, Gunukula SK, Mador MJ. Postoperative outcomes in adult obstructive sleep apnea patients undergoing non-upper airway surgery: a systematic review and meta-analysis. *Sleep Breathing*. 2014;18(3):615–633.

125. Fortis S, Colling KP, Statz CL., Glover JJ, Radosevich DM, Beilman GJ. *Surg Infect*. 2015;16(5):611–617. doi:10.1089/sur.2014.090.

126. Cronin AJ, Keifer JC, Davies MF, Kind TS, Bixler EO. Melatonin secretion after surgery. *Lancet*. 2000;356:1244–1245.

127. De Jonghe A, van Munster BC, Goslings JC, et al. Effect of melatonin on incidence of delirium among patients with hip fracture: a multicentre, double-blind randomized controlled trial. *CMAJ*. 2014;186(14):E547–E556. doi:10.1503/cmaj.140495.

128. Bellapart J, Boots R. Potential use of melatonin in sleep and delirium in the critically ill. *Br J Anaesth*. 2012;108(4):572–580.

129. Bourne RS, Mills GH. Melatonin: possible implications for the postoperative and critically ill patient. *Intens Care Med*. 2006;32(3):371–379.

130. Sultan SS. Assessment of role of perioperative melatonin in prevention and treatment of postoperative delirium after hip arthroplasty under spinal anesthesia in the elderly. *Saudi J Anaesthesia*. 2010;4(3):169–173. doi:10.4103/1658-354X.71132.

131. Artemiou P, Bily B, Bilecova-Rabajdova M, et al. Melatonin treatment in the prevention of postoperative delirium in cardiac surgery patients. *Kardiochirurgia i Torakochirurgia Polska = Polish Journal of Cardio-Thoracic Surgery*. 2015;12(2):126–133. doi:10.5114/kitp.2015.52853.

132. Hanania M, Kitain E. Melatonin for treatment and prevention of postoperative delirium. *Anesth Analg*. 2002;94(2):338–339.

133. Hansen MV, Halladin NL, Rosenberg J, Gögenur I, Møller AM. Melatonin for pre- and postoperative anxiety in adults. *Cochrane Database Syst Rev*. 2015 Apr 9;4:CD009861.

134. Yousaf F, Seet E, Venkatraghavan L, Abrishami A, Chung F. Efficacy and safety of melatonin as an anxiolytic and analgesic in the perioperative period: a qualitative systematic review of randomized trials. *Anesthesiology*. 2010;113(4):968–976

135. Huupponen E, Maksimow A, Lapinlampi P, et al. Electroencephalogram spindle activity during dexmedetomidine sedation and physiological sleep. *Acta Anaesthesiol Scand*. 2008;52(2):289–294.

136. Nelson LE, Lu J, Guo T, Saper CB, Franks NP, Maze M. The alpha2-adrenoceptor agonist dexmedetomidine converges on an endogenous sleep-promoting pathway to exert its sedative effects. *Anesthesiology*. 2003;98(2):428–436.

137. Riker RR, Shehabi Y, Bokesch PM, et al. Dexmedetomidine vs midazolam for sedation of critically ill patients: a randomized trial. *JAMA*. 2009;301(5):489–499.

138. Alexopoulou C, Kondili E, Diamantaki E, et al. Effects of dexmedetomidine on sleep quality in critically ill patients: a pilot study *Anesthesiology*. 2014;121(4):801–807.

7

Situation Awareness

CHRISTIAN M. SCHULZ

SITUATION AWARENESS IN ANESTHESIA

History of Situation Awareness

Military pilots who had limited or no ability to use radar to detect enemy aircraft were among the first who systematically described the importance of adequate situation awareness (SA). These fighter pilots had to intensively observe their surroundings to detect the presence of an enemy aircraft, and then rapidly make an accurate assessment of its position, heading, speed, altitude, and, most important, its intention. Skillful SA enabled them to anticipate the enemies' next actions and to take effective countermeasures and thus, SA ability was the "ace" factor.[1]

Human factors scientists adopted the term *situation awareness* in the late 1980s. They then began to establish a systematic framework that described the process of developing SA and its role for adequate decision-making by individuals or teams in dynamic environments.[2] Additionally, extra- and intra-individual factors were identified that either enhance or hinder the process of developing correct and complete SA. The first empirical studies were published in the domains of aviation and military; later studies were conducted in other dynamic work environments such as nuclear power plants, oil platforms, and healthcare.

SITUATION AWARENESS IN ANESTHESIA: THE FRAMEWORK

In 1995, Gaba introduced the term SA into the field of anesthesia.[3] Later, Fletcher and colleagues embedded SA in the Anaesthetist's Non-Technical Skills (ANTS) framework; since then, it has been considered to be a core principle in crisis resource management (CRM) training.[4,5] Many simulation-based CRM curricula include some focus on behaviors possibly associated with enhanced SA. The cognitive processes involved in the development of SA, however, have been neglected to a certain extent in this approach.

In Endsley's definition, SA is the "the *perception* of elements in the environment within a volume of time and space, the *comprehension* of their meaning, and the *projection* of their status in the near future."[2] Accordingly, SA is subdivided into three hierarchical levels. Perfect SA on the *perception* level is present when someone has completely and correctly perceived the information that is provided in the environment (SA Level I, *perception*). This basic information is then processed and integrated into the working memory in order to arrive at a comprehension of the situation (SA Level II, *comprehension*). A correct understanding of a situation at its present state is a prerequisite for foreseeing and anticipating possible future development of the situation (SA level III, *projection*). Interestingly, Endsley and Gaba published their articles in the same issue of *Human Factors*.[2,3]

In anesthesia, SA represents the degree to which an anesthetist perceives the information in her or his environment, comprehends the patient's situation, and projects the patient's situation into the future.[6] As such, SA can serve as a quantitative measure for specific situations. Anesthetists differ in their abilities to develop adequate SA quickly, and this largely depends on the level of expertise in different categories. Some types of expertise can be learned through training, whereas other types are acquired through work experience. This chapter illustrates the role of SA in anesthesia, and describes factors that have the potential for either enhancing or hindering the development of adequate SA.

The SA Levels: Perception, Comprehension, and Projection

Things can happen quickly in the dynamic environment of an operating theater, and multiple sources of data provide information about the patient's state. A large part of the information is generated by equipment such as patient monitors and anesthesia machines. These variables mostly are on so-called *single-sensor-single-indicators* (SSSI). They consist of a sensor and provide the results of the assessment as numerical and/or graphical values.[7] Other variables are integrated from SSSI data (e.g., parameters describing the compliance or the resistance of the patient's lung). Acoustic signals warn the anesthesiologist when the values are out of predefined limits, if such limits and signals are set. Additional information can be gleaned from the patient through his or her appearance (e.g., cyanosis) and by spoken communication if the patient is conscious. Information about the progress of surgery and complications is acquired when the anesthetist observes the surgical field and seeks information from surgeons. The level of *perception* (SA level I) describes the degree to which this set of information enters the anesthesiologist's working memory for further processing.

At the next level of SA, *comprehension* (SA level II), the perceived information is integrated into working memory in order to understand the patient's state. For example, during induction, the anesthesiologist ventilates by mask and may observe the chest excursions and whether there is end-tidal CO_2 on the monitor. At the same time, haptic information from hands on the ventilation bag and acoustic information from the pulse oximeter may be perceived. This acoustic, visual, and haptic information, if integrated consciously and unconsciously with long-term memory content such as automaticity, medical knowledge, and mental models, allows the anesthesiologist to *comprehend* whether mask ventilation is sufficient or not. Another example is a patient

presenting with hypotension and tachycardia. The anesthesiologist may process this information with a mental model about circulatory shock (which leads to 5 or 6 differential diagnoses). This, in turn, can prompt the search for additional information, and the anesthesiologist will actively look for specific symptoms of the different forms of shock. After integration of this additional information, he or she will *comprehend* the patient's state and come to a diagnosis. The extent to which the anesthesiologist comprehends the patient's situation (SA level II) determines his or her capability to adequately react to a specific diagnosis or problem.

SA on the level of *projection* (SA level III) is the most sophisticated and encompasses the anesthesiologist's estimation of the future development of the patient's state. It is a key factor in the management of rapidly changing, critically ill patients. A good example is the anesthetic care of a bleeding patient who requires transfusion of red blood cell concentrates, fresh frozen plasma, and coagulation factors. In this situation, time is required for diagnostics (including for point-of-care techniques), for ordering, preparing, and receiving appropriate blood products from the blood bank, and for task performance (e.g., establishing sufficient vascular access to permit massive transfusion, and actual administration of blood products). Expert anesthesiologists are aware of these unavoidable time factors and consider the risk for an ongoing hemorrhage early. This knowledge is integrated with current information about the situation on the levels of *perception* and *comprehension* in order to determine what will happen in the next minutes (*projection*). Thus, accurate SA on the level of *projection* is a prerequisite for the proactive management of personnel and material resources.

SA is built in a hierarchical order and entails a process of continuous re-evaluation. Expectation of future events and goals influences the search for information and thus the level of *perception* (top-down goal-directed processing). Alternatively, the anesthesiologist may scan all of the information available at regular intervals and re-evaluate a current diagnosis in order to avoid fixation errors (bottom-up data-driven processing). Regular switching between top-down processing and bottom-up processing is considered to be an important skill for the development of adequate SA. Accuracy of SA on the more basic levels is a prerequisite for the more advanced levels. If an important piece of information is not perceived, is perceived incorrectly, or is forgotten, it is impossible to accurately *comprehend* the situation, which then makes it impossible to *project* the situation into the future.

Long-Term Memory Content Needed for Developing SA

After perception, basic information has to be integrated, and several cognitive mechanisms enable correct, complete, and quick development of SA. These processes require long-term memory content, such as mental models, similar (prototypical) situations that have been experienced earlier, automaticity, and medical knowledge, including guidelines and algorithms.

Mental Models

A *mental model* is structured knowledge in the long-term memory that develops from experience and training over time.[8] Mental models allow for the explanation of elements in the environment and *projections* of their state in the future. They serve as cognitive short-cuts for information processing, and are activated by informational cues that are representative of the model. Mental models therefore significantly accelerate the process of gaining SA on the higher levels. They do not, however, contain information about a specific situation and are not an internal representation of the situation in the working memory. A simplistic example is a mental model in aviation that describes the relationship between speed and lift and serves for integration of basic data about aircraft speed and altitude. In anesthesia, important mental models might include an understanding of pathophysiology and pharmacology.[6]

Well-developed mental models are thus a prerequisite for rapid, accurate information processing and are embedded in the decision-making process. They are less developed or even absent in novices, and thus the cognitive workload of information processing is dramatically increased. This may overwhelm the capacity for processing the basic information, resulting in a lack of SA and, as a logical consequence, in wrong or late or no decisions.

Prototypical Situations

Prototypical situations are episodes that have been previously experienced and are similar to a current situation. The coinciding patterns between a current and a past situation allow developing SA more quickly and with less effort, because much of the information in the prior episode can be recalled. Anesthesiologists with good pattern-matching abilities and a sufficient number of prototypical situations need less cognitive resources for adequate SA. Simulation training probably helps to generate prototypical situations, but whether this effect supports more rapid development of SA in real situations remains uncertain.

Automaticity

Automaticity is another mechanism that allows information to be processed without occupying much capacity in the working memory. Automaticity allows a physical or cognitive task to be performed almost unconsciously, increasing the cognitive resources available for other tasks. When an experienced driver must slow down while driving a car, for example, he or she typically applies the brakes without thinking about which pedal to use. Consider the task of inserting a central line, for example. An anesthesia novice attempting this for the first time will have his or her mind occupied to a high degree with managing eye-hand coordination and effortful attention to each step in the procedure. In contrast, more experienced anesthesiologists will accomplish the task in a more automated manner, which frees the more experienced professional's mind to process additional information about the patient and environment, and thus maintain better SA. Stefanidis et al. demonstrated this effect in a simulated laparoscopy setting[9] and provided evidence that automaticity training is superior to proficiency training.[10]

Medical Knowledge

If mental models, automaticity, and prototypical situations are not well developed or do not cover a given set of information, medical knowledge must be actively recalled in order to process basic data. This process is slower and requires a greater cognitive workload.

Individual Factors

Differences between novices and experts have been used to identify individual factors that hinder or foster the ability to develop SA accurately and quickly.[11,12] There is some evidence (both direct, and indirect via distribution of visual attention) of differences in SA between anesthesia professionals with different levels of experience.[13] Differences in SA can also change within a given professional over time and are influenced, for example, by fatigue,[14] motivation, and perhaps caffeine.[15,16]

Errors on the level of *comprehension* are frequently related to lack of experience, which reflects less automaticity, less developed mental models, and a lower number of prototypical situations.[17] There are also individual differences in the speed of processing and in the capacity of the working memory.

The ability to switch between bottom-up and top-down processing enables more effective development of SA. Top-down processing is goal-driven: once a diagnosis has been made during a critical event, attention focuses on information relevant to the patient's state and therapeutic goals and expectations. During anaphylactic shock, for example, a focused amount of information on hemodynamics and gas exchange is often sufficient to effectively manage the patient. This strategy is successful as long as diagnostic and therapeutic decisions are correct and there are no unexpected problems or new events. To avoid problems from attention narrowing, the expert will switch to bottom-up processing at regular intervals. During this process, the anesthesiologist scans all available data in order to detect changes that might influence the diagnosis, expectancies, or the therapy goal.

Finally, there are differences in anesthesia-specific medical knowledge that must be applied if the mental models are not accurate for a given set of information to be processed.

Team Situation Awareness

Beyond the cognitive processes in individuals, the SA construct also considers processes in teams. Salas defined a team as "a distinguishable set of two or more people who interact dynamically, independently, and adaptively toward a common and valued goal/objective/mission, who have each been assigned specific roles or functions to perform and who have a limited life-span of membership."[18] The SA of individual members overlaps to a certain degree in effective teams. Such an overlap occurs horizontally (e.g., between day and night shift or between physicians in an interdisciplinary team) and also vertically between personnel with different responsibilities.

In order to reach a common treatment goal, two or more healthcare professionals must share the elements of SA that are necessary to make decisions for the completion of their individual tasks. A surgeon who updates the anesthesiologist about the course of surgery enables the anesthesiologist to more accurately project into the future. Similarly, information from the anesthesiologist can influence the surgeon's decisions and actions. However, as the environment becomes more demanding and dynamic, shared information that is not relevant for others causes an increase in cognitive workload without any benefit. Shared SA is therefore defined as "the degree to which team members have the same SA on shared SA requirements" or "the degree to which every team member possesses the SA required for his or her responsibilities."[2]

As illustrated in detail later (see section "Implications"), several mechanisms can be used for sharing SA, including implicit and explicit communication, the use of shared mental models, and shared sources of information (e.g., monitors, surgical field).

Workload

Maintaining SA occupies processing capacities in the working memory. Situations that change rapidly require more working memory capacity to maintain SA. Cognitive workload is also increased in novel or rare situations for which automaticity and mental models are lacking. The increase in cognitive workload compromises SA, which develops more slowly and may remain incomplete, inaccurate or even false. In this way, cognitive overload severely increases the risk for errors, near misses, and patient harm.

Summary

The process of gaining SA is hierarchical and includes the levels of *perception, comprehension*, and *projection*. Current data must be integrated with mental models, automaticity, prototypical situations, and medical knowledge in order to build SA on the more advanced levels of *comprehension* and *projection*. Accurate SA also requires a continuous re-evaluation of information, ideally switching between bottom-up and top-down goal-driven processing. Bottom-up processing prevents relevant information from being missed, while top-down, goal-driven processing directs attention mainly to key sources of information that apply to a given therapeutic goal or problem. Decision-making, performance, and thus patient safety are based on accurate SA. An updated framework has recently been suggested to integrate the anesthetists' non-technical skills and situation awareness (Figure 7.1).[6]

METHODOLOGICAL APPROACHES FOR THE ANALYSIS OF SITUATION AWARENESS

Several tools have the potential to provide qualitative and quantitative assessment of SA in anesthesia. Such assessments may identify promising targets for training and structural interventions to improve SA.

Goal-Directed Task Analysis

The goal-directed task analysis (GDTA) focuses on dynamic information requirements rather than static information. GDTA protocols seek to determine what a professional would *ideally like to know* in order to meet each therapeutic goal, even if that information is not currently available. This approach provides a better understanding of what changes are needed to support SA, regardless of the ways information is acquired in the current system. GDTA can also identify factors that may enhance or impair the development of SA.[19]

The first step of GDTA is to conduct unstructured interviews that focus on the goals

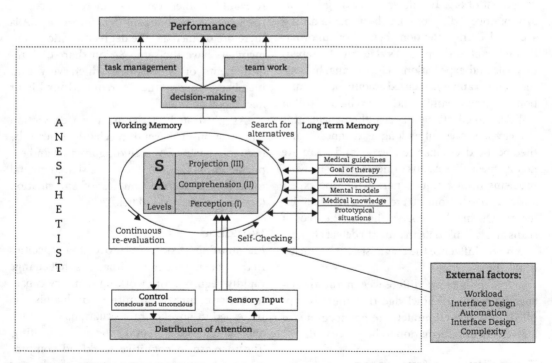

FIGURE 7.1: SA is the indispensable precursor of effective decision-making, task management, and teamwork.

Reprinted with permission from Schulz CM, et al. Situation awareness in anesthesia: concept and research. *Anesthesiology.* 2013;118(3):729–742.

that must be accomplished, the decisions that must be made in order to achieve therapeutic goals, and the information that is required to make appropriate decisions. The interviewer should be familiar with the domain of interest but, at the same time, must be careful to not seek information that only confirms findings from previous interviews. To avoid group thinking, each expert is interviewed individually.

In the next step, interview notes are categorized and organized into a workable preliminary goal structure that accurately represents information requirements. The results can be combined with knowledge from written material such as Critical Incident Reporting Systems (CIRS) to create the initial GDTA. This preliminary goal structure will be used during the introduction to future interviews by asking whether all relevant goals are captured in the preliminary hierarchy. During subsequent interviews, the final GDTA is developed and formatted in a hierarchical fashion to provide an easy trace from goals down to SA requirements (Figure 7.2).

Lastly, the final version of the GDTA is validated with a larger group of experts in order to ensure that the GDTA is complete and accurate. For this purpose, copies of the final GDTA are distributed among the experts with instructions on how to interpret it. The experts are asked to identify missing information or errors, which are then used to correct the GDTA.

GDTA has the potential to systematically identify elements (including new variables) that can enhance individual or team SA. For anesthesiologists, this could go beyond variables in the SSSI design and allow the development of information displays that directly provide higher levels of SA.

Situation Analysis Error Analysis

Adequate SA is the prerequisite for correct decisions and thus performance and patient safety. Decisions based on inaccurate or incomplete SA at any level will be conversely suboptimal or wrong (unless someone is very lucky). SA error analysis systematically identifies sources of errors and their contributing causes, allowing individuals to avoid frequent

SA pitfalls. Error analysis may also be helpful in the design of goal-directed training and structural interventions.

SA Error Taxonomy

Errors on the level of *perception* occur if relevant information is missing or incorrect, or is not perceived due to ineffective distribution of attention or limitations of the working memory. Errors on the levels of *comprehension* arise if correctly perceived information is inadequately processed or if an individual is over-reliant on default values (i.e., the wrong mental model is applied, or medical knowledge is not applied). A *projection* error occurs when a situation is well understood but the future course of actions is estimated incorrectly. Material and human resources may be either overused or not recruited, with either increased costs or potentially deleterious consequences for the patient. For example, an anesthesiologist sees a postpartum hemorrhage (*perception*) and recognizes uterine atony as the most probable cause (*comprehension*) but fails to predict massive hemorrhage and therefore does not mobilize sufficient resources to address all management tasks in a timely way (*projection*). For a more comprehensive understanding, Endsley provides a taxonomy that includes subtypes of errors for each level (Table 7.1).

Analysis of Human Error in Anesthesia: The Incidence of SA Errors

SA errors can have a significant impact on decision-making, decreasing performance and patient safety, and may ultimately lead to patient harm.[17,20]

In an analysis of 2000 critical incidents in the early 1990s, elements of human error were noted in about 80% of cases.[21] Many of these errors fit within the SA framework: "inattention" (12%), "communication problems" (9%), and "monitor problems" (6%) accounted for errors on the level of *perception*. "Inexperience" (11%) and "misjudgment" (16%) are related to lack of mental models, and are therefore errors of *comprehension* and *projection*. Others, such as "haste" (12%), "inadequate preoperative assessment" (7%), and "inadequate preoperative preparation" (4%), intuitively influence or are

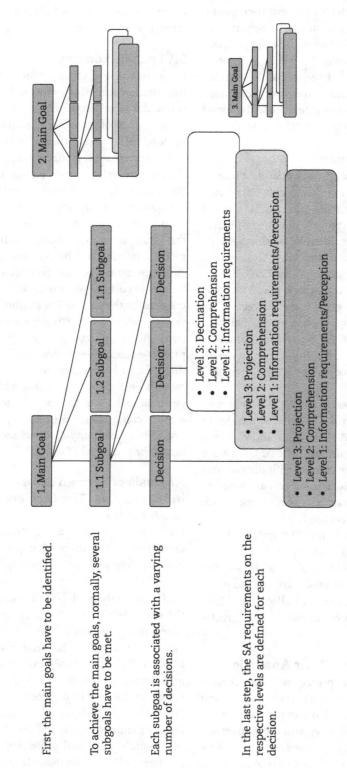

FIGURE 7.2: GDTA is structured hierarchically. For each main goal, associated subgoals, decisions, and SA requirements are identified.

TABLE 7.1. ENDSLEY'S SA ERROR TAXONOMY

SA Level I	Fail to perceive or misperception of information
1.1	Data were not available.
1.2	Data were hard to discriminate or detect (e.g., visual barrier).
1.3	Failure to monitor or observe data
1.4	Misperception of data
1.5	Memory loss

SA Level II	Improper integration or comprehension of information
2.1	Lack or incomplete mental model
2.2	Use of incorrect mental model
2.3	Over-reliance on default values
2.4	Other

SA Level III	Incorrect projections of future trends
3.1	Lack or incomplete mental model
3.2	Overprojection of current trends
3.3	Other

Adapted from Endsley MR, Towards a theory of situation awareness in dynamic systems. *Hum Factors.* 1995;37:32–64; and Endsley MR, A taxonomy of situation awareness errors, in Fuller R, Johnston N, McDonald, eds. *Human Factors in Aviation Operations.* Aldershot, UK: Ashgate; 1995:287–292.

influenced by someone's SA. Taken together, this is consistent with SA errors in 77% of cases, which is similar to findings in aviation.[22]

Two recent studies investigated post hoc anesthesia-related cases from the Closed Claims Project[20] and from the German Critical Incident Reporting System.[17] The first study examined a random sample of 100 anesthesia malpractice claims for death or severe brain damage. Two independent raters found SA errors in 78 claims (78%). Interestingly, SA error claims were more frequently associated with payments on behalf of the anesthesiologist (83%) than other claims (45%, $p < 0.001$).[20] This indirectly reflects that the legal system imposes a responsibility for maintaining SA on the anesthesiologist.

The second study analyzed 200 consecutive cases from the German Critical Incident Reporting System, which is run by the German Society of Anesthesiology and Intensive Care Medicine (DGAI), the Alliance of German Anaesthesiologists (BDA), and the Agency for Quality in Medicine (ÄZQ). The incidence of SA errors was as high as 81.5%, with 38.0% attributable to *perception* (predominantly associated with monitor problems and insufficient communication), and 31.5% attributable to *comprehension* (predominantly lack of experience). Errors on the level of *projection* were much less frequent (12.0%). This study was limited by low inter-rater reliability, probably due to low data quality in self-reported near misses.[17]

Another study explored the incidence of perceptual errors in a setting where participants of varying experience observed a resuscitation video. The authors showed that perceptual errors declined with increasing experience but did not disappear.[23] In summary, these studies provide evidence that SA errors are almost obligatorily involved in the genesis of critical incidents and underline the central role of SA for decision-making. Box 7.1 presents a case from a critical incident reporting system that illustrates how an anesthetist unexpectedly ran into intubation difficulties.

Accurate basic information resulting from the preoperative workup was present (SA level I). However, an accurately integrated mental model of the basic data (ankylosing spondylitis,

---

BOX 7.1   AN EXAMPLE OF A QUALITATIVE ANALYSIS OF SA ERRORS IN A CRITICAL INCIDENT

A patient was scheduled for lung surgery and therefore the use of a double-lumen tube was planned. During premedication visit, the anesthesiologist noticed a big tongue, a Mallampati III score, Morbus Bechterew [ankylosing spondylitis], and reduced mobility of the cervical spine. After bag mask ventilation without any difficulties, the anesthetist intended to conventionally insert a double-lumen tube by direct laryngoscopy. He only saw the top of the epiglottis, indicating Cormack III–IV. The anesthetist was not able to place the tube. Further intentions with a McCoy blade and a long bougie also failed. Evidently, the patient was ventilated by mask intermittently. Finally, the patient's trachea was intubated bronchoscopically with an oral single-lumen tube, which was difficult. In the following a long bougie was used to exchange the single-lumen tube with the double-lumen tube required for surgery. Before, the double-lumen tube was softened using warm water. Otherwise the tube would not have passed the posterior wall of the larynx. After surgery, the patient was extubated without any problems. He did not suffer from any damage.

---

big tongue, Mallampati III, reduced mobility of cervical spine) was absent, demonstrated by the fact that the managing anesthesiologist was obviously surprised by the airway problems after induction of anesthesia. Therefore, the SA error occurred on the level of *comprehension* (SA level II). In the further course of action, the double-lumen tube was softened using warm water and introduced using a long bougie. Warming the tube indicates (1) that the anesthetists knows that the tube becomes softer when it is warm, and (2) that he expects ongoing technical difficulties. However, an airway exchange catheter allowing for oxygenation was not used, and an ongoing traumatization of the airway was risked, both indicating a lack on the level of *projection* (SA level III). Luckily, no further adverse events occurred.

Qualitative analysis is very helpful for the evaluation of individual cases. However, systematic approaches that result in changes at the organizational level are yet to be deployed.

Techniques for the Assessment of SA

A direct, objective measure such as the Situation Awareness Global Assessment Technique (SAGAT) is considered to be the gold standard of SA assessment.[24] SAGAT consists of SA queries that are tailored to different time points in a specific situation and that evaluate each level of SA. This technique is limited to simulator settings because the queries and situation must be pre-scripted, and interruptions are required for completing the queries. Only a handful of studies have applied this technique to healthcare professionals.[25–27]

Post hoc self-ratings, including the Situation Awareness Rating Technique (SART), can be used for the assessment of SA in actual patient care settings. These surveys lack content validity as someone's awareness of *a just experienced* situation is different from SA at different times *during* the evolving event, especially if the situation was resolved under high workload conditions. Online probes of SA in real settings can overcome this disadvantage but are considered to be intrusive.[28]

Most studies investigating the effects of training in anesthesia rely on Fletcher's ANTS scale. Videotapes from simulated incidents or real settings are reviewed to assess behaviors that are believed to reflect the non-technical skills of decision-making, task management, teamwork, and SA. The SA category includes the elements "Gathering Information," "Recognizing and Understanding," and "Anticipating," reflecting the three levels of *perception, comprehension*, and *projection*. For each element, specific behavioral markers are recognized and rated by trained observers. It remains unclear to what degree the presence or absence of these behaviors is related to direct SA measures. Of note, SA is considered to be a skill *besides*—but not *a precursor of*—effective teamwork, team management, and decision-making. This is an important issue to be considered, as future investigations may find a predictive value of SA behavioral markers for the other categories of teamwork, team management, and decision-making. Nevertheless, there is much evidence about the validity and the reliability of the ANTS scale in different settings in anesthesia, and it is the most widespread scale for the assessment of non-technical skills including SA.

Accurate SA is presumed to be a prerequisite for decision-making; thus performance is considered to be an indirect indicator of SA.[25,29] Checklists are common tools for the assessment of performance. They build cumulative scores after the quantification of therapeutic and diagnostic key tasks. Other evaluations time the intervals between the onset, detection, and solution of a problem. Highly realistic simulation scenarios provide standardized test conditions; in the future, simulator outcome itself can provide a valuable marker for performance.[30] These measures, however, only rarely provide insights into the concrete processes that are involved in achieving SA.

IMPLICATIONS

Individual Strategies to Gain and Maintain SA

Even expert anesthesiologists will have significant individual differences in their abilities to maintain SA in a complex and dynamic situation. More difficulties arise when healthcare professionals develop tunnel vision under excessive workload, because this prevents them from reaching the meta-level that allows for an active application of SA strategies. Despite these limitations, it is possible to teach strategies to gain and maintain SA.

A theoretical understanding about how SA emerges from perceptual input and long-term memory content, teammates' SA needs, and common SA pitfalls is an important precondition. This enhances the ability to learn practical techniques and allows a critical review of specific situations, which in turn augments SA behavior.

As has been discussed in the section on individual factors, the ability to switch between top-down goal-directed and bottom-up data-driven processing of information is an important strategy. Such switching toggles between narrowly focused attention on therapeutic goals (on the level of *prediction*) and also minimizes the risk of missing important information on the level of *perception*, or readjustment from an incorrect diagnosis (i.e., fixation/anchoring errors) on the level of *comprehension*. Continual switching between these two modes is considered to be a key feature of SA experts, and can be taught via the "step-back" or "10-seconds-for-10-minutes" techniques. The "step-back" represents a deliberate toggle to the bottom-up approach, to ensure a comprehensive overview of the situation. The "10-seconds-for-10-minutes" metaphorically instructs teams to resist impulsive action, and instead take 10 seconds for decision-making and for planning the next 10 minutes on the basis of what is perceived, comprehended, and predicted. Both techniques require effective self-management in order for clinicians to exclusively reserve time for an active update of both individual and team. Although errors are recognized only in hindsight, these techniques may shorten the interval between error and recognition, and therefore represent a promising antidote to fixation.

Because mental models and prototypical situations enhance SA development, anesthesiologists should aim to refine their mental models and acquire more of them. Prototypical situations are mainly collected during years of work experience, but can be augmented via deliberate practice in simulation training. This is especially true of rare situations that are unlikely to be sufficiently encountered in clinical practice.

Personal communication strategies should aim to increase SA for individuals and teams, ideally without unnecessary increases in workload. This can be achieved through the transfer of basic data on the level of *perception*, but also on the higher level of *comprehension*, and also should include the level of *projection*. As the number of shared mental models within the team and knowledge about the specific SA required for tasks of other team members increases, communication becomes goal-directed and requires less effort. Cross-checking SA further ensures high levels of team SA and avoidance of errors.

Additional strategies include the active management of SA barriers such as fatigue and excessive workload. Although fatigue can often be mitigated through individual effort in routine cases, maintaining SA and decision-making are more difficult in unusual cases or unexpected problems in which innovative thinking is required.[14] This should be borne in mind when considering the effect of sleep deprivation on healthcare professionals, especially if studies focus on routine cases. That is fatigue may indeed impair an anesthesiologist's ability to respond to complex problems when caring for critically ill patients in the middle of the night.

High workload events characterized by dynamic situations and time-related stress can overwhelm the processing capacity needed for accurate SA. This can be managed by delegating manual or cognitive tasks to other team members. This might include a request for more human resources, (e.g., to perform simple manual tasks such as chest compressions) or for cognitive support, (i.e., a more experienced anesthesiologist or a cognitive aid). If possible, the leader should not participate in "hands-on" tasks; this has been shown to improve team performance.[31] Each team member should monitor for cognitive overload and implement countermeasures, such as suggesting different allocation of tasks or recruitment of additional resources.

Design of Training

There is considerable evidence that CRM training improves performance,[32] and SA is a component of most CRM curricula.

The Role of Team Mental Models and Team Monitoring

Considerable research has been done to explore the impact of a shared mental model on team performance.[33–37] For interdisciplinary teams (nurses and physicians, anesthesiologists and surgeons), mental models refer to a common understanding about tasks, technologies, responses to routine as well as rare events, and roles and responsibilities of individual team members. Burtscher et al. showed that similar and accurate team mental models correlated with good team performance during simulated anesthesia induction.[36] *Similarity* has been defined as the degree to which the concepts of two individuals match each other; in contrast, *accuracy* has been defined as the extent to which a team mental model (i.e., the shared concepts among all team members) is consistent with a "gold standard" mental model. Thus, team mental models include the anticipation of other team members' SA needs, allowing each team member to effectively help the others by adjusting his or her own behavior in order to support others during their tasks.[38,39] For example, while a physician is intubating and cannot view the patient monitor, a nurse can report aloud any relevant changes in vital signs. This so-called *mutual performance monitoring* is an important non-technical skill and is a component of good team SA.[40]

Team mental models can be taught and measured.[41,42] Research from other domains suggests that cross training with positional rotations can help strengthen team mental models, and improve team performance by allowing for more implicit coordination (which requires less cognitive processing) rather than explicit communication.[41,43,44–46] The presence of shared mental models enhances contingency planning and group prioritazation on the level of *comprehension* without further need for inter-individual calibration. During a crisis, however, loss of information is minimized by the CRM principle of *explicit* rule-based communication.[42]

Team self-correction can also be used to foster shared mental models. After having worked through a surgical procedure or resuscitation, team members should discuss the things that went well, what could be improved, and how to improve it.[47] This technique should be used in a context of non-blaming culture, facilitated by experienced debriefers.

SA-Oriented Training

A clinician's SA abilities will likely improve over the course of a career without specific SA training. However, specific SA training programs have been successfully implemented in other domains and hold promise for healthcare.[48] Classroom and computer training and simulation environments can be easily adapted to anesthesia.[6] Endsley described a number of skills that improve through SA training and that are relevant to anesthesiology (Table 7.2).[48]

A goal-directed task analysis (GDTA) should be conducted to identify all the factors that may enhance or impair the development of accurate SA before an ideal domain-specific SA training program can be designed.[19] So far, no such GDTA or training design has been done. Hence, it is unknown whether specific SA training for anesthesia personnel would yield more benefit than existing approaches.

In one study of simulation-based training versus classroom-based training or no training, SA was higher in the simulation-trained group than in the classroom or control group. However, no impact on clinical performance was found in any group.[26] The simulation-based training consisted of several severe sepsis cases, and debriefing focused on diagnosis and treatment of sepsis but not on non-technical skills. In other words, although not intended to train SA abilities, this training appears to have boosted the development of shared mental models about sepsis and, moreover, to have created a number of prototypical situations for the participants. Both mental models and prototypical situations significantly facilitate the development of SA, and hence it is not surprising that there was a positive effect on SAGAT scores. In other words, even if simulation-based training is concentrated on diagnosis and treatment instead of non-technical skills, SA can improve.

Patient Handover

When patients are transferred from from one unit to another (including OR, PACU, and ward units), or teams transition from one shift to another, a primary goal of handover communication is to transfer SA across teams. In a recent study about handover communication strategies, the *amount* or *completeness* of information transferred did not contribute to handover quality. Instead, the transferring physician's overall assessment of the patient's state was significantly correlated with

TABLE 7.2. SKILLS THAT IMPROVE AFTER SA TRAINING

Skill	Description
Task management	Ability to deal with the challenges of interruptions, task-related distractions, non-task-related distractions, and overall workload, which poses a significant threat to SA.
Development of *comprehension*	Helping people to properly interpret information to assess the patient's state, importance or severity of tasks and events, including levels of risk, consequences of unexpected events on plans, timing, and other factors that are relevant in anesthesia.
Projection and contingency planning	Anesthesiologists who are good at SA spend much of their time projecting ahead to possible futures and creating contingency plans.
Information seeking and self-checking activities	Individuals with good SA actively seek out the relevant information and are good at checking the validity of their own situation assessments, either with more information or with others.
Basic and higher order cognitive skills	Fundamental psychomotor and communications skills are often deficient in novices and need to be boosted to improve SA, along with meta-cognitive skills such as attention sharing across multiple tasks or information sets.
Training of team SA skills	Includes information sharing both within and across teams, development of shared mental models across teams, and effective communication skills.

Modified from Endsley MR, Robertson MM, Training for situation awareness in individuals and teams, in Endsley MR, Garland DJ, eds. *Situation Awareness Analysis and Measurement*. Mahwah, NJ: Lawrence Erlbaum Associates: 2000.

handover quality.[49] Transfer of SA on the higher levels of *comprehension* and *projection* is essential. This can limit the overall quantity of information to be transferred (and to be processed during handover) and enables the new team to start care in the top-down, goal-driven processing mode that requires less cognitive workload. Moreover, the amount of data that an individual can hold in working memory is limited. From this view, reducing the transfer of basic data to the minimum necessary is advisable during handover.[50]

Design of Information Displays

Patient monitors and ventilator machines are primary sources of data in anesthesia and in intensive care medicine. As stated earlier, most of these parameters are based on SSSI design (i.e., presented as numerical values, in some cases supplemented with graphical curves). As more and more SSSIs have been created over time, the amount of information that must be processed has dramatically increased. Monitoring these variables is a routine but time- and cognition-consuming task, especially during critical events and for novices.[13] Therefore, whether this increase in data corresponds to an increase in SA has been questioned.[7]

In recent years, researchers have intended to improve the presentation of physiologic variables by providing graphical *integration* of data—presenting information on the level of *comprehension*. Others have evaluated novel displays, including head-mounted displays or multisensory outputs such as auditory displays and vibrotactile belts. So far, the results are inconclusive.[27,51-54] This may be because participants were well habituated in using the established control systems, but received only limited training for the newly developed study displays. The resulting bias is hard to eliminate.[7]

Similarly, digital electronic health records (EHR) aim to provide complete and up-to-date information about the patient's history and treatment. These systems ensure that, apart from actual data about vital parameters, all the relevant information can be accessed by healthcare professionals in a single display and in every location in the hospital. Although many of these systems are commercially available, difficulties can arise when historically different documentation systems from different disciplines have to be integrated into one electronic platform. The system should not only provide results from laboratory investigations and body imaging, but also include data about the very recent therapy. An important point of concern is the way in which information is presented in EHR, ranging from a simple chronological data collection to integrated displays that provide information on the levels of *comprehension* and *projection* adapted to the SA needs of the user's task profile. Future efforts should consider the implementation of decision aids and intelligent alarms that indicate deviation from actual guidelines. Recently, an increase in SA and a reduction of task completion time has been successfully demonstrated in experienced ICU nurses that used a novel display integrating information from patient monitor, respirator, infusion pumps, electronic medical record, fluid balance, adverse effects, and medication compatibility.[55]

Organizational Aspects

Results from critical incident and closed claims analysis suggest promising approaches to support the development of accurate SA in individuals and teams. A significant number of *perception* problems arose from inadequate monitoring. This may occur when monitoring is not available (due to unavailability, malfunction, battery problems) or if appropriate monitoring is not used because it is inconvenient or the anesthesiologist is missing a mental model with respect to potential problems (e.g., hypoxia on transport from OR to PACU). In addition to providing sufficient patient monitors for transport and ensuring that battery capacity is sufficient, the implementation of hospital-specific rules and standardized operating procedures for when and how to monitor patients beyond established guidelines can limit the risk of missing information.

Under certain circumstances, there are physical barriers between the anesthesiologist and important sources of information. For example, sterile drapes may obstruct the view onto the surgical field, or the patient monitor may be located behind the anesthesiologist during interventional procedures. Other examples include magnetic resonance imaging suites, where monitors are difficult to view and are generally limited due to interference. In many locations, the anesthesiologist monitors the patient from a control room that may be far from the patient. If the monitor signals are transferred to the observer room, these are high-risk environments because potentially silent information, including circuit disconnections or alterations of blood pressure that are not adequately represented with noninvasive monitoring, may be missed, and it may be difficult to diagnose patient discomfort.

Another important tool is the implementation of checklists. In 2009, Gawande's workgroup demonstrated a decrease in mortality and complications across all participating hospitals in both industrialized and developing countries.[56] The checklist did not depend on individual preferences: anesthesiologists and surgeons were required to complete a "surgical safety checklist" at three specific time points. Most items of the checklist are attributable to the level of *perception*, but some establish SA on the higher levels: "Surgeon reviews critical and unexpected steps, operative duration, and anticipated blood loss"; or "The surgeon, nurse, and anesthesia professional review aloud the key concerns for the recovery and care of the patient." The study concluded that mandatory application of checklists is an important tool to establish SA in teams and that checklists should consider SA on the *comprehension* and *projection* level. The same workgroup also showed a reduction of missed steps from 23% to 6% across several types of simulation scenarios if checklists were made available. This indicates that checklists may at least in part compensate for missing mental models, automaticity, guidelines, and prototypical situations when rare and unexpected events occur. However, the extent of simulation bias is unclear, and this concept has not yet been demonstrated to be beneficial for patient outcome. An anesthesia crisis manual designed as a cognitive aid has recently been published by David Borshoff with support of both the European and American Societies of Anesthesiology (for details, see www.theacm.com.au).[57]

In routine cases, the assignment of an anesthesiologist to a given procedure and patient is based on established curricula during residency, availability according to schedule service, and, sometimes, expertise. Hospitals must also provide a functional backup system to ensure that manual and cognitive assistance is available for complex, non-routine cases. In SA terms, to add SA abilities and to reduce individual workload, additional personnel should be available for unusual and unexpected events. The implementation of regular training programs is also essential. Although the benefits of this approach are obvious, it can be challenging in the setting of high production pressure.

From an institutional or systems perspective, it is not sufficient to provide well-functioning monitoring devices and to order the use of patient checklists. Many interventions to enhance SA are the responsibility of the hospital management. Organizational priorities should include recognizing and mitigating the impact of production pressure on SA, providing an effective and safety-oriented service schedule, ensuring SA-oriented communication, implementation of user-centered information systems (e.g., EHR), and enhancing the healthcare professionals' SA skills.

CONCLUSION

SA in anesthesia describes the extent to which clinicians are aware of the patient's situation, including the *perception* of basic data such as vital parameters, the *comprehension* of the patient's state, and a *prediction* of how the situation will develop. Adequate SA is therefore considered to be a prerequisite for accurate decision-making, task management, and teamwork. Good SA permits appropriate responses to specific situations and to manage human and material resources proactively. Team SA is strong when every team member has both similar and accurate concepts about the situation, allowing team members to effectively help the others by adjusting his or her own behavior to support the tasks at hand. The ability to develop SA quickly and accurately increases with experience through the development of mental models and automaticity. Furthermore, SA skills can be fostered with different training approaches, including techniques for effective sharing of SA among team members.

The hospital management should aim to provide an SA-oriented work environment by reducing barriers of SA and by the implementation of techniques and technologies that enhance SA. This includes providing accurate monitoring equipment, the use of patient safety checklists, and service schedules respecting the effects of fatigue, workload, and the presence of expertise. Future approaches include the development of more user-centered designs of information systems.

REFERENCES

1. Spick M. *The Ace Factor: Air Combat and the Role of Situational Awareness*. Annapolis: US Naval Institute Press; 1988.
2. Endsley MR. Towards a theory of situation awareness in dynamic systems. *Hum Factors*. 1995;37:32–64.
3. Gaba DM, Howard SK, Small SD. Situation awareness in anesthesiology. *Hum Factors*. 1995;37:20–31.
4. Fletcher G, et al. Anaesthetists' Non-Technical Skills (ANTS): evaluation of a behavioural marker system. *Br J Anaesth*. 2003;90(5):580–588.
5. Flin R, et al. Anaesthetists' non-technical skills. *Br J Anaesth*. 2010;105(1):38–44.
6. Schulz CM, et al. Situation awareness in anesthesia: concept and research. *Anesthesiology*. 2013; 118(3):729–742.
7. Kiefer H, Hoeft A. Display of information in the operating room. *Curr Opin Anaesthesiol*. 2010;23(6):772–777.
8. Mathieu J, et al. The influence of shared mental models on team process and performance. *J Appl Psychol*. 2000;85(2):273–283.
9. Stefanidis D, et al. Redefining simulator proficiency using automaticity theory. *Am J Surg*. 2007;193(4):502–506.
10. Stefanidis D, et al. Simulator training to automaticity leads to improved skill transfer compared with traditional proficiency-based training: a randomized controlled trial. *Ann Surg*. 2012;255(1):30–37.
11. Endsley MR. Expertise and situation awareness. In: Ericsson KA, et al., eds. *The Cambridge Handbook of Expertise and Expert Performance*. New York: Cambridge Universitiy Press; 2006:633–651.
12. Endsley MR, Bolstad CA. Individual differences in pilot situation awareness. *Int J Aviat Psychol*. 1994;3(4):241–264.
13. Schulz CM, et al. Visual attention of anaesthetists during simulated critical incidents. *Br J Anaesth*. 2011;106(6):807–813.
14. Harrison Y, Horne JA. The impact of sleep deprivation on decision making: a review. *J Exp Psychol Appl*. 2000;6(3):236–249.
15. Johnson-Kozlow M, et al. Coffee consumption and cognitive function among older adults. *Am J Epidemiol*. 2002;156(9):842–850.
16. Hameleers PA, et al. Habitual caffeine consumption and its relation to memory, attention, planning capacity and psychomotor performance across multiple age groups. *Hum Psychopharmacol*. 2000; 15(8):573–581.
17. Schulz CM et al. Situation awareness errors in anesthesia and critical care in 200 cases of a critical incident reporting system. *BMC Anesthesiology* 2016;16(4).
18. Salas E, et al. Toward an understanding of team performance and training. In: Swezey RW, Salas E, eds. *Teams: Their Training and Peformance*. Norwood, NJ: Ablex; 1992:3–29.
19. Endsley MR, Jones DG. *Designing for situation awareness: An Approach to User-Centered Design*. 2nd ed. London: CRC Press; 2011:147–168.
20. Burden A, et al. *Situational Awareness Errors in Malpractice Claims*. ASA Abstract. New Orleans: ASA, 2014.
21. Williamson JA, et al. The Australian Incident Monitoring Study. Human failure: an analysis of 2000 incident reports. *Anaesth Intens Care*. 1993;21(5):678–683.
22. Jones DG, Endsley MR. Sources of situation awareness errors in aviation. *Aviat Space Environ Med*. 1996;67(6):507–512.
23. Greig PR, Higham H, Nobre AC. Failure to perceive clinical events: an under-recognised source of error. *Resuscitation*, 2014;85(7):952–956.
24. Endsley MR. Direct measurement of situation awareness: validity and use of SAGAT. In: Endsley MR, Garland DJ, eds. *Situation Awareness Analysis and Measurement*. Mahwah, NJ: Lawrence Erlbaum Associates; 2000.
25. Hogan MP, et al. Use of human patient simulation and the situation awareness global assessment technique in practical trauma skills assessment. *J Trauma*. 2006;61(5):1047–1052.
26. Hänsel M, et al. Impact of simulator training and crew resource management training on final-year medical students' performance in sepsis resuscitation: a randomised trial. *Minerva Anesthesiol*. 2012;78(8):901–909.
27. Zhang Y, et al. Effects of integrated graphical displays on situation awareness in anaesthesiology. *Cog Tech Work*. 2002;4:82–90.
28. Endsley MR, Garland DJ, eds. *Situation awareness analysis and measurement*. Mahwah, NJ: Lawrence Erlbaum Associates; 2000.
29. Endsley MR. The role of situation awareness in naturalistic decision making. In: Zsambok CE, Klein G, eds. *Naturalistic Decision Making*. Mahwah, NJ: Lawrence Erlbaum Associates; 1997:269–283.

30. Schulz CM, et al. High-fidelity human patient simulators compared with human actors in an unannounced mass-casualty exercise. *Prehosp Disaster Med.* 2014;29(2):176–182.

31. Cooper S, Wakelam A. Leadership of resuscitation teams: "Lighthouse Leadership." *Resuscitation.* 1999;42(1):27–45.

32. Boet S, et al. Transfer of learning and patient outcome in simulated crisis resource management: a systematic review. *Can J Anaesth.* 2014; 61(6):571–582.

33. Cannon-Bowers JA, Salas E, Converse SA. Shared mental mental models in expert team decision making. In: Castellan NJ, ed. *Current Issues in Individual and Group Decision Making.* Hillsdale, NJ: Lawrence Erlbaum Associates; 1993:221–246.

34. Salas E, Sims DE, Burke CS. Is there a "big five" in the teamwork? *Small Group Res.* 2005;36(5): 555–599.

35. Smith-Jentsch KA, Mathieu JE, Kraiger K. Investigating linear and interactive effects of shared mental models on safety and efficiency in a field setting. *J Appl Psychol.* 2005;90(3):523–535.

36. Burtscher MJ, et al. Interactions of team mental models and monitoring behaviors predict team performance in simulated anesthesia inductions. *J Exp Psychol Appl.* 2011;17(3):257–269.

37. Westli HK, et al. Teamwork skills, shared mental models, and performance in simulated trauma teams: an independent group design. *Scand J Trauma Resusc Emerg Med.* 2010;18:47 .

38. Kolbe M, et al. The role of coordination for preventing harm in healthcare groups: research examples from anaesthesia and an integrated model of coordination for action teams in healthcare. In Boos M, et al., eds. *Coordination in Human and Primate Groups.* Heidelberg: Springer; 2011:75–92.

39. Rico R, et al. Team implicit cordination process: a team knowledge-based approach. *Acad Manage Rev.* 2008;33:163–184.

40. Andersen PO, et al. Identifying non-technical skills and barriers for improvement of teamwork in cardiac arrest teams. *Resuscitation.* 2010; 81(6):695–702.

41. Reynolds R, Blickensderfer E. Crew resource management and shared mental models: a proposal. *J Aviat Aerospace Educ Res.* 2009;19(1):15–23.

42. Petrosoniak A, Hicks C. Beyond crisis resource management: new frontiers in human factors training for acute care medicine. *Curr Opin Anaesthesiol.* 2013;26(6):699–706.

43. Cannon-Bowers JA, Salas E, Blickensderfer E. The impact of cross-training and workload on team functioning: a replication and extension of initial findings. *Hum Factors.* 1998;40(1):92–101.

44. Marks MA, et al. The impact of cross-training on team effectiveness. *J Applied Psychol.* 2002; 87(1):3–13.

45. Volpe CE, Cannon-Bowers JA, Salas E. The impact of cross-training on team functioning: an empirical investigation. *Hum Factors.* 1996;38(1):87–100.

46. Smith-Jentsch KA, et al. Guided team self-correction: impacts on team mental models, processes, and effectiveness. *Small Group Res.* 2008;39:303–327.

47. Blickensderfer E, Cannon-Bowers JA, Salas E. Fostering shared mental models through team self-correction: theoretical bases and propositions. In: Beyerlein M, Johnson D, Beyerlein S, eds. *Advances in Interdisciplinary Studies in Work Team Series.* Greenwich, CT: JAI Press; 1997:249–279.

48. Endsley MR, Robertson MM. Training for situation awareness in individuals and teams. In: Endsley MR, Garland DJ, eds. *Situation Awareness Analysis and Measurement.* Mahwah, NJ: Lawrence Erlbaum Associates: 2000.

49. Manser T, et al. Team communication during patient handover from the operating room: more than facts and figures. *Hum Factors.* 2013; 55(1):138–156.

50. Miller GA. The magical number seven, plus or minus two: some limits on our capacity for processing information. *Psychol Rev.* 1994;101(2): 342–352.

51. Gorges M, Staggers N. Evaluations of physiological monitoring displays: a systematic review. J Clin Monitor Comput. 2008;22(1):45–66.

52. Charabati S, et al. Comparison of four different display designs of a novel anaesthetic monitoring system, the "integrated monitor of anaesthesia (IMA)." *Br J Anaesth.* 2009;103(5):670–677.

53. Liu D, et al. Monitoring with head-mounted displays in general anesthesia: a clinical evaluation in the operating room. *Anesth Analg.* 2010;110(4):1032–1038.

54. Sanderson PM, et al. Advanced auditory displays and head-mounted displays: advantages and disadvantages for monitoring by the distracted anesthesiologist. *Anesth Analg.* 2008;106(6): 1787–1797.

55. Koch SH, et al. Evaluation of the effect of information integration ion dispülays for ICU nurses on situation awareness and task completion time: a prospective randomized controlled study. *Int J Med Inform.* 2013;82(8):665–675.

56. Haynes AB, et al. A surgical checklist to reduce morbidity and mortalitiy in a global population. *N Engl J Med.* 2009;360(5):491–499.

57. Borshoff DC. *The Anaesthetic Crisis Manual.* 1st rev. ed. Perth, Australia: Leeuwin Press; 2013.

8

Creating a Culture of Safety

THOMAS R. CHIDESTER

INTRODUCTION

In 2012, I suffered an attack of acute appendicitis and underwent a laparoscopic appendectomy in a local hospital, performed by a surgeon recommended by my primary care physician. The appendectomy was uneventful. I had no complications and spent a single night in the hospital, and there was minimal scarring. Who should be credited with the successful process and outcome? Should I marvel at the routinization of the procedure by technological advancement? I can commend the surgeon for his skill and the operating room team for anesthesiology and prevention of infection. I can commend the postoperative monitoring and pain management by the nursing staff. But there was more—a discipline of interaction with me as a patient that I interpreted as a culture emphasizing patient safety. Each care team member I spoke with sought to confirm standard information and explore anything that I reported about my condition or state. They did so in a way that reminded me of my extensive experience with aircraft operations and regulatory organizations. Although each team member acknowledged and respected me as an individual, they clearly had in mind standard operating procedures or checklists that would protect me (and themselves) from unrecognized threats to my health or an error in treatment. Front-line caregivers could not develop and implement these techniques on their own or in isolation; doing so requires specific management strategies in the hospital and in the broader healthcare community.

Consider a contrasting event from aviation.[1] A Boeing 757 aircraft making an emergency landing in Chicago departed the paved runway surface as the pilots attempted to avoid the consequences of over-running the end. No one was injured and damage to the aircraft was minimal. But the cause was seemingly simple and avoidable—the main battery had been depleted during flight after a relay failed and some electrical systems switched from generator power to the battery. Depletion of battery power resulted in the loss of some flight instruments, some communication equipment, control trim authority (which reduces the force the pilots must apply to the flight controls), anti-skid braking, and the ability to shut down the engines after landing. Why did this happen? Are the pilots at fault for not landing sooner because they misinterpreted one of several applicable checklists? Is it the fault of the mechanic who reset a circuit breaker on the affected system before departure? Are the maintenance personnel whom the pilots contacted responsible for not understanding the implications of what the pilots told them or not recommending an immediate landing? Is there a problem with the guidance provided to these maintenance personnel by the airline? What about the history of electrical problems on that individual aircraft that were not attributed to the failing relay before this flight? The National Transportation Safety Board (NTSB) determined the probable cause of the incident to be "the failure of an electrical relay due to eroded contacts and the flight crew's decision to continue a flight that was operating on battery power."[1] What, if anything, does the event say about the safety culture of the airline, the industry, or the regulatory and investigatory environment? The incident report offers insight into many of those issues.

Safety culture is a relatively new concept. Its discussion originated with the Chernobyl nuclear accident in 1986, the same year as the Space Shuttle *Challenger* explosion. It focuses on who is responsible, and in what ways, for safety, ranging from individuals and teams performing critical duties on the front lines to the context within which work takes place, and high-level organizational priorities. In perhaps the simplest form, Reason suggested safety culture as a dimension of *concern for production* versus *concern for protection*.[2] This implies that organizations inevitably trade producing goods and services for risk of harm, that those priorities are communicated overtly or subtly to frontline workers, and that trade-offs are sometimes made on the wrong side. From a production perspective, no anesthetic or surgery is without risk, and a completely safe aircraft does not fly. The financial impact of appropriate scheduling can significantly decrease the productivity of an organization. From a protection perspective, the volume of work can exceed the available time, causing workers to rush to meet demands, cutting corners at the expense of safe practice. People can be scheduled to work to unacceptable levels of fatigue. An organization may collect, analyze, and act upon economic performance metrics, while investing relatively little in safety performance metrics. An organization must balance its financial and safety risks in order to survive. But it is more complicated than that. Productivity can be increased through automated tools or advanced preparation of components such as medications. Operations research can lead to targeting critical supplies, actions, or protections that maintain safe performance at a lower cost. In these cases, infrastructure investment is intended to mitigate safety risk at the front line. Complexity implies that safety culture is multidimensional.

DEFINITIONS

The US Agency for Health Research and Quality (AHRQ) defines a sound patient safety culture as demonstrating a commitment to safety at all levels, from front-line providers to managers and executives.[3] This commitment establishes a "culture of safety" that encompasses these key features:

- Acknowledgment of the high-risk nature of an organization's activities and the determination to achieve consistently safe operations;
- A blame-free environment where individuals are able to report errors or near misses without fear of reprimand or punishment;
- Encouragement of collaboration across ranks and disciplines to seek solutions to patient safety problems;
- Organizational commitment of resources to address safety concerns.

They argue that improvements in safety culture are directly tied to error reduction and quality of care.

AHRQ's definition anchors only the positive end of a continuum of culture. Broader definitions vary in their value-driven *versus* action-driven focus. The UK Health and Safety Commission of the Advisory Committee on the Safety of Nuclear Installations (HSC) defined safety culture as "the product of individual and group values, attitudes, perceptions, competencies, and patterns of behaviour that determine the commitment to, and the style and proficiency of, an organization's health and safety management."[4] In this view, values and attitudes drive behavior; in turn, we may measure and develop interventions at all three levels. Alternatively, *safety culture* can be defined as *the product of formal measures taken to minimize risk to an acceptable level (or as low as practical) and to ensure that stakeholders feel secure and in control, and the informal understood priorities of the organization and key subgroups within it.* Formal measures include both actions required or prescribed as "working safely," implementation of physical, organizational, and technical barriers to known risks, and reporting or monitoring systems to detect developing risks. Informal characteristics are manager, leader, and worker perceptions of how employees are to produce work products and prevent accidents and injuries, and the priorities assigned to production and protection activities.[5] In this view, policy and procedure influence practice at the front line, and attitudes and values emerge from process; cognitive constructs of culture are synthesized from behaviors and actions. This perspective may aid in the documentation of positive and negative safety-related behaviors and direct organizations to concrete actions to create or transform a safety culture: managers may communicate values and attempt to persuade attitudes, but they also set policy, define procedures, assure practices, and measure outcomes.

ORIGINS

Antonsen describes the safety cultural approach as the third and newest phase of accident investigation in highly industrialized societies.[5] Accident investigations initially focused on technical failures of equipment and ground structures and systems. This approach was dominant in Western aviation industries through the 1960s, and was highly successful in reducing accident rates. A variety of protective systems and improvements in aircraft functions and navigational capabilities were invented and implemented during this period. Those improvements are paralleled in medical technology. The second phase focused on operator behavior, primarily during the 1970s and 1980s, and led to the study of human factors and crew resource management (CRM) in aviation. This further reduced the accident rate and is reflected in the direct translation of CRM into medical operations.[6,7] The third phase began with the Chernobyl nuclear accident. There were two reports of the investigation. The first attributed the accident to operator error.[8] Investigators characterized pre-accident activities at the plant as prioritizing production over safety measures, allowing procedural violations to become commonplace, and reflecting a complacent belief in risk control, leading to flawed decisions on the day of the accident. However, the second report[9] called those conclusions into question and characterized the accident as being caused by the design of the reactor and implications of the design that were not fully understood by the operators. Both views reinforce a focus beyond the individual or team of front-line employees. The first report extrapolates narrowly to the team of plant operators; the second is a broad examination of reactor design, documentation, and operations processes. Since those reports, safety culture has been raised as a causative or contributing factor in accidents across multiple modes of transportation, in oil and chemical production, and in medicine.

PERSPECTIVES

There are differing perspectives on safety culture that illustrate the need to consider both formal and informal characteristics of an organization. Turner applied a medical model to accidents.[10] If organizations are viewed as living organisms, and accidents, like disease or death, are the ultimate result of an underlying condition, then understanding their early symptoms might improve safety. He described procedural deviations by individual operators as *an organization incubating an accident*. This metaphor presages the transition from a focus on situational factors that lead to inappropriate operator actions to flawed priorities, processes, or procedures in the organization of the workplace.

Perrow offered the strongest version of the formal view of safety culture, arguing that safety and risk are determined by the decisions of those in power, who set priorities, develop procedures, and enforce compliance.[11] Perrow's viewpoint is reflected in the Rogers Commission report on the Space Shuttle *Challenger* accident.[12] The accident resulted from exhaust gases and flame from a solid rocket booster leaking through an O-ring seal and igniting the external liquid fuel tank. Pre-accident experience and post-accident investigation indicated that leakage was more likely at low atmospheric temperatures, and the *Challenger* accident occurred on the coldest launch day experienced in the Shuttle program. The Rogers Commission[12] focused on the decision to launch and its processes, describing it as

based on incomplete and sometimes misleading information, a conflict between engineering data and management judgments, and a NASA management structure that permitted internal flight safety problems to bypass key Shuttle managers.

Vaughn offered a contrasting view of the *Challenger* accident, focusing not on the day of this launch but of organizational change over multiple launches.[13] She cited evidence that solid rocket booster O-rings had leaked on several previous occasions without consequence. As a result, something perceived as catastrophic during design became viewed as moderately probable, but without severe consequence in practice, a process she described as the normalization of deviance. This concept has broad implications for transportation operators and medical professionals; we may come to believe that something is less risky than we thought because we encounter and survive it without incident. Such *bad lessons*[2] will always happen with low-probability events—but successful experience neither changes the underlying probability of occurrence of the hazard nor the severity of its outcome. The ultimate result is informal shortcuts. We must therefore consider not only the positive/negative and overt/covert safety messages from those in power, but also the practices that develop at the front line.

Rochlin, LaPorte, and Roberts observed day-to-day activities in organizations whose business routinely requires high risk (e.g., naval air carrier ships), but who have driven their accident and incident rates to extremely low levels.[14] These *high-reliability organizations* seem to pursue people and processes that are resilient to a variety of hazards, instead of a series of protections for individual hazards. They and several additional authors have summarized the characterics of these workplaces, but Dlugacz and Spath[15] decribe the *cognitive* orientation of workers and managers as involving

- Continuous vigilance to risk, where reports of flawed processes can be made without fear of censure or retribution;
- Efficient and respectful teamwork, where the contribution of every individual is equally valued;

- Effective communication that is democratic and respectful;
- Individual and organizational mindfulness of the potential dangers involved in various processes and functions;
- Ongoing education and training.

This approach suggests greater definition to the informal aspect of safety culture—the orientation that front-line caregivers and their managers should possess. It suggests that medical service organizations consider policy statement, risk assessment, event reporting, and team building to improve safety performance.

There is a growing body of literature about the priorities, policies, processes, and procedures put in place by organizations to manage risk, and the understanding and behavior of the multiple workgroups who carry out an organization's production activities.

CONCEPTS AND DIMENSIONS

In 2010, I was tasked to support the Federal Aviation Administration (FAA) Certificate Management Office overseeing an airline's operations in selecting methods to conduct a safety culture assessment. In doing so, I led a team who examined four approaches to safety culture definition for their common and distinct elements, with the goal of suggesting an overarching set of concepts or dimensions for measurement. We found that each of three approaches to defining component dimensions in transportation[5,16,17] could be sufficiently described using the dimensions of the Safety Culture Indicator Scale Measurement System (SCISMS).[18] Each described a set of similarly defined dimensions to one or more of the high-level and subcomponents, and could be described as more or less comprehensive in its measurement of safety culture. SCISMS is composed of five high-level and 14 subcomponents:

1. *Organizational commitment*: The degree to which the organization prioritizes safety in decision-making, allocates resources to safety management, accepts system delays to mitigate safety problems:

- *Safety values*: Safety values are communicated by leadership and safety performance, managed and monitored to a level comparable to finances;
- *Safety fundamentals*: Compliance with regulated aspects of safety: training, manuals, procedures, maintenance, inter-unit coordination;
- *Going beyond compliance*: Priority is given to non-regulated safety activities: rostering, shiftwork scheduling, fatigue management, scientific risk management.

2. *Operational interactions*: Priority is given to safety and regard for actual risks by operational personnel:
   - *Supervisors/Foremen*: Proactive concern for employee and system safety and ability to convey a safe environment;
   - *Operations Control/Ancillary Ops*: Priority is given to safety by those supporting operations;
   - *Instructors/Training*: Those who provide safety training understand and have adequate access to actual risks associated with operations.

3. *Formal safety indicators*: Procedures and systems for reporting and addressing occupational and process safety hazards:
   - *Reporting system*: Employees have access to, are familiar with, and make use of safety reporting systems;
   - *Response/Feedback*: Appropriate management responses to reported information and dissemination of information to operational personnel;
   - *Safety personnel*: Perceived effectiveness and competence of persons in formal safety roles.

4. *Informal safety indicators*: How employees perceive the fairness of performance management, including rewards and punishments for safe and unsafe actions:
   - *Accountability*: Consistency with which employees are held accountable for unsafe behavior;

- *Employee authority*: Employee involvement in safety decision-making, including proposing and re-engineering ineffective or hazardous work processes;
- *Professionalism*: Employee expectation for peer compliance with procedures and prudent performance.

5. *Safety behaviors and outcomes*: Employee perception of state of safety within the organization:
   - *Perceived personal risk*: Perceived prevalence of deviations from safety standards and attitude toward deviations;
   - *Perceived organizational risk*: Perceived likelihood of negative safety events for the organization.

This level of conceptual definition goes beyond most safety culture parameters in medicine and could represent a step forward in the measurement of current state and the development of interventions.

MEASUREMENT

Each author who has suggested strategies for building an effective safety culture has argued that understanding the current state of an organization should be the first step. A great deal of research effort has therefore been invested in the measurement of safety culture. It can be argued that all concepts are *defined* by how they are measured; even a physical concept such as distance may only be understandable when expressed as the time taken to travel between two points. Safety culture also cannot be described as simply good or bad, but requires the examination of a number of dimensions along which an organization and its workers can be described as more or less tolerant of safety, schedule, and financial risks, disciplined in accomplishing procedures, willing to do more than is required by regulation, and willing to report and correct safety risks.

The AHRQ advocates the use of provider surveys to measure safety culture.[19] They developed four different Patient Safety Culture Surveys for hospitals, medical offices, nursing homes, and pharmacies. The AHRQ website (www.ahrq.gov) also provides benchmarking data relative to other organizations for each category.

Sexton et al. published a Safety Attitudes Questionnaire (SAQ), generalized from their extensive work in aviation.[20] The SAQ is designed to measure a snapshot of safety culture through surveys of front-line worker perceptions. It has been completed by over 10,000 healthcare professionals in over 200 settings in three countries, and its psychometric properties are well documented and benchmarks are available. It provides scores along six dimensions: Teamwork Climate, Safety Climate, Perceptions of Management, Job Satisfaction, Working Conditions, and Stress Recognition.

Transportation industries in general, and aviation specifically, offer techniques for more advanced and detailed surveys and more in-depth and multi-perspective methods. SCISMS[18] uses only an employee survey measurement technique, but it could be used in healthcare in a way that increases depth of analysis. Patankar, Brown, Sabin, and Bigda-Peyton[17] caution that surveys may measure only *safety climate*—the current and temporary state of employee attitudes toward safety. Antonsen[5] has raised concerns about measurement solely by survey, having found that characterization of culture by survey on a North Sea oil platform operation was substantially different and more positive than that obtained through structured interviews following a major incident. This study reports survey, structured interview, and performance observation measurement techniques, which are quite comprehensive, but it was accomplished in North Sea oil production and is not directly transferable to medicine. It could, however, serve as a template to guide research toward more detailed measures.

Abbott and Hiles designed a structured assessment to guide FAA inspectors in their observations and analysis of available data to describe the strengths and weaknesses of an airline.[16] This assessment structures observation by non-members of the operating organization, and is limited to data that an airline provides through regulatory requirements and voluntary programs and concrete and visible characteristics of its safety programs. As a result, it is comprehensive of formal dimensions of safety culture (behaviors and actions), but cannot measure informal dimensions (the beliefs, attitudes, values, and understanding of culture by employees and managers). It could serve as a useful starting point for a medical oversight organization to develop structured observations. Abbott and Hiles highlight one organizing issue that may be relevant for medicine: airlines have increasingly made use of affiliated transportation and maintenance companies and service contractors over the past two decades, just as medical organizations include employees, independent contractors, and physicians. This system may be useful to characterize the impact of affiliated personnel and employees on safety culture.

Patankar, Brown, Sabin, and Bigda-Peyton designed a comprehensive approach that includes formal and informal dimensions.[17] This technique uses multiple measures to assess safety culture, including surveys and interviews of employees of varying workgroups and managers of varying levels, case analysis, field observations, and the examination of organizational "artifacts"—its published materials, such as procedures, manuals, newsletters, brochures, and performance evaluation criteria. The advantages of this technique lie in the use of multiple measures and both quantitative and qualitative analysis, but it requires a significant commitment of effort, time, and cost. This may be the best template for a medical organization seeking to develop a comprehensive strategy for assessment.

Medical organizations seeking to improve their culture have a range of options for measuring their current state. These options include applying readily available survey techniques with accompanying benchmarks and engaging research organizations or consultants to perform multi-method assessments. At the industry level, medicine would likely benefit from further tailoring and broader availability of multi-perspective measurement techniques. Measures that are selected for assessment should be monitored periodically in order to assess the impact of interventions designed to improve safety culture.

CONTROVERSIES

There is significant debate in the literature as to whether safety culture can be independently measured and even as to whether it prevents harm. First, is safety culture separable from the broader culture of the organization? Abbott and Hiles view safety as an inseparable component of organizational culture and suggest instead documenting how the overall organization works, and how safety is considered.[16] Attempting to document a separate safety culture may lead to a narrow examination of the organization in which production remains unexamined except for where it directly impacts safety. Hence, their measurement focuses upon structures, policies, procedures, and practices. Mitchell emphasizes safety as one component of quality of care, along with effectiveness, patient focus, timeliness, efficiency, and equity.[21] The safety component focuses on the prevention of harm in the provision of care. Sumwalt notes that the NTSB has described a number of accidents as "organizational," meaning that the causal or contributing factors include a lack of an organizational culture of safety. "For sociotechnical industries where low probability–high consequence events can transpire, such as aviation, nuclear power, and oil and gas industries, it is essential that organizational culture be aligned with a safety focus."[22] Each of these perspectives suggests caution in the promotion of safety culture—the broader culture of the organization can support or undermine a focus on safety risk and also affect how safety is traded for scheduling and financial risks.

This leads to a second set of questions. What happens when an organization's stated values differ from its incentives? What happens when the informal and formal components of safety culture conflict? Formal statements of value for safety in the context of an organization investing its resources and rewarding employees solely by production metrics are unlikely to advance the safety culture. For example, what happens if an airline publishes guidelines that require pilots to abandon unstable approaches, but also publishes each month the number of missed approaches and their cost in additional fuel burn and missed passenger connections? Encouraging stabilized approaches accepts the production costs of not attempting risky landings to avoid the costs of a landing accident. Many of the former are worth a single of the latter in lives, property, dollars, and damage to the airline's reputation. Which does the airline value in the messages it puts forth? Examples of efforts to improve culture in medical settings demonstrate how emphasizing action at multiple levels of the organization, along with changes to front-line procedures and norms, appears to be linked to improvement in safety outcomes.

A third set of questions raises concern about the about potential harm to patients caused by avoiding risk. Reason's reference to the trade-off of production and protection functions may have special meaning in medicine.[2] In transportation, a decision to delay, divert, or cancel an operation out of safety concern inconveniences passengers, may cascade into larger system-level delays, and imposes costs for both customers and the organization. Such a decision rarely results in injury or loss of life, with the exception of operations transporting perishable medications or transplantable organs, for example. But in medicine, attempting to avoid error, risk of complication, malpratice, or unintended consequence can bring with it a decision not to treat, or to use a less effective treatment. This can result in a worse outcome that is caused by the natural progression of injury or disease. Arnstein discussed this issue in the context of analgesic use to treat chronic pain among older patients:[23]

> The medical management of pharmacologic treatment for pain in older adults is often suboptimal, ranging from failing to use analgesics for patients with considerable pain to exposing older adults to potentially life-threatening toxicities, overdoses, or drug interactions.

Focusing solely on the risks of medications ensures that the patient will experience pain.

Similarly, treatment teams can reach an impasse when choosing appropriate therapy for patients with multiple comorbidities; meanwhile, each condition continues its natural course. Arnstein argues for balancing efficacy and safety in pain management; discussions about safety *versus* efficacy among care providers may need to be more prominent in discussions of safety culture. Whether made explicit or not, treatment decisions balance efforts to *do good* and to *prevent harm*. Our discussion of safety culture, focused on preventing error and managing threats, and in turn an organizational effort to promote patient safety, may obscure potential trade-offs with effectiveness. The optimal culture most likely makes these compromises prominent and deliberate. Efforts to publish standards of care for specific diseases and conditions are consistent with this type of discussion at the professional and specialty level. Advocates of full disclosure would make explicit to the patient the risks being balanced and the potential outcomes of each course of action (e.g., the discussion of condition, objectives of treatment, alternatives, and risks by the American College of Physicians[24]).

CREATING SAFETY CULTURE AT THE ORGANIZATIONAL LEVEL

Many of the chapters of this book describe management actions that serve to create an effective safety culture. To the extent that a hospital, clinic, or anesthesiology practice pursues patient safety and quality management functions, it establishes *formal measures to minimize risk to an acceptable level (or as low as practical) and to ensure that stakeholders feel secure and in control.* This would include quality management, standardization of procedures, advancing training through simulation and crisis resource management, patient outcome monitoring, and systemic corrective action processes. To the extent that an organization trains, monitors, and provides process feedback, it influences *the informal understood priorities of the organization and key subgroups within it.*

Wilson[25] suggested that medical practices wishing to improve safety culture should

- Undertake a baseline cultural survey of the practice;
- Undertake a risk assessment to identify potential risks to patients and staff;
- Appoint a risk manager for the practice;
- Develop effective leadership (i.e., lead by example, perceived as sincerely committed to safety);
- Encourage team working—build ownership of patient safety at all levels and exploit the unique knowledge that employees have of their own work;
- Develop a structured approach to safety;
- Ensure effective communication with the team and patients;
- Learn lessons from complaints and mistakes—remember we will all make mistakes (to err is human), but the key is to learn from those mistakes and ensure that systems are robust so that errors are less likely to happen;
- Ensure that staff are trained to competently undertake the roles assigned to them.

McCarthy and Klein reported the implementation of a comprehensive safety initiative in a multi-location health provider organization that resulted in an 80% reduction in serious events across its system, including misdiagnoses, medication errors, hospital-acquired infections, wrong-site surgery, and falls resulting in serious injury.[26] This program included conducting a baseline assessment, clearly communicating safety as a core value, defining and reinforcing general safety practices, simplifying and providing checklists for standard procedures, implementing root cause analysis of events, requiring unit responses to analysis recommendations, and implementing a just culture approach to investigation and discipline. As part of the general safety practices, the organization identified "red rules": procedures requiring redundant verification of patient identification for administration of blood, blood products, and high-risk medications. Their *just culture* approach ensured that employees would not be disciplined for honest mistakes that may identify systemic risk. Disciplinary action was reserved for willful misconduct, incurring unacceptable risk, or repeated unsafe acts. Initial moderate (though short-of-expectation) success offered solutions for Abbott and Hiles's concern for mixed workforces.[16] The hospital system was composed of employees and physicians who were affiliated by admitting and surgical privileges; initial efforts had focused only on the employees. Physicians were engaged by naming "safety champions" across employment status and specialty. They were given training equivalent to that of the hospital system's employees, having them participate in "safety rounds," and encouraging them to influence both physician and employee team members.

Several of the interventions used by McCarthy and Klein's initiatives made use of extended human resources technical functions in large organizations that may be a challenge for smaller facilities.[26] Development of procedures, including identifying general safety behaviors and tasks in need of checklists, often are based in sound job task analysis by practitioner category. Task analyses describe the core activities accomplished by each professional group and identify abilities to be selected and knowledge and skills to be trained. A small organization may not be able to conduct these kinds of analyses on their own, but there are good templates in the literature. For example, Phipps, Meakin, Beatty, Nsoedo, and Parker developed a hierarchical task analysis for operating room anesthesia, after which they applied a human error taxonomy to each step, creating descriptions of the errors that could take place.[27] Smaller organizations may consider adapting previously published task analyses, standard procedures, and training modules, if a customized comprehensive approach is beyond their means.

As with measurement, the transportation industry's experience in culture change might successfully translate to medicine. Standardization of procedures has been pursued in aviation since the 1930s,[28] creating a substantial body of research that may be useful to medicine. Developing procedures for standard tasks may require standardization of flows (initiation of procedures, configuration change, and sequencing of events) and checks of equipment and interfaces, may require deliberate division of performing versus monitoring and checking duties, and may require well-organized documentation and reference materials to be available to work teams. Degani and Weiner[29] published an excellent starting point for studying procedures, which has been cited by several subsequent medical researchers. White, Trbovich, Easty, and Savage made use of this technique to examine checklist effectiveness for preventing medication errors.[30]

Developers of CRM-like approaches to training care teams may benefit from concepts and teaching methods involving situation awareness, communication, team function, and threat and error management (TEM).[31] For example, Endsley has argued that situation awareness requires knowledge of state or data (e.g., blood pressure, pulse, oxygen saturation), its relationship to targets (high, low, trend relative to goal), and its projected impact on the planned sequence of action (e.g., continue course, stop to stabilize, or terminate a surgical intervention).[32] Many interventions in aviation have branched from this concept, and they are readily applicable to anesthesia and to other areas in medicine with adaptation. Stiegler, Chidester, and Ruskin suggested a TEM approach to analyzing and preventing threats and errors in anesthesia.[33] Nemeth offers an excellent guide for translating progress in transportation to initial and continuing medical training.[34]

Process monitoring, to include error reporting, sample auditing, and data stream analysis, has advanced a great deal in the transportation industry. Medicine has established processes for the equivalent of investigating accidents and lesser incidents through morbidity and mortality review conferences and root cause analysis. The majority of airlines have established Aviation Safety Action Programs (ASAP), allowing most employee groups to report any safety concern they observe without fear of reprisal, even if they inadvertently caused the issue.[35] At the industry level, the National Aeronautics and Space Administration operates the Aviation Safety Reporting System (NASA ASRS)[36] on behalf of the FAA, which grants transactional immunity for reported safety events, and has established a model Patient Safety Reporting System (PSRS)[37] in collaboration with the Veterans Administration. Reporting systems are recognized as important to most safety culture transformation interventions in medicine and require a disciplined approach to event analysis, such as root cause analysis,[38] the Human Factors Analysis and Classification System (HFACS),[39] or TEM.[31] Line-Oriented Safety Audits (LOSA)[40] accomplish sample audits of team performance by training a small group of observers who are subject matter experts to a standard set of ratings, then having them observe performance of multiple teams, providing de-identified, non-jeopardy feedback referenced to benchmarks. This approach is conceptually generalizable to the operating room. Process monitoring in aviation involves the routine download and analysis of flight data (Flight Operations Quality Assurance, FOQA).[41] FOQA analyses make use of data de-identified under rules negotiated among the airline, its unions, and the FAA, and seek to identify situations in which an aircraft operates outside its typical or desired flight envelope. This enables early identification of practices that might otherwise be detected only following an accident. Most automated equipment in medicine is similarly capable of storing large amounts of data during surgery or recovery. The Anesthesia Quality Institute has begun storing complete anesthesia records. This could lead to routine integration and analyses across events and patients. In the interim, patient outcome monitoring may be a reasonable substitute, though it makes use of higher order data.

A discussion of monitoring requires a discussion of its use in discipline. Although the US Agency for Health Research and Quality[3] mentioned blame-free culture, McCarthy and Klein made reference to the concepts of accountability and justice.[26] This controversy is a developing art and science across industries. The Government of Ireland Commission on Patient Safety and Quality Assurance[42] states the issue succinctly:

> Although much has been said in recent years about the need to create a "fair and just culture" in order to foster openness and honesty, there is also an argument which supports the holding to account of those whose competence and performance has fallen below what might reasonably be expected of them.

An opportunity to disclose can reinforce unsafe acts rather than remedy systemic risk if it is treated by a workforce as a "get out of jail free" card for procedural or regulatory noncompliance. The purpose of reporting systems is to receive an early warning to prevent future, potentially catastrophic events. A non-punitive approach must balance the risks of not knowing about a potential hazard and maintaining professional accountability.[43]

The issue of fatigue in a 24-hour workplace is common to transportation and medicine, among other industries. All humans become more prone to error as a function of time since awakening, time on duty, and time of day. Those risks are predictable using computer-based systems, and may be controlled by scheduling decisions by organizations and disciplined application by front-line personnel. Building a safety culture requires some form of fatigue risk management. In US, aviation, rest and duty-time regulations for pilots were revised in 2011. At that time, the FAA offered guidance for building Fatigue Risk Management Systems (FRMS).[44] Ground transportation has similarly revised hours of service rules.[45] The Accreditation Council for Graduate Medical Education issued duty hours for graduate residents in 2003 and revised them in 2011.[46] Given the difficulty in establishing regulations and standards, organizations working to improve safety culture might pursue a local FRMS. Programs used in the aviation industry could be used for guidance, referencing the FAA's advisory circular.[47]

The international movement toward Safety Management Systems (SMS) in aviation might be construed as institutionalizing safety culture transformation. "SMS is the formal, top-down business approach to managing safety risk, which includes a systemic approach to managing safety, including the necessary organizational structures, accountabilities, policies and procedures."[48] SMS creates formal structures within operating and regulatory organizations, implementing a disciplined approach to safety-related decision-making and requires policy, risk management, assurance, and promotion processes. Larger medical service providers may wish to consider this approach to culture improvement.

CREATING SAFETY CULTURE AT THE FRONT-LINE EMPLOYEE LEVEL

What do organizations with strong safety cultures expect of their front-line workers? McCarthy and Klein emphasized safety habits in the form of an error-prevention toolbox, red rules, checklists, and recognizing and reporting safety issues.[26] The toolbox they deployed at Santara Healthcare is reproduced as Box 8.1.

These responsibilities have analogs in the transportation industry. While procedural discipline is fundamental to aviation operations, feedback loops identifying procedural inadequacy emerged in the development of monitoring and reporting systems in the 1990s. McCarthy and Klein's call for a questioning attitude is analogous to a TEM mindset.[26] TEM suggests that most adverse events can be described in terms of risks or challenges present in an operational environment (threats) and the actions of specific personnel that potentiate or exacerbate those threats (errors). While most accident sequences begin with some provocation in the operating environment, every flight and every surgery are presented with some number of hazards. Only the risks that the team recognizes and mitigates separate an accident chain from a routine outcome. Surgeons, anesthesiologists, nurses, aids, and technicians should remain alert for developing threats and should position themselves to catch and correct any mistakes. The latter is a secondary function of procedures and checklists—we do and then we review. Importantly, some risks are constant, but many are contingent upon the situation and vary by phases of activity. This regularity may be used to predict and prevent error.[33,49]

BOX 8.1   SENTARA HEALTHCARE'S ERROR-PREVENTION TOOLBOX

1. *Pay attention to detail*: Follow the "stop, think, act, review" (STAR) method to focus attention and think before initiating a critical task.
2. *Communicate clearly*: Use repeat-backs and ask clarifying questions to ensure that you understand requests.
3. *Have a questioning attitude*: "That doesn't mean challenge everything," Burke said. "It means if I'm not certain about exactly what you want me to do, ask for clarification." It also means employees should heed their intuition. If something doesn't seem right, "Take time to figure out why ... Then go to an external source to get verification," whether that source is a person, a textbook, or an online resource.
4. *Hand off effectively using an "5P" checklist*: To ensure that all elements of a successful transfer are followed, the handoff should identify the "5Ps": patient/project, plan, purpose, problems, and precautions.
5. *Never leave your wingman*: This phrase, adopted from military aviation (which plays a prominent role in the local culture), refers to the need for peer checking and peer coaching as appropriate.

Reproduced with permission from The Commonwealth Fund, ©2001.

Two additional expectations of individual front-line professionals should be part of an effective safety culture. First is a commitment to lifetime skill acquisition and maintenance. Medicine is evolving rapidly; providers must work to keep up with innovation. Second, fatigue management at the organization level requires the cooperation of individual front-line personnel. Duty-hour limits and fatigue risk management systems will not be effective if time planned for sleep and recovery is used for other purposes. Alertness management must be perceived as a shared responsibility. One could argue that recent progress is revolutionary in perceiving alertness as anything other than an individual responsibility. A sound safety culture will expect both organizational and individual responsibilities to be fulfilled.

CONCLUSION: INTERVENING TO BUILD A SOUND SAFETY CULTURE

To understand the current state of an organization's safety culture, we must assess the priorities, processes, and procedures put in place by organizations to manage risk, and the understanding and behavior of the multiple workgroups who carry out an organization's production activities. To improve a culture, actions are required throughout the organization. The literature suggests the following:

- Assess current state using a benchmarked survey, followed by focus groups, case analysis, field observations, and examination of organizational artifacts, where survey results fall below benchmark or incident history suggests concern.
- Communicate safety as a core value by managers at all levels in a methodical and sustained manner, acknowledging areas where improvement is needed.
- Establish feedback systems, including adverse event and safety concern reporting, process audits, and patient outcome monitoring.
- Develop, publish, promote, and monitor compliance with standardized procedures by workgroup and task,

accompanied by best practices that span workgroups, such as "safety toolkits."
- Develop, deliver, and maintain training supporting policies, procedures, and best practices.
- Align reward systems with safety performance outcomes.
- Assess and report safety progress to the workforce alongside economic progress, communicating an appropriate balance of concern for safety and production.

From this perspective, transforming and maintaining a sound safety culture require a sustained process. However, it is an investment that yields returns in patient outcomes, which can in turn improve productivity and profitability of service provider organizations.

REFERENCES

1. National Transportation Safety Board. *Incident Report CHI08IA292.* Washington, DC: National Transportation Safety Board; 2010.
2. Reason J. *Managing the Risks of Organizational Accidents.* Aldershot, UK: Ashgate; 1997.
3. US Agency for Health Research and Quality. *Patient Safety Primers: Safety Culture.* October 2012. http://psnet.ahrq.gov/primer.aspx?primerID=5.
4. Health and Safety Commission. *Third Report: Organizing for Safety: Advisory Committee on the Safety of Nuclear Installations.* London: HSE Books; 1993.
5. Antonsen S. *Safety Culture: Theory, Measurement, and Improvement.* Burlington, VT: Ashgate; 2009.
6. Helmreich R. On error management: lessons from aviation. *BMJ.* 2000;320(7237):781–785.
7. Howard S, Gaba D, Fish K, Yang G, Sarnquist F. Anesthesia crisis resource management training: teaching anesthesiologists to handle critical incidents. *Aviat Space Environ Med.* 1992;63:763–770.
8. International Nuclear Safety Advisory Group. *Summary Report on the Post-Accident Review on the Chernobyl Accident. Safety Series No. 75-INSAG-1.* Vienna: International Atomic Energy Agency; 1986.
9. International Atomic Energy Agency. *The Chernobyl Accident: Updating of INSAG-1. Safety Series 75-INSAG-7.* Vienna: International Atomic Energy Agency; 1993.
10. Turner B. *Man-Made Disasters.* London: Wykeham; 1978.

11. Perrow C. *Normal Accidents: Living with High-Risk Technologies*. New York: Basic; 1984.

12. Rogers Commission. *Report of the Presidential Commission on the Space Shuttle Challenger Accident*. Washington, DC: National Aeronautics and Space Administration; 1986.

13. Vaughn D. *The Challenger Launch Decision: Risky Technology, Culture, and Deviance at NASA*. Chicago: University of Chicago Press; 1997.

14. Rochlin G, LaPorte T, Roberts K. The self-designing high-reliability organization: aircraft carrier flight operations at sea. *Naval War Coll Rev.* 1987;40:76–90.

15. Dlugacz Y, Spath P. High reliability and patient safety. In: Spath P, ed. *Error Reduction in Healthcare: A Systems Approach to Improving Patient Safety.* 2nd ed. San Francisco, CA: Jossey-Bass; 2011:35–57.

16. Abbott K, Hiles J. *Review of Corporate Culture Philosophies, Policies, Procedures and Practices.* (Unpublished).

17. Patankar M, Brown J, Sabin E, Bigda-Peyton T. *Safety Culture: Building and Sustaining a Cultural Change in Aviation and Healthcare.* Burlington, VT: Ashgate; 2012.

18. von Thaden T, Gibbons A. *The Safety Culture Indicator Scale Measurement System (SCISMS), Technical Report HFD-08-03/FAA-08-02.* Savoy: University of Illinois, Human Factors Division; 2008.

19. US Agency for Healthcare Research and Quality. *Surveys on Patient Safety Culture.* July 2012. http://www.ahrq.gov/professionals/quality-patient-safety/patientsafetyculture/.

20. Sexton J, Helmreich R, Neilands T, Rowan K, Vella K, Boyden J, ... Thomas E. The Safety Attitudes Questionnaire: Psychometric properties, benchmarking data, and emerging research. *BMC Health Serv Res.* 2006;6(44):1–10.

21. Mitchell P. *Defining Patient Safety and Quality Care.* March 4, 2008. Retrieved from United States Agency for Health Research and Quality: http://www.ahrq.gov/professionals/clinicians-providers/resources/nursing/resources/nursesh-dbk/MitchellP_DPSQ.pdf.

22. Sumwalt R. *The Role of Organizational Culture, Safety Culture, and Safety Climate in Aviation and Aerospace Safety.* October 12, 2012. Retrieved from National Transportation Safety Board: http://www.ntsb.gov/doclib/speeches/sumwalt/Sumwalt_121007b.pdf.

23. Arnstein P. Balancing analgesic efficacy with safety concerns in the older patient. *Pain Manag Nurs.* 2010;11(Suppl 2):S11–S22.

24. American College of Physicians. *ACP Ethics Manual.* 6th ed. January 9, 2014. Retrieved from Center for Ethics and Professionalism: http://www.acponline.org/running_practice/ethics/manual/manual6th.htm#informed.

25. Wilson J. How to create a patient safety culture. *Sessional GP.* 2012;4:12–13.

26. McCarthy D, Klein S. Sentara Healthcare: making patient safety an enduring organizational value. In *Keeping the Commitment: Progress in Patient Saftey.* Commonwealth Fund, publication 1476, vol. 8, 2011:1–19.

27. Phipps D, Meakin G, Beatty P, Nsoedo C, Parker D. Human factors in anaesthetic practice: insights from a task analysis. *Br J Anaesthesia.* 2008;100(3):333–343.

28. Schamel J. *How the Pilot's Checklist Came About.* September 10, 2012. Retrieved from atchistory.org: http://www.atchistory.org/History/checklst.htm.

29. Degani A, Weiner E. Cockpit checklists: concepts, design, and use. *Hum Factors.* 1993;35: 345–359.

30. White R, Trbovich P, Easty A, Savage P. Checking it twice: an evaluation of checklists for detecting medication errors at the bedside using a chemotherapy model. *Qual Saf Health Care.* 2010;19:562–567.

31. Helmreich R. Error management as organisational strategy. *Proceedings of the IATA Human Factors Seminar.* Bangkok: International Air Transport Association; 1998:1–7.

32. Endsley M. Situation awareness in aviation systems. In: Wise J, Hopkin V, Garland D, eds. *Handbook of Aviation Human Factors.* New York: Taylor & Francis; 2010:12:1–12:22.

33. Stiegler M, Chidester T, Ruskin K. Clinical error management. *Int Anesth Clin.* 2013;51:22–36.

34. Nemeth C. *Improving Healthcare Team Communication: Building on Lessons from Aviation.* Aldershot, UK: Ashgate; 2008.

35. Federal Aviation Administration. *Aviation Safety Action Program.* April 11, 2013. http://www.faa.gov/about/initiatives/asap/.

36. National Aeronautics and Space Administration. *Aviation Safety Reporting System.* October 2013. http://asrs.arc.nasa.gov/.

37. National Aeronautics and Space Administration. *Patient Safety Reporting System.* October 2013. http://psrs.arc.nasa.gov.

38. US Agency for Health Research and Quality. *Root Cause Analysis.* October 2012. Retrieved from Patient Safety Primers: http://psnet.ahrq.gov/primer.aspx?primerID=10.

39. Wiegmann DA, Shappell SA. *A Human Error Approach to Aviation Accident Analysis: The Human Factors Analysis and Classification System.* Burlington, VT: Ashgate; 2003.

40. Federal Aviation Administration. *Line Operations Safety Audits. AC-120-90.* Washington, DC:

Federal Aviation Administration; 2006. http://rgl.faa.gov/Regulatory_and_Guidance_Library/rgAdvisoryCircular.nsf/list/AC%20120-90/$FILE/AC%20120-90.pdf.

41. Federal Aviation Administration. *Flight Operational Quality Assurance (FOQA)*. March 19, 2013. http://www.faa.gov/about/initiatives/atos/air_carrier/foqa/.

42. Commission on Patient Safety and Quality Assurance. *Building a Culture of Patient Safety*. Dublin: Government of Ireland; 2008.

43. Marx, D. *Patient Safety and the "Just Culture": A Primer for Health Care Executives*. April 17, 2001. Retrieved from Agency for Healthcare Research and Quality: http://psnet.ahrq.gov/resource.aspx?resourceID=1582.

44. Federal Aviation Administration. *Press Release—FAA Issues Final Rule on Pilot Fatigue*. December 21, 2011. http://www.faa.gov/news/press_releases/news_story.cfm?newsId=13272.

45. Department of Transportation. *Summary of Hours-of-Service (HOS) Regulations*. December 27, 2011. Retrieved from Federal Motor Carrier Safety Administration (FMCSA.DOT.GOV): http://www.fmcsa.dot.gov/rules-regulations/topics/hos/index.htm.

46. Accreditation Council for Graduate Medical Education. *ACGME Duty Hours*. July 2011. http://www.acgme.org/acgmeweb/tabid/271/GraduateMedicalEducation/DutyHours.aspx.

47. Federal Aviation Administration. *AC 120-103A—Fatigue Risk Management Systems for Aviation Safety*. May 6, 2013. http://www.faa.gov/regulations_policies/advisory_circulars/index.cfm/go/document.information/documentID/1021088

48. Federal Aviation Administration. *Safety Management System*. February 5, 2010. Retrieved from Aviation Safety: http://www.faa.gov/about/initiatives/sms/.

49. Merritt A, Klinect J. *Defensive Flying for Pilots: An Introduction to Threat and Error Management*. December 12, 2006. Retrieved from FlightSafety.ORG: http://flightsafety.org/files/tem_dspt_12-6-06.pdf.

PART II

Clinical Applications

9

Adverse Event Prevention and Management

PATRICK J. GUFFEY AND MARTIN CULWICK

INTRODUCTION

"We cannot fix what we do not know."

Preventing adverse events requires an understanding of current practice, and then strategies to influence that practice so as to produce the desired result. This typically requires learning from previous adverse events or "near misses," and then adjusting the system to prevent adverse events from occurring again.

A *patient safety incident* is defined by the World Health Organization as *an event or circumstance, which could have resulted, or did result, in unnecessary harm to a patient*.[1] A *near miss* is defined as *an incident that did not reach the patient but reasonably could have*.[1,2] Most medical errors are multifactorial, and many individual errors must usually align in order to cause harm.

There are two approaches to reducing adverse events and harm to patients. The first approach is reactionary, and consists of analysis, dissection, and changes designed to prevent the same (or a similar set of) circumstances from resulting in harm. The second approach is to proactively analyze changes or systems, sometimes before they are implemented, for opportunities to improve the system and decrease the error rate. A failure mode and effects analysis (FMEA) is an example of one such tool.

FREQUENCY

It is difficult to estimate the incidence of adverse events in healthcare because of its diverse nature and because there are few comprehensive reporting systems. Standardizing the definition of an adverse event is also difficult, so estimates of adverse event rates may vary from study to study, depending upon the definition used. The US Department of Health and Human Services reported that 1 in 7 of 1 million Medicare beneficiaries discharged from the hospital (13.5%) experienced an adverse event. A study that used the ICD-10-AM code as a marker reported that 5.3% of hospital separations (when a patient leaves a hospital because of discharge, death, or transfer) were associated with an adverse event.[3] The rate of events for same-day separations was much lower than that of overnight separations (1.4%–1.8% compared with 9.4%–10.7%). Emergency admissions were also associated with a higher rate of adverse events (9.1%) than were non-emergency admissions (3.8%).

Healthcare professionals voluntarily strive to reduce adverse events with a variety of interventions, including systems changes, implementation of new technology, and the adoption of human factors principles to clinical practice. Government initiatives have been implemented with the goal of reducing adverse events, as well regulatory changes to attempt to improve safety (e.g., the Patient Safety and Quality Improvement Act of 2005).[4] Individual patients who have been harmed may pursue litigation that includes punitive damages. The extent to which this might prevent adverse events is unclear, however, and may have unintended consequences such as increasing healthcare costs and reducing voluntary event reporting.

PREVENTION

Human error is ubiquitous. Humans make mistakes—very reliably and frequently. According to the landmark Institute of Medicine report, approximately 100,000 people in the United States die each year due to preventable medical error.[5] Many of these deaths were due to human error that the system did not prevent. Several fundamental strategies can be used to decrease the probability of adverse events. The most important intervention is to create a safety culture (see Chapter 8). If the goal is to create a healthcare environment where death due to preventable errors is eliminated, the answer cannot be to eliminate human error—but rather to refine our systems such that human error cannot reach the patient.

The next step is to understand and learn from past events, which allows improvements in the system. In order to achieve these goals, there must be an effective detection mechanism, the data collected must be analyzed, and changes then must be enacted in order to prevent the recurrence of similar incidents in the future. Ensuring that the preventive mechanisms are effective requires an objective way of determining that the desired outcome has been achieved. Several methodologies can facilitate this task, but many of them provide statistics that are used to benchmark an organization and do not offer effective methods to achieve improvement.

The first step in preventing adverse events is detection and the subsequent collection of data. This initial detection is usually undertaken by one of the healthcare professionals involved in the event, or alternatively by the patient or his or her friends and family. Data may also be collected by registries, audits, incident monitoring, research, and medico-legal resources that include closed legal cases and findings of the medical examiner or pathologist. The anesthesia closed claims database, for example, contained 8954 legal settlements or court judgments as of June 2011.[6] Unfortunately, much of this "data" has failed to effectively improve outcomes. In some cases, especially events associated with minor harm, the data might be recorded in the patient record but not analyzed by the organization. Near misses might not be reported at all. It has been widely established in other industries (e.g., manufacturing) that a culture that tolerates minor adverse events may ultimately result in a major or potentially catastrophic adverse outcome.[7,8]

INCIDENT REPORTING

Voluntary incident reporting is widely used to report near misses as well as cases of harm. Voluntary reporting to a central repository can take many forms, ranging from highly complex electronic systems to a paper form. The most important element is that the system is reliably used to report cases of harm or near misses. Several studies have suggested that incident-reporting systems only capture a small subset of the data.[9–11] For instance, Cullen found that reporting of adverse drug events was highly unreliable and variable across a 1300-bed tertiary hospital.[12] Another problem associated with voluntary reporting is that healthcare professionals report events at different rates. Milch, for example, found through analysis of 92,547 reports across 26 hospitals that physicians were the least likely to report a case of harm to a patient.[13]

Despite these problems, it is possible to increase the use of reporting systems and to access this data. Systems that are well designed, easy to use, and customized to the specialty can result in higher rates of use.[10,14,15] For example, when a reporting system was customized to the needs of anesthesiologists at two major academic medical centers, reporting increased by two orders of magnitude compared to the baseline hospital system.[14] Box 9.1 (Disincentives for Reporting Adverse Events)[10,11,15–18] and Box 9.2 (Features of a Successful Incident Reporting System) illustrate some of the reasons that reporting systems are not used adequately, and methods to increase reporting.[15]

ANALYSIS

The goal of analysis is to find latent errors and system errors that might cause a problem to recur. Although human errors are a frequent component of an adverse event, there is often an underlying latent error, which then makes the human error more likely. Solving latent errors in the system is a far more effective strategy than simply trying to address the human errors.

Various tools have been used to analyze and manage hazards and incidents in healthcare,

---

BOX 9.1   DISINCENTIVES FOR REPORTING ADVERSE EVENTS

Poor education about what constitutes an event
Concern over legal or credentialing consequences
Personal shame
Fear of implicating others
Time-consuming processes
Systems that are difficult to access
Lack of anonymity
Potentially discoverable information
Slow infrastructure
Arduous, poorly designed interfaces
Lack of feedback and follow-up, no perceived value to the department

Adapted from

Leape LL, Reporting of adverse events. N Engl J Med. *2002;347(20):1633–1638.*

Taylor JA, et al., Use of incident reports by physicians and nurses to document medical errors in pediatric patients. Pediatrics. *2004;114(3):729–735.*

Guffey P, Culwick M, Merry A, Incident reporting at the local and national level. Int Anesthesiol Clin. *2014;52(1).*

Kaldjian LC, et al., Disclosing medical errors to patients: attitudes and practices of physicians and trainees. J Gen Intern Med. *2007;22(7):988–996.*

---

including forms of root cause analysis (RCA) or apparent cause analysis (ACA). The Joint Commission on Accreditation of Healthcare Organizations requires an RCA to be performed for all adverse events that reach the patient and cause severe temporary harm requiring intervention, permanent harm, or death (*sentinel events*).[19] The relationship between hazards, barriers, and incidents, which may be identified in one or more RCAs, may, however, be complex and difficult to represent in a concise manner. Moreover, root cause analysis can be very time-consuming and is not an appropriate method for analyzing the majority of events and near misses that are reported to a voluntary registry. Most important, solutions that are proposed to prevent recurrence of the event may not be robust, and follow-up of their impact is rare.[20] A number of cognitive aids have been developed to show the causes of an incident, including the use of

---

BOX 9.2   FEATURES OF A SUCCESSFUL INCIDENT REPORTING SYSTEM

Secure and non-discoverable data
Quick entry time (less than one minute) and ease of use
Accessibility of the system
The capture of both near misses and incidents of patient harm
An option of anonymity for near misses
Data searchable by the department QI committee
Summary reports to department and hospital

Reprinted with permission from Guffey, P, Culwick M, Merry A, Incident reporting at the local and national level. Int Anesthesiol Clin. *2014;52(1).*

causal trees.[20] The results of an RCA should ideally be depicted in a diagram, so that the accident trajectory can be understood. Diagrams for depicting the accident trajectory include the *Swiss cheese model*,[21] *causal trees*,[20] and more recently, *bow-tie diagrams*.[22,23]

Bow-Tie Diagrams and Analysis

James Reason[2] first proposed the use of diagrams showing accident trajectories; these subsequently became known as the *Swiss cheese model*.[21] The *Swiss cheese model* illustrates the path by which a hazard progresses to an incident due to an alignment of deficiencies in safety or preventive barriers. For example, a Swiss cheese diagram of intra-operative hypertension might include the potential barriers to the development of intra-operative hypertension.

Figure 9.1 shows an abstract *Swiss cheese diagram* for intra-operative hypertension. Under ideal circumstances, a number of barriers, represented by the grey slices, would prevent the risks of hypertension being propagated to an episode of intra-operative hypertension. One or more number of holes might, however, appear in these barriers, as shown on the right-hand side of the diagram, as a result of omissions or events. If all of the barriers fail, intra-operative hypertension might occur.[22] In this model, the layers of cheese represent the system, and the holes represent failure modes.

Figure 9.2 shows an example of some of the latent risks for intra-operative hypertension, as well as the barriers that might be used to prevent an incident from occurring. There are multiple potential parallel paths, each of which

would require its own Swiss cheese diagram. The Swiss cheese model cannot easily be used to guide management of the incident; this may result in incomplete analysis and resolution of the event. Although it is better to prevent an adverse event from occurring, it is important to consider the recovery component because there may still be an opportunity to avoid harm or to reduce the consequences of the adverse event by appropriate and timely management.

A causal tree and an event tree can be fused to create a *bow-tie diagram*, which pictorially takes the shape of a bow tie (Figure 9.3 a,b). The left side of the diagram is similar to multiple Swiss cheese paths and provides an easy way to represent latent risks and to associate these risks with barriers that prevent progression to a critical incident. A box at the center of the diagram, known as the Top Event, contains the name of the event that is being analyzed. The right-hand side shows the management options in the recovery controls. It also shows possible consequences that occur if the recovery controls are unable to prevent progression of the event. Each of the boxes in the diagram represents a concept and provides an overall picture of the risks, the barriers that might be deployed to avert these risks, and the management of the Top Event if these barriers are circumvented.

Although preventing future harm through a systems-based change is ideal, this may not always be possible. In some cases, prevention relies in whole or in part upon human memory, which is both imperfect and unreliable in stressful circumstances. Pictures are easier to recall for many people than protocols,

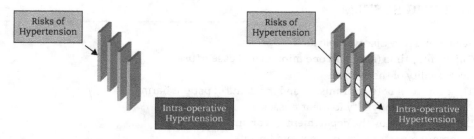

FIGURE 9.1: Swiss cheese diagram.

Adapted from Reason J, *Human Error*. New York: Cambridge University Press; 1990. Used with permission from Culwick M. Web based anaesthetic incident reporting system [WEBAIRS]: new methods to analyze and manage critical incidents (Presentation). The Australian and New Zealand Annual Scientific Meeting, Perth, Western Australia, 2012.

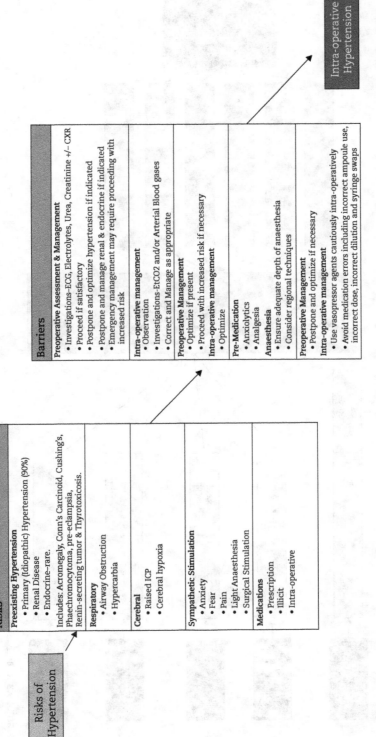

FIGURE 9.2: Latent risk diagram.

Used with permission from Culwick M. Web based anaesthetic incident reporting system [WEBAIRS]: new methods to analyze and manage critical incidents (Presentation). The Australian and New Zealand Annual Scientific Meeting, Perth, Western Australia, 2012.

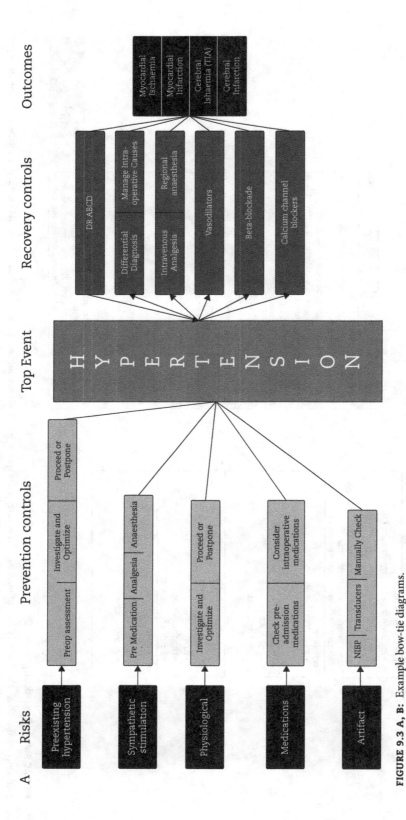

FIGURE 9.3 A, B: Example bow-tie diagrams.

Used with permission from Culwick M. Web based anaesthetic incident reporting system [WEBAIRS]: new methods to analyze and manage critical incidents (Presentation). The Australian and New Zealand Annual Scientific Meeting, Perth, Western Australia, 2012.

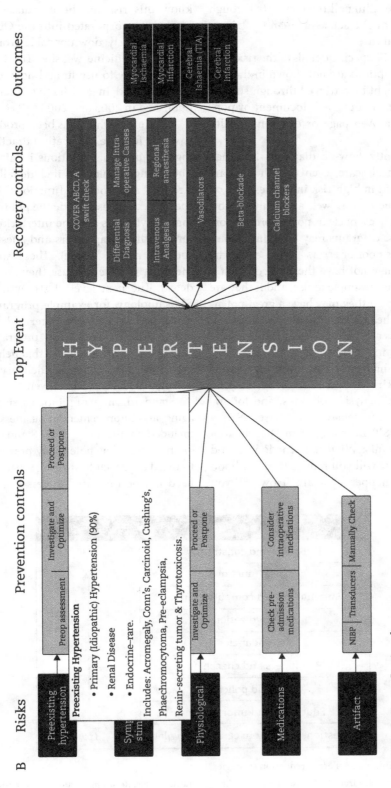

FIGURE 9.3 A, B: Continued.

however, so recalling all the concepts through the diagram might act as a memory trigger during clinical care.

Although the specific details of the risks and management options are not shown in the diagram, they might be retrieved through supplementary tables in a printed document or pop-up boxes on a Web page or electronic health record.

Until recently, bow-tie diagrams have had little use in healthcare, even though they are commonly used in high-risk industries (e.g., oil and gas production) as well as highly reliable industries such as nuclear power production. However, these diagrams may have limitations. If the design is poor or errors are present in the design, they may not have the desired result.[23] They are, however, simple to use, and if they are properly designed they may have a great potential for use in healthcare. Bow-tie diagrams can also be used as a cognitive tool in risk management, for teaching, and in clinical practice.

The Learning from Defects Tool, developed at John Hopkins Medicine in 2004, may be helpful in the analysis, solutions, and follow-up.[24] The Comprehensive Unit-Based Safety Program (CUSP) Learning from Defects Tool covers four points: What happened? Why did it happen? How will you reduce the likelihood of this defect happening again? How will you know this risk has been reduced? This tool has been incorporated into the CUSP toolkit, which is freely downloadable from the John Hopkins Medicine website. The CUSP methodology, how to use it, and how to validate it are described in articles by Peter Pronovost published in 2005 and 2006.[24,25]

Figure 9.4, which has been produced by the Institute for Safe Medication Practices, groups together potential solutions in nine themes.[26] The strongest solutions include fail-safes, constraints, and forcing functions (anesthesia-specific examples include the pin index system for gas cylinders and the interlocking controls for anesthetic vaporizers and anesthetic gases such as nitrous oxide). These solutions are the most reliable because they are difficult to defeat. The next level of strength makes use of technology, for example programmable syringe pumps and computerized medication orders. These devices and programs can include built-in safety checks that help to prevent the wrong dose, the wrong delivery rate, or the wrong drugs from being given.

Standardization of protocols, standard packaging, and improvement in business process are included in the next level. Standardization is often criticized as potentially preventing a customized approach to treating a patient, but this need not be the case. Process standardization

Error-Reduction Strategy	Power (leverage)
Fail-safes and constraints	High
Forcing functions	
Automation and computerization	
Standardization	
Redundancies	
Reminders and checklists	
Rules and policies	
Education and information	
Suggestions to be more careful or vigilant	Low

FIGURE 9.4: Rank-order of error-reduction strategies.

Reprinted with permission from the Institute for Safe Medication Practices, 2006. Report medication errors or near misses to the ISMP Medication Errors Reporting Program (MERP) at 1-800-FAIL-SAF(E) or online at www.ismp.org.

can be considered as consistent delivery of a particular method or therapy so that the team is familiar with the equipment that might be required and the steps of the process.

Checklists and double-check systems should in theory be a strong process, but they require that the staff be focused and careful when they are used. It is also possible that routine violations might compromise the effectiveness of checklist and double-check systems.

Rules and policies are often perceived as protecting the organization while doing little to prevent adverse events because the rule or policy is seldom integrated at the point of care. Healthcare systems typically have a large number of rules and policies. Moreover, it is too difficult for the average person to recall from memory all of the rules and policies that might apply to the task at hand. In order to be effective, rules and policies should be combined with a standardized process or a computerized system that either educates or informs the user at the point of care. Forcing functions are ideal if they are clinically possible.

Education and information can help to prevent adverse events in the short term. As time passes and memories fade, however, the message might be forgotten unless ongoing efforts are made to reinforce them.

Simply telling a person to be more vigilant is the least effective way to improve safety, for several reasons. This method assumes that the person who was involved in an event was not being vigilant. Telling someone to be more careful implies that someone was to blame and therefore ignores latent factors; this is antithetical to a good safety culture. If a person was involved in an adverse event, he or she is likely to be inherently vigilant in the future and possibly overcautious. Finally, this method does not necessarily inform anyone else who was not directly involved, and may suffer from the same memorability issues as rules and policies. Unfortunately, rules, policies and telling people to be more vigilant are the most common methods employed because they are inexpensive and easy to deploy.

Planning is the next practical step in preventing adverse events because it facilitates anticipation of a possible adverse event, allowing a practitioner to formulate a plan to avoid it. Planning might include a written treatment plan when the patient is first admitted to a hospital and a verbal briefing or time-out before starting a procedure in the operating room. A plan should include not only an outline of desired steps, but one or more contingency plans that deal with possible deviations from the desired course. The main plan and contingencies are often named Plan A, Plan B, Plan C, and so on. A plan should be discussed for each adverse event that might be likely to occur during a high-risk procedure.

MANAGEMENT

Management of an adverse event can be split into the four phases of mitigation, immediate management, refractory management, and follow-up. The knowledge and skills used to manage these four phases may either be tacit or codified. *Tacit knowledge* is defined as something that is difficult to write down or explain. This might apply to knowledge such as "what do you do when the oxygen saturation falls?" There may be multiple subconscious reactions learned by experienced anesthesia professionals that are based on other factors (e.g., the type of procedure, recent events, and other abnormal parameters). This may be difficult to write down or explain as an algorithm. Alternatively, there may be tacit or learned skills that require dexterity, such as laryngoscopy or vascular access in a patient with poor veins. *Explicit knowledge* is defined as knowledge that can be easily expressed or verbalized. Examples of explicit knowledge include an algorithm for managing a difficult airway or a checklist for desaturation. Cognitive aids such as mnemonics, algorithms, diagrams, and emergency manuals can be used in the management of a critical event, while guidelines might assist with follow-up after the adverse event.

Mitigation

Mitigation is the management of an ongoing adverse event to prevent or minimize harm to the patient. The response depends on the urgency of the situation. It is sometimes possible to start mitigating an adverse event when warning signs of an impending crisis first appear. An adverse event that does not reach the patient because of early mitigation is defined as a *near miss*.

A good plan can help the professional to anticipate an adverse event, and also enables him or her to determine that there has been a deviation from the plan that requires further action. This in turn allows the contingency plan to be activated. As a result, an impending adverse event can be recognized more quickly, and a pre-formulated contingency plan invoked to mitigate further development of the incident. This may not prevent the adverse event from occurring, but it may help to mitigate the severity of the outcome.

Consider, for example, unanticipated hemorrhage during a surgical procedure. During the pre-procedure briefing, the surgeon indicates that the expected blood loss will be less than 500 cc, so there was no need for a type and cross. If the surgical blood loss exceeds 500 cc and the bleeding is not under control, a blood sample should be sent for blood type and screen. If then the blood loss exceeds 1000 cc, the appropriate blood components should be cross-matched. When blood loss exceeds 2000 cc or the hemoglobin level falls below a predetermined value, transfusion could be considered. Finally, if blood loss is greater than the patient's circulating blood volume, the massive transfusion protocol is initiated. The precise triggers should be set for an individual patient while the concept is that of escalating the care and management.

Mitigation often involves the immediate application of tacit knowledge and often begins even before a working diagnosis is made. The mnemonic *CAB* is commonly used to guide the initial management of a critical event. CAB is well known and stands for *circulation, airway*, and *breathing*. This involves determining cardiac and perfusion status, checking that the airway is clear, managing airway obstruction, and checking that ventilation is adequate. This mnemonic has been extended to include additional steps, becoming DR ABCD. The *D* of *DR* is checking for and managing any danger to the responder or the patient. The *R* directs the

clinician to check for a patient response (i.e., gentle shaking and shouting to see if there is a response) The last *D* of DR ABCD is to check for drugs (prescribed or otherwise) as a cause of the event.

In summary, mitigation usually involves three steps. Attempting to prevent the event from getting any worse, attempting to improve the situation, and making a diagnosis so that further management can be targeted to a specific cause.

Immediate Management

This step follows mitigation and starts with the targeted management of a presumed diagnosis. The word *presumed* is used because the mode of presentation of the event might lead to an incorrect working diagnosis. This is not a reflection on the skill or decision-making of the responder, merely an acknowledgment that it is often not possible to make the correct diagnosis until the event has evolved. During the initial management, therefore, one must accept that initial pathways might not be ideal. Until a definitive diagnosis is made (and possibly even afterward), the responder should be aware of alternative possibilities and be prepared to change the working diagnosis.

Anaphylaxis provides a good example of the need to continually evaluate the working diagnosis. This event may initially present with bronchospasm, and the bronchospasm might be treated according to a specific management protocol,[27] but other causes of bronchospasm should be considered and excluded while this treatment is commenced. At the first stage of bronchospasm the blood pressure might be normal; the patient might eventually reach a second stage and become hypotensive. The working diagnosis of anaphylaxis is made and treatment is begun. If, however, the patient becomes more difficult to ventilate, a final diagnosis of tension pneumothorax might then be considered, which takes into account the bronchospasm, the fall in blood pressure, and the progressive difficulty in ventilation. In a different situation, the correct diagnosis might be either bronchospasm or anaphylaxis, but this example highlights the importance of keeping an open mind during the immediate management of an adverse event.

Refractory Management

Refractory management begins after the initial management fails to produce the desired response or fails to control the progression of the adverse event. If a "call for extra help" has not already been made, this is the stage where consultation or "calling for help" is appropriate or possibly mandatory. Management strategies or interventions are escalated, while at the same time alternative diagnoses are considered. Escalation might include more aggressive use of the current therapies or the introduction of more powerful therapies. If they have not already been placed, invasive monitoring devices could be inserted and further investigations could be performed. Refractory management might include transfer to an intensive care unit and ongoing management over several days. A good example for the refractory management of anaphylaxis is available from the Australian and New Zealand Anaesthetic Allergy Group (ANZAAG).[28]

Follow-up

This includes follow-up and management of the residual clinical conditions, learning from outcomes, improvements in patient safety, risk management, and medico-legal considerations. The most important follow-up is reporting to an event registry because this can trigger studies that lead to prevention of the initial event. The reporting may be through an incident report, morbidity and mortality process, or other means—but a sign of a strong safety culture is that cases of harm or near misses are always reported and evaluated for improvement.

SUMMARY

Adverse events are an unfortunate reality of caring for patients in our current healthcare system. Preventing and mitigating these events is an important part of quality improvement. First, an understanding of the events and how often they are occurring is critical to planning improvements. Incident reporting systems are one way of gathering this information. Then,

events should be categorized and analyzed for improvement. The bow-tie diagram is one tool for this purpose. Interventions should be chosen that are the most effective, such as forcing functions and standardization. Once an event has occurred, there are four phases to management. A clear understanding of each of these phases will allow for the best result. Consideration should be given to the caregivers as well as the patient when managing and resolving adverse events.

- Preventing adverse events starts with an understanding of current practice, and then considers strategies to influence that practice to the desired result.
- Incident reporting is the most common way to track adverse events.
- Prevention requires strong analysis of events and recognition of both latent (system) and human causes.
- Interventions have different degrees of effectiveness, ranging from highly effective forcing functions, to marginally effective encouraging statements.
- There are four steps to event management: mitigation, immediate management, refractory management, and follow-up.

REFERENCES

1. Conceptual Framework for the international classification for patient safety. WHO/IER/PSP/2010.2. January 2009, pp. 21–24. http://www.who.int/patientsafety/taxonomy/icps_full_report.pdf.
2. Reason J. *Human Error.* New York: Cambridge University Press; 1990.
3. Australian Institute of Health and Welfare. Hospital performance: adverse events treated in hospitals. 2015. http://www.aihw.gov.au/haag11-12/adverse-events/.
4. *The Patient Safety and Quality Improvement Act of 2005.* Rockville, MD: Agency for Healthcare Research and Quality; 2008.
5. Kohn LT, Corrigan J, Donaldson MS. *To Err Is Human: Building a Safer Health System.* Washington, DC: National Academy Press; 2000.
6. Metzner J, et al. Closed claim's analysis. *Best Pract Res Clin Anaesthesiol.* 2011 Jun;25(2):263–276.
7. Heinrich HW. *Industrial Accident Prevention: A Scientific Approach.* New York: McGraw-Hill; 1950.

8. Bird F, Germain G. *Loss Control Management: Practical Loss Control Leadrship*. Det Norske Veritas; 1996.

9. Kaldjian LC, et al., Disclosing medical errors to patients: attitudes and practices of physicians and trainees. *J Gen Intern Med*. 2007;22(7):988–996.

10. Leape LL. Reporting of adverse events. *N Engl J Med*. 2002;347(20):1633–1638.

11. Taylor JA, et al. Use of incident reports by physicians and nurses to document medical errors in pediatric patients. *Pediatrics*. 2004;114(3): 729–735.

12. Cullen DJ, et al. The incident reporting system does not detect adverse drug events: a problem for quality improvement. *Jt Comm J Qual Improv*. 1995;21(10):541–548.

13. Milch CE, et al. Voluntary electronic reporting of medical errors and adverse events: an analysis of 92,547 reports from 26 acute care hospitals. *J Gen Intern Med*. 2006;21(2):165–170.

14. Guffey P, et al. Design and implementation of a near-miss reporting system at a large, academic pediatric anesthesia department. *Paediatr Anaesth*. 2011;21(7):810–814.

15. Guffey P, Culwick M, Merry A. Incident reporting at the local and national level. *Int Anesthesiol Clin*. 2014;52(1).

16. Rowin EJ, et al. Does error and adverse event reporting by physicians and nurses differ? *Jt Comm J Qual Patient Saf*. 2008;34(9):537–545.

17. Kaldjian LC, et al. Reporting medical errors to improve patient safety: a survey of physicians in teaching hospitals. *Arch Intern Med*. 2008; 168(1):40–46.

18. Kaldjian LC, et al. Disclosing medical errors to patients: attitudes and practices of physicians and trainees. *J Gen Intern Med*. 2007; 22(7):988–996.

19. Williams PM. Techniques for root cause analysis. *Proceedings (Baylor Univ Med Center)*. 2001;14(2):154–157.

20. Wu AW, Lipshutz AK, Pronovost PJ. Effectiveness and efficiency of root cause analysis in medicine. *JAMA*. 2008 Feb 13;299(6):685–687.

21. Reason J. Human error: models and management. *BMJ*. 2000 Mar 18;320(7237):768–770.

22. Culwick M. Web based anaesthetic incident reporting system [WEBAIRS]: new methods to analyze and manage critical incidents (Presentation). The Australian and New Zealand Annual Scientific Meeting, Perth, Western Australia, 2012.

23. Pitblado R, Weijand P. Barrier diagram (bow tie) quality issues for operating managers. *Proc Safety Prog*. 2014;33:355–361. doi: 10.1002/prs.11666.

24. Pronovost PJ, et al. A practical tool to learn from defects in patient care. *Jt Comm J Qual Patient Saf*. 2006 Feb;32(2):102–108.

25. Pronovost PJ, et al. Implementing and validating a comprehensive unit-based safety program. *J Patient Saf*. 2005 Mar;1(1).

26. Institute for Safe Medication Practices. https://www.ismp.org/newsletters/ambulatory/archives/200602_4.asp.

27. Looseley A. Management of bronchspasm during general anesthesia. *Updates Anaesth*. 2011;18–21. http://e-safe anaesthesia.org/e_library/14/Bronchospasm_during_anaesthesia_Update_2011.pdf.

28. Australian and New Zealand Anaesthetic Allergy Group (ANZAAG). Management Resources. http://www.anzaag.com/Mgmt%20Resources.aspx.

10

Complex Systems and Approaches to Quality Improvement

LOREN RISKIN AND ALEX MACARIO

Change is not made without inconvenience, even from worse to better.

—RICHARD HOOKER (1554–1600)

INTRODUCTION

Physicians and other perioperative caregivers always try to provide safe and high-quality care, so an event that causes harm or an adverse outcome is often doubly challenging for the clinician. Despite everyone's best intentions, unsafe, inefficient or low quality care does occur.[1] Improving healthcare has proven to be a challenging task that requires the introspection and dedication of all providers and institutions, as well as the design and implementation of programs to ensure high-quality, safe patient care.

This chapter explains the science behind quality improvement (QI) initiatives, beginning with a discussion of the ultimate goals of this movement. It will then briefly cover the history of QI development, the universal elements of a successful QI project, and barriers to systems and individual change. The chapter then concludes with an explanation of quality measurement, frequently used quality measurement tools, and anesthesia-specific applications.

THE GOALS OF PATIENT SAFETY AND QUALITY IMPROVEMENT

Healthcare quality has been defined as "the degree to which health services for individuals and populations increase the likelihood of desired health outcomes and are consistent with current professional knowledge"[2] (Box 10.1).

The Institute of Medicine's (IOM) landmark publication in 1999, *To Err Is Human: Building a Safer Health System*, estimated that between 44,000 and 98,000 Americans die annually from preventable medical error. More recent estimates suggest that there are approximately 564,000 annual inpatient injuries in the United States alone (1.5% of all inpatient admissions)[3] with 210,000 to 400,00 errors contributing to premature death.[4] The subsequent IOM report, *Crossing the Quality Chasm: A New Health System for the 21st Century*, laid out the following six aims for improvement in healthcare.[6] Care should be

1. *Safe*: in addition to being the intention of the caregiver, safety must be designed into the system to avoid injuries to patients from care that is intended to help them.
2. *Effective*: care should not overuse or underuse services and should align with the best available scientific knowledge.
3. *Patient centered*: care should be respectful of and responsive to an individual patient's culture, values, social context, and specific needs.
4. *Timely*: care should be given in an appropriate time frame, without unintended or detrimental delays.
5. *Efficient*: the system should seek to reduce unnecessary waste of supplies,

---

BOX 10.1   COMMON TERMS AND THEIR DEFINITIONS

Quality of care—the degree to which healthcare services for individuals and populations increase the likelihood of desired health outcomes and are consistent with current professional knowledge.[5]

Efficacy—the extent to which a specific drug or treatment works under the best possible conditions; the ability to produce a desired or intended result.

Efficiency—a measure of whether healthcare resources are being used to get the best value for money. It is the ratio of the output to the inputs of any system. An efficient system or person is one who achieves higher levels of performance (outcome, output) relative to the inputs (resources, time, money) consumed.

Patient safety—the prevention of errors and adverse effects to patients associated with healthcare.

Value—healthcare outcomes achieved per dollar spent.

Source: Porter ME, Teisberg EO. Redefining Health Care: Creating Value-Based Competition on Results. Boston: Harvard Business School Press, 2006.

---

equipment, capital, ideas, time, or opportunities.

6. *Equitable*: care should not discriminate or be variable based on race, ethnicity, gender, location, or socioeconomic status.

Accordingly, patient safety is a single, albeit complex, part of overall healthcare quality. Indeed, patient safety and overall quality improvement are closely related, and substantial overlap can blur distinctions between the fields. Although the concept of value is not included directly in the Institute of Medicine's goals for improvement, it is an inherent component of both effective and efficient care. *Value* is the quality of healthcare divided by the cost of care provided. Highly effective healthcare can still be of low value if cost is increased by inefficiencies in the system. Although they are inherently different, patient safety, quality improvement, and value are all aligned goals within healthcare, and measures designed to improve one goal will be successful when they also improve the others.

A BRIEF HISTORY OF QUALITY IMPROVEMENT

Medical professionals have long focused on improving the lives of individual patients, but it took time to adopt the widespread systemic changes necessary to ensure better outcomes across populations. Several successful examples of individuals pioneering widespread healthcare change exist in the 1800s. Florence Nightingale, for example, was an English nurse who linked unsanitary conditions in an Istanbul hospital to wounded soldiers' mortality. By instituting measures such as hand washing, instrument sanitization, and regular linen laundering, mortality decreased from 60% to 1%. Still, formal approaches to quality improvement did not develop until the twentieth century.

Dr. Earnest Codman, a surgeon at Massachusetts General Hospital in the early twentieth century, is considered the father of modern quality improvement in healthcare. He was the first to institute a regular Morbidity and Mortality conference, he started the first bone tumor registry in the United States, and he initiated a three-step approach to quality assurance called the "End Results System of Hospitalization Standardization Program." Tracking individual patients on pocket cards, Codman used measures to evaluate problems with patients, the healthcare system, or clinicians, and suggested means of preventing recurring bad outcomes. He believed that physicians should follow every patient long enough to determine whether treatment had been successful and should then use this information to guide treatment decisions in the future. In 1914, his hospital rejected Codman's plan for evaluating clinicians and terminated his privileges, at which time he founded his own hospital. He published the outcomes of his personal practice in book form and remained a fervent supporter of transparency and outcomes tracking.

Although Codman's efforts to track and improve outcomes "brought him mostly ridicule, poverty and censure"[6] during his lifetime, his End Results System was adopted by the American College of Surgeons, which used his ideas to establish minimum standards for hospitals. The current system of hospital accreditation in the United States, the Joint Commission (formerly the Joint Commission on Accreditation of Healthcare Organizations [JHACO], founded in 1951), was a direct result of Codman's work. Although he received little recognition for his contributions during his lifetime, Codman is now recognized as the first person to implement healthcare outcomes management.

Quality improvement in medicine was then further defined from outside the field in the following decades. While Codman focused largely on poor outcomes and departure from standards on the part of individuals, American industry began to recognize the importance of the institution in creating consistent quality. Standardization and consistency began to replace price as the predominant determinant of sales and competition. W. Edwards Deming and his forerunner Walter Shewhart, both physicists, sought to increase the efficiency of industry through the standardization and streamlining of manufacturing processes, error opportunity reduction, data-driven change, and a cultural commitment to improvement[7] (Box 10.2). Deming developed a System of Profound Knowledge that consisted of the following four components, designed to aid the understanding of key aspects of any system requiring change:

BOX 10.2   W. EDWARD DEMING'S 14 POINTS

1. Create constancy of purpose toward improvement of product and service.
2. Adopt the new philosophy.
3. Cease dependence on inspection to achieve quality. Eliminate the need for inspection on a mass basis by building quality into the product in the first place.
4. End the practice of awarding business on price alone; instead, minimize total cost by working with a single supplier, building loyalty and trust.
5. Improve constantly and forever every process or planning, production, and service.
6. Institute training on the job.
7. Adopt and institute leadership; the aim of supervision should be to help people and tools do a better job.
8. Drive out fear, so that everyone may work effectively for the company.
9. Break down barriers between staff areas, so that people may work as a team.
10. Eliminate slogans, exhortations, and targets for the workforce asking for zero defects. Eliminate work standards (quotas) and management by numeric goals; substitute leadership.
11. Remove barriers that rob the hourly worker of his [or her] right to pride of workmanship.
12. Remove barriers that rob people in management and in engineering of their right to pride of workmanship. Abolish the annual rating system.
13. Institute a vigorous program of education and self-improvement.
14. Put everybody in the company to work to accomplish the transformation.

Reprinted with permission from Deming WE, Out of the Crisis, pp. 23–24, © 2000 Massachusetts Institute of Technology, by permission of The MIT Press.

1. An appreciation of a system;
2. An understanding of variation;
3. The psychology of change;
4. A theory of knowledge.

Deming and Shewhart suggested a continuous cycle of improvement, linking change to outcome evaluation and reaction. Deming's work is credited with creating the post–World War II economic boom in Japan and revolutionizing international manufacturing and business. Healthcare gradually adopted these elements of system change, as they were shown to be successful in other industries, and as the need for healthcare improvement became increasingly apparent.

In 1966, Dr. Avedis Donabedian, a physician dedicated to the study of healthcare quality, published "Evaluating the Quality of Medical Care."[8] This seminal article described a replicable model relying on the study of structure, process, and outcomes to determine the quality of care provided. Donabedian posited that quality can be measured based on who provides care (structure), what care is provided and how (process), and the end results of treatment (outcomes). Quality was viewed not just as a matter of technical or clinical skill, but also as a function of culture, team psychology, and leadership. His model was widely accepted and has become a crucial component of later efforts to improve quality of care.

A multitude of both broad-reaching and field-specific healthcare agencies and institutions have emerged over the last 50 years. The Institute of Medicine (IOM) was established by the National Academies of Science in 1970 and is dedicated to evaluating and improving healthcare in the United States. The Agency of Healthcare Research and Quality (AHRQ, formerly the Agency for Health Care Policy and Research) was established in 1989 by the Department of Health and Human Services to examine trends in misuse and overuse of care and to make recommendations for equitable care guidelines. AHRQ currently develops programs with a goal of increasing healthcare safety, access, efficiency, and affordability.

The National Committee for Quality Assurance (NCQA) is another organization that measures healthcare quality. Founded in 1990, NCQA manages physician, health plan, and medical group accreditation using standards developed around many of Deming's ideas. They published the first Health Plan Report Card in 1993, using data from the Healthcare Effectiveness Data and Information Set. This publication was the first to compare the effectiveness of delivered care on a health-plan level.

The need for quality improvement and patient safety in healthcare has become pressing over the last several decades, resulting in significant growth in the number and size of contributing organizations. Founded in 1984, the Anesthesia Patient Safety Foundation (APSF) was the first medical specialty organization to focus specifically on patient safety. Its mission was that "no patient shall be harmed by anesthesia." The National Patient Safety Foundation (NPSF) was created in 1996, with the goal of partnering with patients and families to advance patient safety and healthcare worker safety, "thereby creating a world where patients and those who care for them are free of harm" through education and research support. In 1991, the Institute of Healthcare Improvement (IHI) was founded, focused on cultivating and disseminating ideas in patient safety through leadership training and education. The National Quality Forum (NQF) was created in 1999 and is geared toward defining, measuring, and reporting on healthcare quality in the United States. The NQF is most widely known for listing 27 "never events" (e.g., an operation being performed on the wrong patient) and 30 "safe practices" (e.g., standardized abbreviations) that are commonly used as indicators of quality and safe practice.

Quality improvement and patient safety continue to play prominent roles in the national and international healthcare landscape. Although healthcare began as a "cottage industry" with individual practice patterns guiding treatment, it has grown into a highly complex system, encompassing large corporations that provide a wide spectrum of services.

ELEMENTS OF SUCCESSFUL QUALITY IMPROVEMENT AND PATIENT SAFETY WORK

Before addressing the various techniques used to improve quality and safety, this chapter will discuss the overarching elements that are necessary for such techniques to be successful.

The success of any QI program requires a sophisticated understanding of the current system. The prevailing culture, availability of resources, organizational structure, and beliefs of crucial individuals cannot be ignored. An institution that has not developed a culture supportive of change will not respond to sudden or drastic improvement efforts; an institution with scarce resources may not be able to implement large-scale changes or use the technological advantages that may be available to a wealthier institution; a new process that may have otherwise been successful can quickly fail if a key thought leader openly refuses to support it. Any QI initiative must therefore be individually tailored from the ground up to meet the local needs and situation of an institution or department.

A successful QI program requires a team approach. A single individual is rarely in a position to completely understand a complex healthcare system, or to have the individual relationships necessary to gain cooperation from every stakeholder. Process improvements nearly always occur across multiple fields and affect multiple groups within an institution; therefore, representation from all domains increases the chance of success. Change should ideally be driven by contributions from all levels of staff and all stakeholders. Teamwork is also required because QI efforts require creativity; complex problems nearly always have complex solutions that may affect many individuals and work processes. Developing ideas as a group and involving persons who are familiar with the environment and workflow are more likely to lead to appropriate and resourceful problem-solving, as well as adoption and compliance with the change.

Effective quality management also requires continuous review of the process that is to be improved, as well as long-term follow-up, accountability, and data-driven change. Continued monitoring and follow-up are necessary to ensure that the changes that were implemented remain in place, because compliance with new workflows and processes often decreases over time.[9] Ongoing evaluation is also important to ensure that changes lead to the desired effect and to detect unwanted consequences. Management teams should ideally use data markers and other quantified outcomes to measure objective improvement reliably. A successful QI team takes accountability for the changes made, measuring them until they have been ingrained as part of the institutional culture and workflow. These changes are ideally driven by a prospective desire for improved healthcare quality, and not a reactionary, retrospective need to correct deficient care. This chapter will cover both proactive and retroactive techniques for quality improvement, because recognizing and reacting to poor care is an important part of quality management.

IMPROVING CARE: QUALITY IMPROVEMENT VERSUS RESEARCH

Healthcare professionals seek to improve care not just for an individual patient, but for an entire population; this goal has traditionally been the purview of scientific research.[10] QI projects were rarely discussed outside institutional boundaries, but they are increasingly viewed as publishable research.[11] The recent increase in the volume of papers reporting the results of QI projects stems from both the traditional motivation of faculty to publish and institutional pressures to demonstrate excellence in order to increase market share, to facilitate accreditation, and to secure funding.

The growing emphasis on QI research has blurred the distinctions between quality improvement and scientific clinical research. Both use patient data to answer important questions about patient disease states and healthcare processes, analyzing data with the ultimate goal of improving patient care and outcomes. Data may be acquired in the same fashion, whether a project is intended for research or QI. Publication aids in the dissemination of ideas and the repeatability of results, and allows authors the benefits of carefully processing their work. Despite these similarities, it is critical to determine at the beginning whether a given project is intended to be quality improvement or scientific research. Failure to distinguish between the two during the design phases of a project may ultimately prevent the results from being used in the manner intended and may preclude publication if appropriate consent was not obtained.[12] A QI project may be considered to be research when it involves a change in practice, affects patients and assesses their outcomes, employs randomization or blinding, or exposes patients to additional risks.[13]

QI has historically been differentiated from research by the intent behind the work. Quality improvement projects in the first half of the twentieth century were limited to retrospective attempts to understand why a mishap had occurred and to prevent a future occurrence. In contrast, most research projects gathered data with a prospective, double-blinded clinical trial. The US government has defined research as "systematic investigation … designed to develop or contribute to generalizable knowledge" about health and healthcare.[14] QI projects are undertaken to improve current processes; they are "an assessment, conducted by or for a QI organization, of a patient care problem for the purpose of improving patient care through peer analysis, intervention, resolution of the problem and follow-up."[15] QI projects seek to gather confidential data intended for internal review, whereas data produced by research is anonymized and generally published in a scientific journal. As a result, QI initiatives have traditionally not been subject to the same oversight requirements as scientific research and are often exempt from internal review board (IRB) approval and patient consent (Table 10.1).

TABLE 10.1. COMPARISON OF TRADITIONAL QUALITY IMPROVEMENT VERSUS TRADITIONAL RESEARCH (RANDOMIZED CLINICAL TRIAL)

Standard Research	Quality Improvement
Treatment is assigned to the patient at random.	Treatment is selected by the physician-patient care team for best outcome.
A group is assigned control status to establish treatment effects.	No control or placebo group, though a retrospective analysis may be done to establish gains or control for baseline variations.
Participants and caregivers are blinded as to which treatment patients receive, if any.	Participants and caregivers are aware of the individual treatment given and its possible effects and side effects.
Informed consent and internal review board approval are mandatory.	Informed consent and internal review board approval are generally not necessary.
Outcomes are analyzed in a blinded fashion.	Outcomes are evaluated in the context of known treatment modalities.
Data are often derived from multiple organizations.	Data are organization specific.
Goal of advancing scientific knowledge and extrapolating or generalizing to larger patient groups	Scope specific to local problem through local process improvement with goal of decreasing negative outcomes
Typical dissemination is attempted to the national or global scientific community.	Typical dissemination is attempted at a unit or institutional level.
Develops new interventions	Applies interventions into practice
Not a necessary requirement for existence as a healthcare system; limited to research institutions	Crucial component of caregiving in every healthcare institution

Quality improvement is adaptive over time; it does not follow rigid protocols, but instead is responsive to data as it becomes available. QI projects are designed around the needs of the host institution. QI is an essential, necessary component of care for a healthcare organization, whereas scientific research is not an inherent requirement. Despite these differences, however, it can be difficult to draw a sharp line between research and QI because both may target groups of patients for selective changes, with the goal of overall health improvement. Although there is no globally accepted standard to determine which types of projects fall into a given category, some guidelines do exist,[16,17] and the threshold for consulting an IRB or ethics board should be low.

BARRIERS TO HEALTHCARE CHANGE

There are substantial hurdles to creating meaningful change at the institutional and individual levels within the healthcare professions. Changing organizational behavior is always a difficult task, and it is particularly challenging in healthcare because of the complexity of the system and the number and educational levels of the stakeholders. In order to manage a QI project successfully, it is important to first identify the barriers to change (Box 10.3).

Quality improvement must be incorporated into the culture of a healthcare system. An organization that does not hold quality and safety among its core values is unlikely to foster an environment of improvement, regardless of the dedication of individual staff. Institutional interest and dedication to continuous quality improvement and patient safety create a culture of meaningful change. Institutions must have a structure in place through which to assess the safety and efficiency of healthcare processes and establish availability of both resources and leadership. The ability to collect and analyze data in a systematic fashion is critical to removing barriers to QI projects and to assessing the effectiveness of change. The availability of resources is not in and of itself sufficient to create quality, but an organization that does not dedicate at least some personnel or funds toward improvement has little hope of success. Similarly, improvement projects that lack strong, local administrative backing, visible champions, and long-term follow-up are unlikely to succeed. Moreover, most individuals find change difficult on a personal level; most diets fail, as do many improvement initiatives. Traditional methods of spurring behavioral change in healthcare professionals, such as requiring increased vigilance or compliance with a new treatment algorithm, have largely failed.[18] Thousands of new treatment recommendations that are intended to

---

BOX 10.3   BARRIERS TO INSTITUTIONAL CHANGE

Lack of resources (such as dedicated improvement personnel, equipment, funds), or a hesitancy to utilize such resources

Lack of strong, local leadership engagement or support

Undervaluing quality and safety as core values

Cultural complacency, lack of motivation for change

Skepticism from staff or leadership

Insufficient emphasis on importance or use of measures

Overloaded workforce

Uncertain roles or structure within improvement and safety projects, a lack of accountability

Poor communication or an inability to convey expectations

Lack of a structure through which to assess the safety and efficiency of healthcare processes

Lack of awareness of deficits

Inability to collect and analyze data in a systematic fashion.

improve care quality and safety have been developed, yet there is little data to support that publication in peer-reviewed journals alone leads to change in practice. Healthcare practitioners will not initiate or maintain improvements to care unless they can overcome personal barriers; these must be identified before they can be effectively removed.

Barriers to individual change include the following:

- lack of awareness of guidelines or clear expectations;
- lack of motivation;
- lack of personal accountability;
- lack of available data or evidence that new changes will be positive;
- lack of sufficient skills;
- lack of resources, including time or bandwidth.

Each stakeholder must understand what needs to be changed and why; it is difficult to sustain successful change without being aware of the pertinent deficits. Overcoming resistance to change requires objective data or anecdotal evidence that the current process has deficiencies. Motivating factors may be internal, such as the drive and desire to provide excellent care, or external, through the use of incentives for achieving certain benchmarks or penalties for failing to do so. Individuals must believe that the change will create value or benefit, and they must be provided with a means of successfully changing their practice or workflow, commensurate with their abilities. Support from peers or an initiative champion is often necessary.

There are many approaches that can be used to identify and overcome barriers to change, which have met with variable and sometimes unpredictable degrees of success.[19] Brainstorming can be used to identify potential barriers, while real or perceived barriers can be discovered through observations, surveys, interviews, and audits. Implementation efforts can then be directly targeted at specific barriers, for example, by providing additional educational resources or training if a lack of guideline awareness is present, or by

appointing a prominent champion if there is a perceived lack of leadership.

SELECTED TOOLS TO EXAMINE AND MITIGATE RISK

Institutions and individual departments can use a variety of tools to examine and mitigate the risk of patient harm. A specific strategy is ideally based on specific circumstances, including the ability to access data, whether a retrospective or prospective approach is required, the availability of resources, and the familiarity of personnel with the chosen technique.

Informal Approaches

Improvement processes have historically been approached in an ad hoc fashion that does not use formal scientific methodology as part of the attempt to change organizational and professional behavior. Trial and error, adopting another healthcare professional's or institution's success, and a top-down institutional mandate are the three most commonly used unscientific approaches to manage change.

Just as healthcare looks for data- and evidence-driven medicine rather than a trial and error approach to care, it also has moved away from trial and error as an improvement method. Trial and error offers several advantages: its informal nature allows quick, flexible change, and it is often used by personnel at the point of care who are most familiar with that component of the system. Approaches developed by trial and error are not systematically measured, however, which can hinder an institution's ability to learn from both positive and negative changes. Improvement by trial and error precludes building knowledge about the system, which in turn decreases the ability to measure change and to learn from mistakes.

Adopting a QI practice that has been developed by another practitioner or institution is common throughout the healthcare industry. Medical training has historically been constructed as an apprenticeship, in which clinicians learn to care for patients by observing and then imitating senior physicians. It is, therefore, not surprising that many institutions have sought to improve the quality of care by importing the techniques and practices of other, more successful hospitals. Although this technique may be effective, it also fails to take into account the foundations for success at the institution that developed the practice. If, for example, a given hospital has demonstrated improved rates of hand hygiene by placing sanitizing gel in convenient locations, simply mimicking this practice may not necessarily increase hand washing at a different hospital. The successful hospital might have had fewer available sinks, while the second hospital did not educate providers about hand hygiene or had a poorly developed culture of safety. An effective response to a quality deficit requires an individualized analysis of the root cause of the problem, which facilitates a targeted intervention.

Many institutional and national mandates serve as the basis for ongoing patient safety and QI initiatives. Institutional mandates that are developed and enforced by managers are rarely sufficient to create sustained improvement in practice. Institutional mandates can be imposed on a wide scale, but are unlikely to be effective without the appropriate engagement of QI leaders and an understanding of barriers to change. For example, hand hygiene has been the prominent focus of many top-down mandates, and every healthcare professional understands that hand washing prevents infections, but overall compliance has not reached target rates. A new guideline or policy that is developed and implemented without determining the barriers to success is unlikely to result in prolonged quality improvement or safety change.

In more recent years, QI methods "generally emphasize the importance of identifying a process with less-than-ideal outcomes, measuring the key performance attributes, using careful analysis to devise a new approach, integrating the redesigned approach with the process, and reassessing performance to determine if the change in process is successful."[20] As improvement methods have transitioned from quality assurance into the science of quality improvement, more formalized methods of evaluating and creating systems improvement have emerged. Some of the most common— Deming's System of Profound Knowledge and the Model for Improvement, Lean, Six Sigma, Healthcare Failure Modes and Effects Analysis, and Root Cause Analysis—will now be examined in more detail.

Deming's System of Profound Knowledge and the Model for Improvement

W. Edwards Deming, one of the fathers of improvement science, described a System of Profound Knowledge, components of systems knowledge that create the foundation for improvement.[21] These components include *appreciation of a system, knowledge of variation, theory of knowledge,* and *psychology.*

- *Appreciation of a system* requires a thorough understanding of an organization as an interconnected system with many stakeholders. By viewing improvement in the context of an entire interdependent system, rather than as individual disconnected or discrete departments and individuals, the institution can work as a whole toward a shared aim.
- *Knowledge of variation* is the understanding of the range and the causes of variation in a process. Variation can be due to *common causes* that are inherent variations within the system, or *special causes* that are external and uncontrollable. Understanding whether common or special causes are responsible for variation allows improvement leaders to target only that variation over which they have influence.
- *Theory of knowledge* requires that personnel who lead improvement projects test their theories and hypotheses to develop a better understanding of the system. Change is more likely to result in improvement when leaders have experience and knowledge of the area they wish to change.

- *Psychology* requires that those involved in process improvement understand the concepts of human nature and how human psychology creates incentives and barriers to change. Improvement leaders should understand the people who are involved in the process, including how they may react to or resist change, and should use individual differences to optimize their approaches. Deming was largely opposed to more common incentives, such as bonuses and merit ratings, and instead focused on intrinsic motivators, including pride in quality performance and teamwork.

Deming drew from the work of his colleague Walter Shewhart while developing the System of Profound Knowledge. He also developed the Plan-Do-Study-Act cycle,[22] which was incorporated into the Model for Improvement by Associates in Process Improvement.[23]

The Model for Improvement (Figure 10.1) is a straightforward and simple tool that is divided into two parts and has been used successfully in healthcare improvement.[24] In the first part, three fundamental questions are asked:

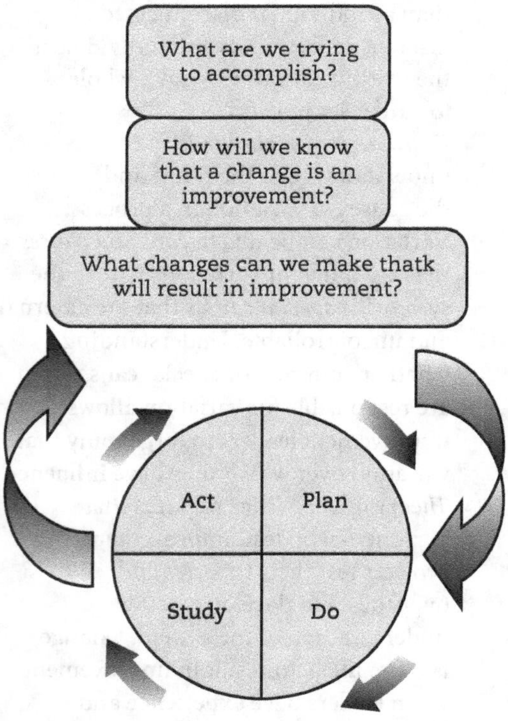

1. *Aim*: What are we trying to accomplish? An aim statement should be specific, identifying how much improvement is needed, when, and who will work toward it. For example, "We will reduce our central line infection rates" is not as effective as "We will reduce our central line-associated bloodstream infection (CLABSI) rates in our cardiac intensive care unit by 90% in the next 8 months."

2. *Measures*: How will a change be identified as an improvement? Measurement is a crucial step in QI to determine that changes are achieving the stated aims. Improvement projects rely on the following three types of measures: *outcomes measures*, which directly indicate the quality of the process being examined; *process measures*, which are surrogate markers for quality; and *balance measures*, which indicate that a change is having unintended consequences. From the preceding example, the incidence of CLABSI would be an outcome measure, daily documentation of the indication for a central line or total number of central line days could be process measures, and time spent on central venous catheter insertion or the number of patients requiring catheter replacement might be balance measures.

3. *Changes*: What changes will result in improvement? The team develops ideas that may result in success. Identifying options for change may include techniques such as brainstorming, critical thinking, and outlining of the current system; comparing current practice to "best practices" through benchmarking; using new technology; or using a new or outside perspective. The Institute for Healthcare Improvement offers a list of 72 change concepts,[25] which are generalized

FIGURE 10.1: Three crucial questions to defining the goals and process of QI. They may be answered in any order.

approaches that may stimulate specific ideas for change that are applicable to various situations.[26]

These three questions may be answered in any order, but are crucial to defining the goals and process of QI.

During the second stage, improvement teams translate the ideas generated during the first stage into actions using the Plan-Do-Study-Act (PDSA) cycle. The quality improvement team plans a test and predicts its results before implementing the change. The data are then studied and compared to the predicted result to assess whether the change resulted in the desired improvement. This new information is then used to develop the next test. Teams may expand the scope and scale of a positive intervention or move to a new intervention if the original change was shown to be ineffective. Changes should first be implemented and tested on a small scale and widely disseminated only after several PSDA cycles.

Six Sigma and Lean

Although it has been used by thousands of healthcare organizations, Deming's Model for Improvement is only one of several effective frameworks. Six Sigma's DMAIC (for Define, Measure, Analyze, Improve, Control) and Lean (also called Lean Enterprise or Toyota Production Systems) are also widely used for QI initiatives.

Six Sigma is a QI model that grew out of Japanese manufacturing after World War II.

It was initially applied by Robert Galvin at Motorola, and is based on reducing variation and defect rate, thus redefining the concept of "acceptable quality." Sigma is the Greek letter signifying standard deviation, with *Six Sigma* representing a rate of 3.4 defects per one million opportunities. A six-sigma process is therefore one that allows for defects only 0.0003% of the time.* The Six Sigma methodology, DMAIC, consists of the following five steps:

1. *Define*: Outline the process clearly, identifying the stakeholders and their needs, the process capabilities, and the project objectives.
2. *Measure*: Quantify defects and gather data on which to evaluate improvement efforts.
3. *Analyze*: Perform an in-depth assessment of the conditions leading to defects using Pareto analysis, process flow diagrams, fish-bone diagrams, process measures, and other analytical tools (Box 10.4).
4. *Improve*: Allocate resources to define and test changes aimed at reducing defects.
5. *Control*: Monitor the new process carefully to ensure that performance is maintained.

These steps can be repeated as necessary to improve the quality of care. Six Sigma is data-driven and focuses on measurement and analysis instead of instincts. Its overall success in defect reduction, customer satisfaction, and increased profitability has led to widespread use among major companies, including General Electric, Texas Instruments, and Boeing Aircraft.

Lean methodology, initially used in the production of Toyota automobiles, has some overlap with Six Sigma methodology, but differs in that Lean methodology is driven by the identification of consumer (i.e., patient) needs and seeks to improve value through the elimination of unnecessary waste.[27] Lean uses root cause analyses of negative events to improve quality and prevent similar errors while examining workflow to maximize efficiency and value. Application of Lean methodology

---

* Anesthesiology is currently the only specialty to have reduced serious defects to rates that are close to 3.4 per million opportunities. In the 1970s, anesthesia-related deaths occurred at rates of 1 in 10,000 to 20,000, representing 25 to 50 deaths per million cases (Ross AF, Tinker JH, Anesthesia risk. In Miller RD, ed. *Anesthesia*, 4th ed. New York: Churchill-Livingston, 1994). After decades of ongoing practice improvement through increased availability of monitors, new techniques, the development of widespread practice guidelines, an increased culture of safety, and other systematic approaches to harm reduction, anesthesiology has achieved six sigma (Lunn JN, Devlin HB, Lessons from the confidential enquiry into perioperative deaths in three NHS regions. Lancet. Dec 12 1987;330 (8572):1384–1387).

BOX 10.4   SEVEN BASIC TOOLS OF QUALITY: SO NAMED BECAUSE THEY REQUIRE LITTLE STATISTICAL BACKGROUND ON THE PART OF THE USER

Cause-and-effect diagram (also known as a "fishbone" or Ishikawa diagram): a visual representation of factors contributing to a negative outcome, in which contributing events are placed on spokes leading toward said outcome. Visually, this diagram breaks down (in successive layers of detail) root causes that potentially contribute to a particular effect (Figure 10.2).

Check sheet: form used to collect data through tallying in a grid. This provides a structured way to collect quality-related data as either a rough means for assessing a process or as an input to later analyses.

Control chart (also known as a Shewhart chart or process-behavior chart): typically used for time-series data, this chart visually displays trends and whether a process is controlled or should undergo a formal examination for quality problems. Data is charted over time and a mean is calculated, with a horizontal line drawn across time at the mean value. Upper and lower limits are created based on the threshold at which process variation is unlikely to be natural or at goal outputs.

Histogram: a graphical representation of the probability of given values through the distribution of numerical data. This chart depicts the frequencies of an observation occurring within a range of values.

Pareto chart: a chart containing both a bar and a line graph, where individual values are represented in descending order by bars, and summation values are represented by the overarching line. This chart is useful for visualizing the most common components or contributing factors to an outcome.

Scatter plot: a visual aid for identifying linear or nonlinear relationships between two variables, in which data are displayed as points along Cartesian coordinates.

Flow chart or run chart: a visual aid or diagram for representing a workflow, algorithm or process. Steps are shown in boxes and variables are written along arrows that link the boxes together, illustrating actions or events.

---

in healthcare requires an understanding of the concept of quality care and good outcome from the patient's point of view, or job satisfaction from the professional's point of view. A *value stream* then outlines the typical steps involved in care and examines which steps enhance quality rather than increasing inefficiencies. The ideal state can also be mapped and compared to the current state, and efforts are made to improve flow, efficiency, and value.

Healthcare Failure Modes and Effects Analysis

Failure modes and effects analysis (FMEA) is a prospective, formalized evaluation of the potential for failure or bad outcome within a system. FMEA is used to eliminate known or potential errors within a system, design, process, or service before they occur.[28] Originally used in the US military, FMEA has also been used heavily by the National Aeronautics and Space Administration (NASA). This technique attempts to identify every way that a given process could fail, estimating the probability and consequences of each failure, and then taking actions to protect against such failure. This process was adopted for use in healthcare by the Veterans Affairs (VA) National Center for Patient Safety. Healthcare failure modes and effects analysis (HFMEA) uses a multidisciplinary team in a similar fashion to evaluate healthcare processes to improve risk assessment and mitigation.[29]

HFMEA consists of the following five steps:

1. Clearly define the topic of analysis.
2. Assemble a multidisciplinary team that includes members with domain expertise.
3. Begin mapping processes, elucidating and numbering each step and substep in the care process.
4. Conduct a hazard analysis. This involves identifying potential causes of failure, scoring each failure mode using the hazard scoring matrix, and working through a decision-tree analysis. Listing all possible failures and scoring them based on likelihood of occurrence and severity of outcome allow the team to make educated decisions on which failure modes should be addressed. Changes should be targeted at minimizing the likelihood and severity of bad outcomes.
5. Develop and implement actions that will rectify opportunities for failure and follow outcome measures to assess their effectiveness.

Root Cause Analysis

Root cause analysis (RCA), sometimes called *systems analysis*, is a technique for investigating a problem that has already occurred, understanding how it happened, and preventing future occurrences. RCA was first developed for analyzing engineering mishaps and is a formalized investigation that is used to identify trends and to evaluate both overt and latent risks and vulnerabilities. RCA is typically used in the healthcare setting after a single poor outcome or episode of poor quality care has been identified (e.g., wrong-site surgery, retained foreign body, or unrecognized need for increase in the level of care). Bad outcomes are rarely the result of a single person or an isolated faulty process, and RCA is an effective tool for examining how multiple otherwise harmless faults within a complex system can align to cause harm. RCA assumes that a single individual is rarely at fault, and seeks to discover latent system vulnerabilities, instead of placing blame on specific individuals. This technique examines the system for faults that allowed a reasonable person making reasonable decisions to experience an undesired outcome. Multiple causative factors can influence clinical practice and increase the likelihood of medical errors, and several may be involved at any given time, including the institutional context, organizational and management factors, work environment, team factors, individual staff members, task factors, and patient characteristics.[30]

RCA begins with creation of a multidisciplinary team that includes personnel trained in RCA. Some institutions also include care providers and patients who were involved in the inciting event. The team then works together to establish what should have happened and then determine what actually occurred. Factors leading up to the negative outcome are then determined. One useful tool for outlining contributing factors is a *fishbone diagram*, sometimes called an Ishikawa or "cause and effect" diagram, in which causative factors are visually displayed (Figure 10.2). Typically, the "spine" of the diagram is an arrow leading to the negative outcome, while the "ribs" coming off the spine are thematic groupings of the contributing factors. It is important to evaluate contributing events that occurred earlier in the care process. Causal statements can then be written, linking the identified cause to its effects and then to the negative outcome. Ineffective safety processes and gaps in safe care can be elucidated by asking why a negative event could occur.

Once the cause of an adverse outcome has been thoroughly examined, the RCA team generates clear and concise recommendations to prevent recurrence. Recommendations can be varied in breadth and should be clearly targeted at the causative factors. Actions should address all of the root causes, be designed to reduce the risk of recurrence of the adverse event, and be specific, measurable, achievable, realistic, and timely.[31] Findings must then be shared with leadership and improvement teams that are able to make the necessary changes to prevent further harm. Action plans must be monitored for effectiveness.

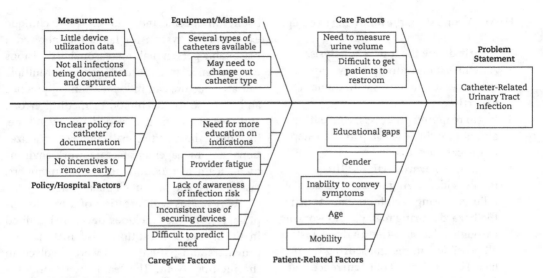

FIGURE 10.2: Sample cause-and-effect (fishbone) diagram.

RCA analysis can also be done in aggregate, as it is in the VA Health System, grouping similar episodes into simultaneous RCAs that assess trends.[32] Grouping analysis can be both an efficient use of resources and allow the assessment of common vulnerabilities across institutions. The Joint Commission requires an institution to perform an RCA after all sentinel events and then develop and implement a plan to reduce future risk of similar events.[33] Like all improvement methods, the success of RCA depends upon the team members and their efforts.

There are many options and variations available for institutions wishing to pursue quality. Choosing a framework can be based on many metrics, including applicability to the exact process requiring improvement and user familiarity. Studies have shown that the use of a standard framework by an institution is more important than the specific type that is being used.[34] Regardless of the tool used, the following elements remain essential for success: fostering and sustaining a culture of change and safety, developing and clarifying an understanding of the problem, involving key stakeholders, testing change strategies, and continuous monitoring of performance and reporting of findings to sustain the change.[35]

CONCLUSION

Improving quality in healthcare and creating patient safety are a complex process, made more so by the inherent complexities of the current healthcare system. The last century has seen both the beginnings and tremendous growth of this critical field. Leaders and organizations have emerged and a multitude of techniques and frameworks have joined the healthcare landscape. Increased provider and institutional awareness of quality improvement science will be essential to our national care deficit.

REFERENCES

1. Institute of Medicine. Kohn LT, Corrigan JM, Donaldson MS, eds. *To Err Is Human: Building a Safer Health System.* Vol. 627. Washington, DC: National Academies Press; 1999.
2. Lohr KN, Schroeder SA. A strategy for quality assurance in Medicare. *N Engl J Med.* 1990;322:1161–1171 [p. 1161].
3. Van Den Bos J, Rustagi K, Gray T, Halford M, Ziemkiewicz E, Shreve J. The $17.1 billion problem: the annual cost of measurable medical errors. *Health Aff.* 2011;30(4);596-603.
4. James JT. A new, evidence-based estimate of patient harms associated with hospital care. *J Patient Safety* 2013;9(3):122–128.
5. Institute of Medicine. *Crossing the Quality Chasm: A New Health System for the 21st Century.* Washington, DC: National Academies Press; 2001.

6. Mallon B. *Ernest Amory Codman: The End Result of a Life in Medicine.* Philadelphia: W. B. Saunders; 1999.

7. Luce JM, Bindman AB, Lee PR. A brief history of health care quality assessment and improvement in the United States. *West J Med.* 1994;160:263–268.

8. Donabedian A. Evaluating the quality of medical care. *Milbank Mem Fund Q.* 1966;44(Suppl):166–206.

9. Institute for Healthcare Improvement (in collaboration with Richard Scoville, IHI Improvement Advisor), Cambridge, MA. http://www.ihi.org/resources/Pages/Tools/ImprovementProjectRoadmap.aspx. Accessed February 2, 2016.

10. Jennings B, Bailey MA, Bottrell M, Lynn J. *Health Care Quality Improvement: Ethical and Regulatory Issues.* Garisson, NY: Hastings Center, 2007.

11. Reinhardt AC, Ray LN. Differentiating quality improvement from research. *Appl Nurs Res.* 2003;16(1):2–8.

12. Morris PE, Dracup K. Quality improvement or research? The ethics of hospital project oversight. *Am J Crit Care.* 2007;16(5):424–426.

13. Shortell SM, Bennet CL, Byck GR. Assessing the impact of continuous quality improvement on clinical practice: what it will take to accelerate progress. *Milbank Q.* 1998;76(4):593–624.

14. US Code of Federal Regulations, 45 CFR.46.102 (d).

15. Centers for Medicare & Medicaid Services. *Quality Improvement Organization Manual.* Chapter 16, Health care quality improvement program. http://www.cms.hhs.gov/manuals/downloads/qio110c16.pdf. Accessed October 25, 2014.

16. Lynn J, Baily MA, Bottrell M, et al. The ethics of using quality improvement methods in health care. *Ann Intern Med.* 2007;146(9):666–673.

17. Newhouse RP, Pettit JC, Poe S, Rocco L. The slippery slope: differentiating between quality improvement and research. *J Nurs Adm.* 2006; 36(4):211–219.

18. Grol R, Grimshaw J. From best evidence to best practice: effective implementation of change in patients' care. *Lancet.* 2003;362(9391):1225–1230.

19. Baker R, Camosso-Stefinovic J, Gillies C, Shaw EJ, et al. Tailored interventions to overcome identified barriers to change: effects on professional practice and health care outcomes. *Cochrane Database Syst Rev.* 2005;3(3). http://onlinelibrary.wiley.com.laneproxy.stanford.edu/doi/10.1002/14651858.CD005470.pub3/epdf. Accessed April 4, 2016.

20. Shojania KG, McDonald KM, Wachter RM, et al. *Closing the Quality Gap: A Critical Analysis of Quality Improvement Strategies.* Vol. 1: *Series Overview and Methodology.* Rockville, MD: Agency for Healthcare Research and Quality; August 2004. AHRQ Publication No. 04-0051-1.

21. Deming WE. *Out of the Crisis.* Cambridge, MA: MIT Press; 1986.

22. Deming WE. *The New Economics for Industry, Government, Education.* 2nd ed. MIT Press: 2000.

23. Langley GJ, Nolan KM, Nolan TW. *The Foundation of Improvement.* Silver Spring, MD: API Publishing; 1992.

24. Langley, Nolan KM, Nolan K, Norman C, Provost L. *The improvement guide: A practical guide to enhancing organizational performance.* San Francisco, CA. 1996.

25. Institute for Healthcare Improvement. *Using Change Concepts for Improvement.* http://www.ihi.org/knowledge/Pages/Changes/UsingChangeConceptsforImprovement.aspx. Accessed October 20, 2014.

26. Nolan TW et al. *Reducing Delays and Waiting Times Throughout the Healthcare System.* 1st ed. Boston: Institute for Healthcare Improvement; 1996.

27. Sahney VK. Generating management research on improving quality. *Health Care Manage Rev.* 2003;28(4):335–347.

28. Croteau RJ, Schyve PM. Proactively error-proofing health care processes. In: Spath PL, ed. *Error Reduction in Health Care: A Systems Approach to Improving Patient Safety.* Chicago, IL: AHA Press; 2000:179–198.

29. DeRosier J, Stalhandske E, Bagin JP, et al. Using health care failure mode and effect analysis: the VA National Center for Patient Safety's Prospective Risk Analysis System. *J Qual Improv.* 2002;28(5): 248–267.

30. Vincent CA, Taylor-Adams S, Stanhope N. Framework for analyzing risk and safety in clinical medicine. *BMJ.* 1998:316:1154–1157.

31. NHS National Reporting and Learning Service. RCA investigation tools: guide to investigation report writing. September 2008. http://www.nrls.npsa.nhs.uk/resources/?entryid45=59847. Accessed October 20, 2014.

32. Joint Commission. Using aggregate root cause analysis to improve patient safety. *Jt Comm J Qual Patient Saf.* 2003;29(8):434–439.

33. Joint Commission. *2003 Hospital Accreditation Standards.* Oakbrook Terrace, IL: Joint Commission Resources; 2003.

34. Boaden R, Harvey G, Moxham C, Proudlove N. *Quality Improvement: Theory and Practice in Health Care.* University of Warwick Campus, Coventry, UK: NHS Institute for Innovation and Improvement; 2008.

35. Barton, A. Patient safety and quality: an evidence-based handbook for nurses. *AORN Journal.* 2009;90(4):601–602.

11

Crisis Resource Management and Patient Safety in Anesthesia Practice

AMANDA R. BURDEN, JEFFREY B. COOPER, AND DAVID M. GABA

INTRODUCTION

Despite ongoing efforts to improve patient safety, medical errors persist. In the United States in 1999, the Institute of Medicine estimated that each year between 44,000 and 98,000 people die as a result of medical errors.[1] Recent studies estimate that the true number of premature deaths associated with preventable harm to patients may be far greater, with more than 400,000 such deaths occurring each year.[2] Many of these deaths are not the result of inadequate medical knowledge and skill, but rather occur because of problems involving communicating and managing the situation and team.[1-6] The operating room is a dynamic and complex environment; critical events can happen without warning. When these events occur, the anesthesiologist must lead an interprofessional team whose members have varying levels of training while at the same time caring for a critically ill patient.[5-9] At any time, one or more factors, including patient comorbidity and procedural or equipment challenges may combine, ultimately leading to a crisis that threatens the patient's well-being or life. Anesthesiologists must manage rapid changes in the patient's status, along with often incomplete information about the situation, while leading this team. They are frequently required to make decisions quickly, in a rapidly evolving situation where there is no room for error.[5,6,8-9] Crisis resource management (CRM) provides tools that help the anesthesiologist and the team manage the critical situation.[5,6,8,10]

HISTORY OF CRISIS RESOURCE MANAGEMENT

Aviation

Crew resource management (originally *cockpit resource management*) is a paradigm that was first designed in an effort to improve aviation safety by helping flight crews prepare for and mitigate serious events in flight.[11] Crew resource management training grew out of a National Aeronautics and Space Administration (NASA) workshop that was convened to consider data from the National Transportation Safety Board (NTSB) that identified human error and failures of communication, decision-making, and leadership as the primary causes of air transport accidents.[4,11] Crew resource management specifically focuses on interpersonal communication, leadership, and decision-making in the cockpit. Although it retained the pilot's command and leadership of the team, it was intended to foster a less authoritarian culture, in which first officers (i.e., the copilot) and flight engineers (i.e., a crew member specifically responsible for monitoring and controlling aircraft systems) were encouraged to question the captain (pilot) and offer suggestions for the management of the situation.[11,12] The NTSB first recommended requiring crew resource management training for airline crews in 1979.[13,14] United Airlines was the first airline to provide such training for its cockpit crews in 1982; by the 1990s it had become a global standard.[12] While originally involving only the flight crew, it later evolved to include other members of the aircraft crew.[4,11]

Over the last three decades, these training concepts have been adopted and adapted for application to a wide range of activities where personnel must make dangerous time-critical decisions; among these are nuclear power, fire-fighting, and healthcare.[15-17]

Healthcare: Anesthesiology at the Forefront

In 1978, Cooper et al. first described the causes of anesthesia-related errors and patient injuries;[3] this early research into error and human factors helped to catalyze a national patient safety movement.[10] Cooper's research was one of the influences that led to the formation of the Anesthesia Patient Safety Foundation (APSF), which funded simulation research, specifically the creation of physiologic patient simulators.[16,18] Inspired by Cooper's research and funded by the APSF, David Gaba and colleagues at Stanford University were the first to recognize that anesthesiology, like fields such as aviation and nuclear energy, was also a complex and dynamic environment.[5-9] In part inspired by the book *Normal Accidents*,[19] Gaba had begun to consider physician decision-making during patient emergencies.[7,9] He adapted crew resource management to the anesthesia environment, and called it *anesthesia crisis resource management* (ACRM—as anesthesia professionals would better relate to the concept of crisis management than "crew" management).[5,6,8,9]

CRM skills are difficult to incorporate into clinical practice. To ingrain these behaviors, CRM must be repeatedly practiced in situations that approximate actual conditions under which the behaviors will be used. Beginning in the fall of 1990, Gaba and his group established simulation-based courses to teach these skills to anesthesia trainees and experienced anesthesiologists.[17,20] Believing that learning is best accomplished by creating an emotional component, they created as much realism as was reasonably achievable. This team has conducted a variety of CRM courses continuously for the past 25 years, at several simulation centers in the Stanford complex. Ultimately, they, along with others, adapted this discipline to other

healthcare domains as *crisis resource management* (CRM).[5,6,8,9,17,20]

In February 1994, the Boston Anesthesia Simulation Center (BASC), a collaboration of the hospitals affiliated with Harvard Medical School (HMS), became the first dedicated center to teach CRM. CRM principles and scenarios were replicated via a collaboration between Jeffrey Cooper at HMS and Gaba and colleagues at Stanford.[21] BASC has evolved into the Center for Medical Simulation and has continued the ACRM program; all Harvard anesthesia faculty participate in a one-day course every 2 years as a requirement for a substantial reduction in their malpractice premium and also as required for hospital credentialing.[22]

CRISIS RESOURCE MANAGEMENT PRINCIPLES

CRM is designed to focus the attention of individuals and the entire team on factors that improve patient safety by reducing the causes of adverse events and improving responses to evolving events. Although medical knowledge and technical skills are essential components of patient care, nontechnical skills such as leadership, communication, and situation awareness are equally critical for the safe care of the patient, especially during a critical event.[5,6,23] To manage the crisis effectively, the anesthesiologist must manage the full situation. Gaba describes a set of principles and actions that comprise effective CRM (Figure 11.1). These principles are composed of actions that focus the team on the effective coordination of all activities in response to an evolving event. It is expected that many of these principles (e.g., effective communication) will carry over to routine activities in ways that will make the initiation of an event less likely. The set of CRM principles most recently described by Gaba are summarized in the next sections.

Know the Environment

One of the prerequisites of crisis resource management is to know the resources that are available, including personnel, equipment, and cognitive aids. Knowing who can be asked for help, who is available at different times, and how to mobilize that help quickly are essential even

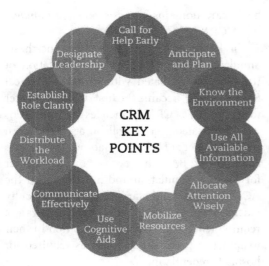

FIGURE 11.1. Key Points of Anesthesia Crisis Resource Management.

before the crisis develops. It is equally important to know what equipment is available and where it is, and also how to operate that equipment. Especially when equipment is infrequently used, it must be kept in working order, and members of the team must be familiar with its operation. Knowing about the availability and operation of these resources can make a desirable outcome more likely and also help to make a crisis less stressful for the care team.

Anticipate and Plan

Vigilance is an essential tenet of the practice of anesthesiology; anticipating and planning are critical elements of that practice. The team should plan for and consider the requirements of the anticipated procedure in advance. A well-formulated anesthetic plan can help to avoid problems as well as guide management if a critical event emerges. The goal of the team is to explore potential crises and their management, with the aim of avoiding those that are predictable.

Throughout the procedure, it is imperative to maintain awareness of every change that occurs in the environment.[23-26] This is termed *situation awareness* and is discussed in Chapter 7. It is easy to fall behind if the situation changes rapidly. If the patient seems to be failing quickly, it is essential to catch up, which may require asking the surgeon to pause

the procedure until help arrives and while the problem is managed. By planning ahead, it is possible to identify potential helpers and to plan the case with the surgical team, making a critical event more manageable if it does occur and helping to maintain a calmer atmosphere for the team.

Call for Help Early

Calling for help is the sign of a strong and competent anesthesia professional. It is critical to call for help at the earliest sign of a problem in order to make a difference in the patient's care, especially in an emergency, or if the patient's condition is deteriorating and is unresponsive to interventions. Another person can see things that might have been missed, as well as providing additional physical resources to perform critical tasks.[27,28] It can be useful to call for someone who can help to think through the patient's diagnosis and treatment options, to administer medications, or to perform emergent interventions (e.g., perform chest compressions or achieve vascular access). Calling for help early is particularly challenging for many professionals because it could be construed as a sign of indecision or weakness, but it can be the element that determines success or failure in preventing an adverse event.

Designate Leadership

A designated effective leader is essential to a well-functioning team during a critical event. The leader's role is to take command of the team, coordinate the overall management of the event, communicate about the patient's physiologic status, and distribute of the workload. To fulfill these leadership functions, the anesthesiologist must have good technical knowledge and skills and must remain calm and organized. An important part of the leader's role is to articulate the full plan so the team has a shared mental model of the patient's situation and plan and will then be able to follow the plan. Although the team leader is ultimately responsible for making decisions, other people in the room may have critical information; the leader should solicit and accept information from other team members whenever possible. It is not possible to see or know everything that is happening in the case, and another member of the team may have information that is essential to a good outcome. Being open to receiving communication from the other team members will help ensure that all available information about the case can be incorporated into the plan. Disagreement about the optimal care elements should not be about *who* is right, but about *what* is right *for the patient.*

Followership

Other members of the team must be mindful followers, listening to the team leader's and others' communications, and completing the tasks that they have been assigned. A team member must also pay close attention to the situation and must be assertive if the leader might lack important information or may be making an incorrect decision. The patient's safety depends upon everyone working together to arrive at an accurate diagnosis and plan. While it is the leader's job to coordinate the patient's care, everyone on the team is responsible for the patient's safety.

Use All Available Information

The volume of information that must be comprehended and integrated during a critical event adds considerably to the complexity of anesthetic care. Medical information must be collected from a variety of different sources, and that information must then be correlated with the patient's vital signs and the clinical impression in order to understand the patient's status and arrive at the correct diagnosis. It is also essential to deliberately seek out information that does not fit the original picture of the situation in an effort to avoid fixating on an incorrect diagnosis.

Establish Role Clarity

Creating a well-functioning team begins before the team is needed; this is hard work and requires the full participation of all team members. The leader should mentally review what he or she needs from the team and should plan to brief the team members when or as they arrive. Role ambiguity is a source of stress for the team. Role clarity (i.e., each person knowing his or her role and responsibilities) is therefore a prerequisite for effective team performance. Team members who know the plan and their role are more likely to be effective, and team coordination is made easier. During a crisis, team members commonly feel tense; effective, periodic briefing of the team as to the situation and the plan can focus and calm them. After the situation resolves, debriefing about the event and the teamwork is a learning opportunity. Respect for the team members and being explicit about what needs to be done and who needs to do it will improve team function, increasing the likelihood of a satisfactory patient outcome.

Allocate Attention Wisely

Attention is a limited resource; it is important to maintain vigilant assessment of the anesthetized patient at all times, especially during a critical event. During a crisis, tasks must be prioritized and reprioritized as the patient's condition evolves. It is also important to alternate between focusing on details and focusing on the big picture. There will be points at which the details of a specific problem require close attention (e.g., a difficult intubation), but one should then refocus attention on the big picture and re-evaluate the patient's overall status. At least one anesthesia professional should be assigned to monitor the patient's condition at all times. If the crisis becomes more challenging, the tasks may become more complex; it may be necessary to mobilize additional resources to complete the tasks and care for the patient.

Distribute the Workload

During a crisis, whenever possible, the team leader should delegate tasks or specific responsibilities in order to avoid becoming fixated on a single component of patient management.[29]

The leader should define the tasks, verify that they are properly carried out, and review changes in the patient's situation. If possible, the team leader should remain free of manual tasks in order to observe, gather information, and delegate tasks. In a high-functioning team, the leader should not have to direct every team action, but team members should inform and confirm the plan with the leader before spontaneously performing a task. It is common during crises for a handful of people to be overworked while others do nothing. A crisis is not a good time for inexperienced people to attempt to perform critical skills; experienced individuals should perform the most critical tasks. The leader should assign specific tasks to specific people according to their expertise and skills. Ideally, the leader should avoid performing manual tasks when possible so that she or he is able to observe the evolving situation and direct the team.

Mobilize Resources

Mobilizing resources requires time and planning. The team leader must therefore request personnel and resources that could help as early as possible in the evolution of the crisis. Operating room "resources," such as personnel, equipment, and cognitive aids (e.g., emergency manuals or checklists) should all be employed to help assure the safe care of the patient. Knowledge and skills, and the leader's knowledge of his or her strengths and weaknesses, are the most important resources. Whatever resources are available should be used; a crisis should not be managed alone when there are people available who could help.

Communicate Effectively

Clear, closed-loop communication is critical in crisis situations. Good teamwork depends on full communication and a shared mental model so that every team member knows what is happening and what is planned. Effective communication can help ensure that everyone on the team knows the patient's condition, what needs to be done, and what has already been done. Communication can be especially difficult during a crisis, and messages are communicated only when they are received (Figure 11.2). It is therefore important to address people directly, acknowledge that information was heard, and confirm when a task is completed using closed-loop communication.

Closed-loop communication (CLC) is an important part of CRM.[30,31] CLC is a transmission model in which verbal feedback is critical and helps ensure that the team members understand and will act on the message. CLC involves three steps: (1) the sender transmits a message, (2) the receiver accepts the message

and acknowledges its receipt, and (3) the sender verifies that the message has been received and interpreted correctly (i.e., the loop is closed).[30,32] In other high-hazard industries (e.g., aviation), CLC is required for any communication that contains critical information, such as requesting permission to enter an active runway. Unfortunately, its use is variable in operating room cultures. Training and emphasis on making CLC a normal behavior is challenging but critical for adverse event recovery.[33] It is also essential to make communication as *complete* and *clear* as possible and to relay all relevant information, while avoiding unnecessary details that may lead to confusion. Sufficient time should be allowed for team members to ask questions, and those questions should be answered as completely as possible.

Use Cognitive Aids

There are many forms of cognitive aids or emergency manuals (EM). These EMs are especially important for situations when things must be done in a specific order and skipping a step could lead to disastrous results (e.g., omitting dantrolene while treating a patient with malignant hyperthermia). EMs should be used to help assure that critical steps are not missed. Using EMs is common in other industries and is likely to help the team accomplish every important step in diagnosis and treatment. Using these EMs to assure correct dosages and steps in a crisis demonstrates responsibility, not a lack of knowledge. There is a growing trend toward use of EMs in anesthesia and perioperative medicine.[34] Several forms of emergency lists have been promulgated.[35-37]

Establish Situational Awareness and a Shared Mental Model

Anesthesiology is a dynamic process and is especially so during a crisis. What is correct now may be wrong in the next minute; every piece of information might change a situation. Some parameters might also change slowly over time. Subtle changes are hard to perceive; at times these cues are barely above the threshold of perception.[25] Situational awareness is essential as the patient's condition is continuously re-evaluated (Chapter 7). Conversely, changes in the patient's condition may require an alternate strategy. Continually investigate to assure that the patient's main problem and the factors that are most likely to cause harm are correctly diagnosed. One must remain skeptical about the diagnosis, periodically re-evaluating other options in order to recheck the mental model of the situation. After re-evaluating the situation, it might be necessary to define new priorities and goals, adapting to the changing environment and to the new situation. New priorities should be communicated to the team, while asking for team members' views.

Call for Help Early
• Call for help early enough to make a difference
• Err on the side of getting more help
• Mobilize early personnel with special skills if they may be needed

Designate Leadership
• Establish clear leadership
• Inform team members who is in charge
• 'Followers' should be active in asking who is leading

Anticipate and Plan
• Plan & prepare for high work-load periods during low work-load periods
• Know were you are likely headed during the crisis and make backup plans early

Know the Environment
• Maintain situational awareness
• Know how things work and where things are
• Be aware of strengths and vulnerabilities of environment

Establish Role Clarity
• Determine who will do what
• Assign areas of responsibility appropriate to knowledge, skills, and training
• Active followers may offer specific roles

Use All Available Information
• Monitor multiple streams of data and information
• Check and cross check information

Distribute the Workload
• Assign specific tasks to team members according to their abilities
• Revise the distribution if there is task overload or failure

Allocate Attention Wisely
• Eliminate or reduce distractions
• Monitor for task saturation & data overload
• Avoid getting fixated
• Recruit others to help w/ monitoring

Mobilize Resources
• Activate all helpful resources including equipment and additional personnel

Communicate Effectively
• Command and request clearly
• Seek confirmation of request (close the loop)
• Avoid "thin air" statements
• Foster input and atmosphere of open information exchange among all personnel

Use Cognitive Aids
• Be familiar with content, format and location
• Support the effective use of cognitive aids

FIGURE 11.2. Crisis Resource Management Key Points.

TEACHING AND LEARNING CRISIS RESOURCE MANAGEMENT SKILLS

CRM elements may seem obvious. Using and applying them is not. CRM skills must be taught in a setting where participants have the opportunity to learn and deliberately practice these skills in order to effectively implement them in a real patient crisis.[5,6] Failure to perform critical CRM actions and behaviors often proves to be the pivotal factor in severe negative outcomes.[1,2,5-8,38] These omissions have been identified as the leading cause of medical errors, morbidity, and mortality in repeated Joint Commission sentinel event reports.[39]

To improve CRM competence it is important to reflect on these principles and even seek out education to improve performance. After dealing with an unexpected event, it is beneficial to take a few minutes to review CRM performance after the fact.[5,6]

There is an increasing number of simulation centers[40] that offer CRM courses for anesthesiologists. These courses include the opportunity to practice CRM key points in a simulated crisis.[5,6,9,16,21,41,42-47] The simulation courses that are an element of the Practice Performance Assessment and Improvement component of Maintenance of Certification in Anesthesiology (MOCA® Part 4) all have a mandate from the American Board of Anesthesiology to address and teach CRM principles.[48-50] Participants in the courses work through medical/technical actions and decisions and CRM practices in highly realistic environments. During video-assisted debriefings, emphasis is placed on using CRM principles to improve patient safety.[48-50] These courses are available to all anesthesiologists. They are outstanding opportunities to be prepared for managing critical events, especially for those providers for whom such events are not usually encountered.

Teaching Crisis Resource Management

Team training is essential to improve communication and the ability to work together when things are not going well. For anesthesia, and healthcare in general, many different versions

of CRM or "team training" have been created. ACRM has been widely followed, adapted, and altered by groups of instructors around the world.

Several other standardized team training curricula with similar, if not quite the same, approaches are available in the United States, especially over the last 10 years. These include (but are not limited to) MedTeams (adapted from US Army rotorcraft safety experience);[51,52] TeamStepps (developed by the Department of Defense's Patient Safety Program in collaboration with the Agency for Healthcare Research and Quality);[53] and the US Department of Veterans Affairs Medical Team Training program.[54]

Crisis Resource Management and Patient Safety

While errors in healthcare have been identified as a leading cause of morbidity and mortality,[1,2] there is no formal required training for healthcare personnel aimed at improving CRM skills. CRM is also not yet a standard part of medical training. There is only scant evidence that CRM training improves patient outcomes,[55,56] but practicing for urgent situations has strong face validity. That validity has been sufficient motivation for requirements for such training in aviation and nuclear power. In these arenas, as in healthcare, there is also no level 1 or 2 evidence (randomized trials)[57] that CRM training prevents accidents or saves lives. It is unlikely that this evidence will ever be available, as the lives of pilots and power plant operators are at stake; hence they are unlikely to volunteer to serve in the control group. As Gaba earlier commented, "... no industry in which human lives depend on the skilled performance of responsible operators has waited for unequivocal proof of the benefits of simulation before embracing it. ... Neither should anesthesiology."[58] The same comment can be made about CRM training in general, with or without simulation.

REFERENCES

1. Kohn LT, Corrigan J, Donaldson MS. *To Err Is Human: Building a Safer Health System.* Washington, DC: National Academy Press, 1999.

2. James, JT. A new, evidence-based estimate of patient harms associated with hospital care. *J Patient Safety*. 2013:9(3):122–128.

3. Cooper JB, Newbower RS, Long CD, McPeek, B. Preventable anesthesia mishaps: a study of human factors. *Anesthesiology*. 1978;49(6), 399–406.

4. Helmreich RL, Merritt AC, Wilhelm JA. The evolution of crew resource management training in commercial aviation. *Int Journ Aviat Psych*. 9(1):19–32.

5. Gaba DM, Fish KJ, Howard SK. *Crisis Management in Anesthesiology*. New York: Churchill Livingstone; 1994

6. Gaba DM, Fish KJ, Howard SK, Burden AR. *Crisis Management in Anesthesiology*. 2nd ed. Philadelphia: Elsevier; 2014.

7. Gaba D, Evans D, Patel V: Dynamic decision-making in anesthesiology: cognitive models and training approaches. In: Evans, David A. and Patel, Vimla L, eds., *Advanced Models of Cognition for Medical Training and Practice*. Berlin: Springer-Verlag: 1992:122.

8. Gaba DM, Howard SK, Fish K, et al. Simulation-based training in anesthesia crisis resource management (ACRM): a decade of experience. *Simul Gaming*. 2001;32:175–193.

9. Howard SK, Gaba DM, Fish KJ, et al. Anesthesia Crisis Resource Management Training: teaching anesthesiologists to handle critical incidents. *Aviat Space Environ Med*. 1992; 63:763–70.

10. Cooper JB. Towards patient safety in anaesthesia. *Ann Acad Med*. 1994;23:552–557.

11. Cooper GE, White MD, Lauber JK. *Resource Management on the Flightdeck: Proceedings of a NASA/Industry Workshop*. NASA CP-2120 1980. Moffett Field, CA: NASA-Ames Research Center.

12. United Air Lines, Inc. McDonnell-Douglas DC-8-61, N8082U, Portland, Oregon: December 28, 1978. National Transportation Safety Board. December 28, 1978. 9 (15/64).

13. National Transportation Safety Board. http://www.ntsb.gov/safety/mwl/Pages/was2.aspx. Accessed April 27, 2015.

14. Woods D, Johannesen L, Cook R, Sarter N. *Behind Human Error: Cognitive System, Computers, and Hindsight*. Wright Patterson Air Force Base, Crew Systems Ergonomics Information Analysis Center, 1994.

15. Diehl, Alan. Crew resource management . . . it's not just for fliers anymore. *Flying Safety*. USAF Safety Agency, 1991: 73–79.

16. Cooper JB, Taqueti VR. A brief history of the development of mannequin simulators for clinical education and training. *Qual Saf Health Care*. 2004;13(Suppl 1):i11–i18.

17. Gaba D. Anaesthesiology as a model for patient safety in healthcare. *Br Med J*. 2000;320:785–788.

18. Anesthesia Patient Safety Foundation. www.apsf.org. Accessed May 18, 2015.

19. Perrow C. *Normal Accidents: Living with High-Risk Technologies*. Princeton, NJ: Princeton University Press; 1984.

20. Gaba DM. The future vision of simulation in health care. *Qual Saf Health Care*. 2004;13(Suppl 1):i2–10.

21. Cooper JB. Patient safety and biomedical engineering. In: Kitz RJ, ed., *This Is No Humbug: Reminiscences of the Department of Anesthesia at the Massachusetts General Hospital*. Boston: Department of Anesthesia and Critical Care, Massachusetts General Hospital; 2002:377–420.

22. Hanscom R. Medical simulation from an insurer's perspective. *Acad Emerg Med*. 2008;15:984–987.

23. Gaba DM, Howard SK, Small SD. Situation awareness in anesthesiology. *Hum Factors*. 1995;37(1): 20–31.

24. Manser T. Teamwork and patient safety in dynamic domains of healthcare: a review of the literature. *Acta Anaesth Scand*. 2009;53(2): 143–151.

25. Endsley MR. Design and evaluation for situation awareness enhancement. In: *Proceedings of the Human Factors Society*, 32nd Annual Meeting, Santa Monica, October 24–28, 1988:97–101.

26. Schulz CM, Endsley MR, Kochs EF, Gelb AW, Wagner KJ. Situation awareness in anesthesia: concept and research. *Anesthesiology*. 2013;118 (3):729–742.

27. Sutcliffe KM, Lewton E, Rosenthal MM. Communication failures: an insidious contributor to medical mishaps. *Acad Med*. 2004; 79(2):186–194.

28. Larsen MP, Eisenberg MS, Cummins RO, Hallstrom AP. Predicting survival from out-of-hospital cardiac arrest: a graphic model. *Ann Emerg Med*. 1993;22(11):1652–1658.

29. DeKeyser V, Woods D, Masson M, Van Daele A. Fixation errors in dynamic and complex systems: descriptive forms, psychological mechanisms, potential countermeasures. Technical Report for NATO Division of Scientific Affairs; 1988.

30. Burke CS, Salas E, Wilson-Donnelly K, et al. How to turn a team of experts into an expert medical team: guidance from the aviation and military communities. *Qual Saf Health Care*. 2004; 13:96–104.

31. Salas E, Wilson KA, Murphy CE, et al. Communicating, coordinating, and cooperating when lives depend on it: tips for teamwork. *Jt Comm J Qual Patient Saf*. 2008;34:333–341.

32. Wilson KA, Salas E, Priest HA, et al. Errors in the heat of battle: taking a closer look at shared cognition breakdowns through teamwork. *Hum Factors*. 2007;49:243–56

33. Prabhakar H, Cooper JB, Sabel A, Weckbach S, Mehler PS, Stahel PF. Introducing standardized "readbacks" to improve patient safety in surgery: a prospective survey in 92 providers at a public safety-net hospital. *BMC Surgery.* 2012; 12(1):8.

34. Goldhaber-Fiebert SN, Howard SK. Implementing emergency manuals: can cognitive aids help translate best practices for patient care during acute events? *Anesth Analg.* 2013; 117(5):1149–1161.

35. Emergency Manuals Implementation Collaborative. http://www.emergencymanuals.org/free-tools .html. Accessed May 23, 2015.

36. Stanford Anesthesia Cognitive Aid Group. http://emergencymanual.stanford.edu/. Accessed May 23, 2015.

37. Project Check Ariadne Labs: A Joint Center at Brigham and Women's Hospital & the Harvard School of Public Health. http://www.projectcheck.org/crisis.html. Accessed May 23, 2015.

38. Lingard L, Espin S, Whyte S, Regehr G, Baker GR, Reznick R, Bohnen J, Orser B Grober E. Communication failures in the operating room: an observational classification of recurrent types and effects. *Qual Safe Health Care.* 2004;13(5):330–334.

39. Joint Commission on Accreditation of Healthcare Organizations. Joint Commission International Center for Patient Safety. Communication: a critical component in delivering quality care. http://www.jointcommission.org/topics/patient_safety.aspx. Accessed April 24, 2015.

40. Rall M, Van Gessel E, Staender S. Education, teaching and training in patient safety. *Best Pract Res Clin Anaesth.* 2011;25(2):251–262.

41. Blum RH, Raemer DB, Carroll JS, Sunder N, Feinstein DM, Cooper JB. Crisis resource management training for an anaesthesia faculty: a new approach to continuing education. *Med Educ.* 2004;38(1):45–55.

42. American Society of Anesthesiologists Simulation Education Network. http://education.asahq.org/Simulation-Education. Accessed May 25, 2015.

43. CRICO/RMF. High risk areas: obstetrics. http://www.rmf.harvard.edu/high-risk-areas/obstetrics/index.aspx. Accessed May 25, 2015.

44. The Doctors' Company. http://www.thedoctors.com. Accessed May 25, 2015.

45. Orasanu J, Connolly T, Klein G, Orasanu J, Calderwood R, Zsambok C. The reinvention of decision making. In: Klein G, Orasanu J, Calderwood R, Zsambok CE eds., *Decision Making in Action: Models and Methods.* Norwood, NJ: Ablex; 1993:3.

46. Manser T. Teamwork and patient safety in dynamic domains of healthcare: a review of the literature. *Acta Anaesth Scand.* 2009; 53: 143–51

47. Salas E, Rosen MA, King H. Managing teams managing crises: principles of teamwork to improve patient safety in the emergency room and beyond. *Theor Issues Ergon Sci.* 2007; 8:381–394.

48. McIvor W, Burden AR, Weinger MB, Steadman RS. Simulation for maintenance of certification in anesthesiology: the first two years. *J Contin Educ Health Prof.* 2012;32(4):236–242.

49. Weinger MB, Burden AR, Steadman RH, Gaba DM: This is not a test!: misconceptions surrounding the maintenance of certification in anesthesiology simulation course. *Anesthesiology.* 2014; 121:655–659.

50. Steadman RH, Burden AR, Huang YM, Gaba DM, Cooper JB. Practice improvements based on participation in simulation for the maintenance of certification in anesthesiology program. *Anesthesiology.* 2015 May;122(5):1154–1169.

51. Small SD, Wuerz RC, Simon R, Shapiro N, Conn A, Setnik G. Demonstration of high fidelity simulation team training for emergency medicine. *Acad Emerg Med.* 1999;6:312–323.

52. Morey JC, Simon R, Jay GD et al. Error reduction and performance improvement in the emergency department through formal teamwork training: evaluation results of the MedTeams project. *Health Serv Res.* 2002;37:1553–1581.

53. Clancy CM, Tornberg DN. TeamSTEPPS: assuring optimal teamwork in clinical settings. *Am J Med Qual.* 2007;22: 214–217.

54. Dunn EJ, Mills PD, Neily J, Crittenden MD, Carmack AL, Bagian JP. Medical team training: applying crew resource management in the Veterans Health Administration. *Jt Comm J Qual Patient Saf.* 2007;33:317–325.

55. Wayne DB, Didwania A, Feinglass J, Fudala MJ, Barsuk JH, McGaghie WC. Simulation-based education improves quality of care during cardiac arrest team responses at an academic teaching hospital: a case-control study. *Chest Journal.* 2008;133(1):56–61.

56. Andreatta P, Saxton E, Thompson M, Annich G. Simulation-based mock codes significantly correlate with improved pediatric patient cardiopulmonary arrest survival rates. *Pediatr Crit Care Med.* 2011;12(1):33–38.

57. OCEBM Levels of Evidence Working Group. *The Oxford 2011 Levels of Evidence.* Oxford Centre for Evidence-Based Medicine. http://www.cebm.net/index.aspx?o=5653.

58. Gaba DM. Improving anesthesiologists' performance by simulating reality. *Anesthesiology.* 1992;76(4):491–494.

12

Quality in Medical Education

VIJI KURUP

INTRODUCTION

Continuing medical education is now universally accepted as a standard of excellence. Few standards have been developed to guide medical education programs, however, and techniques that are effective for teaching and learning are not widely understood or integrated into medical education. One possible reason for this is that few educational studies are published in the medical literature; most are published in education- or psychology-themed journals. Furthermore, expertise in medicine is still assumed to be sufficient to be a good teacher. Although a few gifted educators may be able to motivate students, many teachers do not have significant insight into educational theory, and they struggle to keep their students motivated.

Several recently published reviews examine the state of the art in medical education.[1] The quality of evidence in educational research has, however, been called into question.[2] This chapter will discuss the known evidence to define quality in terms of the *teacher*, the *learner*, and the *process*. The primary focus will be on interactive learning and simulation in particular. Finally, practical examples will show how to integrate evidence-based education in a residency training curriculum.

THE TEACHER

Although it is difficult to describe the characteristics of an effective teacher, most learners can identify a good teacher when they encounter one. Interestingly, one study concluded that faculty and residents differed in their definition of the essential attributes of an effective teacher.[3] In the survey conducted among family medicine practitioners and residents, both faculty and residents considered enthusiasm to be important. Resident physicians, however, placed more value on the teacher being non-judgmental and clinically competent and valued scholarly activity and perception as a role model less. Faculty rated "being a role model" as important. Also, residents felt that it was important for faculty to "respect their autonomy" to be an effective clinical teacher, whereas faculty placed the least importance on this trait. The problem is universal, with studies from different cultural backgrounds showing similar results. A qualitative study from South Africa identified the following attributes of a good teacher:[4]

1. Teacher's familiarity with subject knowledge;
2. Speaking clearly;
3. Eye contact with learner;
4. Being approachable even outside class;
5. Encouraging questions to clarify knowledge;
6. Sharing learning outcomes with learners before the session.

For clinical teachers, the supervision of trainees is an important task. There is general agreement in the literature that supervision should include educative, supportive, and administrative functions. Supervision helps trainees gain skills faster and can result in behavioral changes faster, but the quality of the relationship also determines the effectiveness of supervision.[5,6] Kilminster defined *supervision* as including monitoring, guidance, and feedback in the personal, professional, and educational development of the trainee.[7] He emphasized that helpful supervisory behaviors include giving direct guidance on clinical work, linking theory and practice, engaging in joint problem-solving, and offering feedback and reassurance to trainees. Genniss and Genniss conducted a study in an outpatient clinic and found that faculty frequently thought that a given patient's level of acuity was higher when they saw the patients themselves than when hearing a resident's assessment of the patient. This resulted in frequent changes in diagnosis and management.[8] Several studies suggest that the competence of teachers and the relationship between the teacher and learner contribute significantly to the way in which future clinicians work as members of a team and as caring professionals.[9] The problem, then, is to find a way to identify the characteristics of effective teachers and to determine whether these attributes can be taught to faculty. Menachery et al. identified eight characteristics of physicians that are associated with high learner-centered scores for educators:[10]

1. Proficiency in giving lectures/presentations;
2. Helping learners to identify resources to meet their own needs;
3. Proficiency in eliciting feedback from learners;
4. Frequently attempting to detect and discuss emotional responses of the learners;
5. Frequently reflecting on the validity of feedback from the learners;
6. Identifying available resources to meet teacher's learning needs;
7. Having given an oral presentation related to education at a national/regional meeting;
8. Letting the learners know how different situations affect the teacher.

Researchers have also looked at the self-evaluation of teachers and have found that knowledge of subject matter, professional identity, motivation, enthusiasm, and communication skills were felt to be important attributes of an effective teacher.[11,12]

Few studies have explored the question of whether good teaching can be learned or comes from innate talent. Branch et al. implemented a longitudinal faculty development program designed to enhance humanistic teaching at five medical schools. They compared responses from students taught by these faculty compared to controls on a 10-item questionnaire on humanistic teaching practices[13] and found a statistically significant difference between the participants and matched controls. The learning program included experiential methods such as role-play, practice, and feedback. This study suggests that faculty development efforts can play a role in improving the institutional quality of teaching.

THE PROCESS

Modern healthcare is a complex system with multiple institutions, large teams of professionals, and sometimes conflicting regulations governing the care of each patient. Physicians must incorporate a multitude of skills to negotiate even routine patient care. The rapidly evolving state of the healthcare system requires learners to sustain their medical knowledge, and also to develop a special set of cognitive skills to become "forward thinkers." Physicians completing their training must understand basic medical concepts; use this information in the clinical setting for patient care; stay current with latest developments in the field, articulate a plan of care to patients, colleagues, and peers; and have the skills and tools to continue self-directed learning after graduation.

Over the past two decades, there has been a shift from a teaching-centered model to a learning-centered one, while the integration of technological tools has led to the use of blended learning in anesthesia education[14] (Figure 12.1). The introduction of new teaching and learning methods were accompanied by calls for the assessment and personalization of lesson plans to accommodate different learning styles. Learning has also changed because duty-hour restrictions limit the number

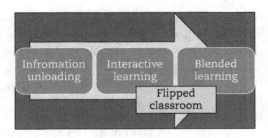

FIGURE 12.1: Evolution of content delivery.

of hours that resident physicians now spend at work or in educational activities.[15] A number of residency teaching programs are therefore turning to a *flipped classroom* model to use the resident-faculty interaction time more effectively.[16,17] This technique makes use of an online format to present basic facts related to remembering and understanding information. The face-to-face interaction time between students and faculty is then used for the analysis and synthesis of information. Prunuske et al. showed that students who watched an online lecture do better on questions addressing lower order cognitive skills, while there was no difference between the groups in questions related to higher order cognitive skills.[18] Students were better able to assimilate material related to higher order cognitive skills when it was presented face to face. Based on this evidence, the author uses the *flipped classroom* model for anesthesia resident didactics, presenting basic information on a topic before the session in multiple formats to the learners, who come to class familiar with the basics; in-class activities are designed around team-based learning, are interactive, and promote student engagement with the material (Figure 12.2).

Adverse events occur in the greatest numbers at the beginning of an academic year.[19] For example, Haller et al. examined more than 19,000 anesthetics involving 93 trainees and found that the rate of adverse events was higher in the first month of the academic year as compared to the rest of the year. This excess risk decreased progressively and disappeared after the fourth month. Because anesthesiology requires a significant number of technical skills, an argument can be made for the use of simulation to teach technical skills at the beginning of training. There has been a significant growth in the use of simulation for training resident physicians, especially for teaching technical skills. Simulation offers an environment where learners can practice a skill many times in succession and can make errors without causing patient harm.

The next logical question is whether skills practiced in simulation translated into the clinical setting. Hall et al. recruited 36 paramedic students with no prior experience in endotracheal intubation into a study in which they were randomized to intubations on a patient simulator or on human subjects in the operating room. He then assessed their intubations and complication rate on 15 intubations in the operating room and found no difference between the groups in rate of intubation on first attempt as well as complications.[20] This suggests that it might be possible to overcome at least the adverse events from errors during

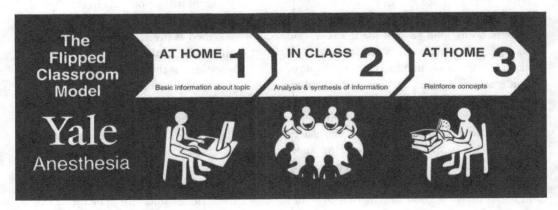

FIGURE 12.2: Graphic of the *flipped classroom* model used in the Yale Anesthesiology Residency curriculum.

technical procedures by having residents practice technical skills on a mannequin before their encounter with patients. Given the current trends toward increasing public scrutiny, decreased tolerance of medical errors, and reluctance on the part of patients to receive care from novice learners, simulation may help to bridge a gap. Performance of a technical skill involves progression from the cognition phase to the integration phase and finally to automation, where the skill is performed without the need to think about the steps involved.[21] This has led to the proposal for using simulation to make learners into "pre-trained novices" before encountering live patients.[22] In one institution (Yale University), residents are exposed to technical training in simulator for insertion of peripheral intravenous catheters, intra-arterial catheters, and central venous catheters during orientation, before their contact with patients.

Simulators have also been used to teach transesophageal echocardiography (TEE), which has traditionally required training on high-acuity patients undergoing cardiovascular surgery. A study of post-training test scores between resident physicians in their first year of anesthesia training who were randomized to training on a TEE simulator *versus* American Society of Echocardiography/Society of Cardiovascular Anesthesiologists guidelines and other conventional resources found higher scores among the study group compared to the control group.[23]

Feedback and motivation, in addition to repetitive practice, are required to improve learner performance.[24] Moreover, multiple short sessions have been demonstrated to be better than one long session for the retention of skills.[25] The use of simulation for formative and summative assessments is still the topic of considerable debate, while its use for introducing cognitive aids for crisis management has gained popularity.[26] A number of studies have been done to evaluate the effect of the use of cognitive aids in a simulator involving anesthesia residents.[27,28] Ideally, a cognitive aid should be readily available at the point of care, and should have a good design that provides clinicians dealing with a stressful situation an "easy to understand and follow" sequence of steps that will aid in the diagnosis of a condition or the treatment of a problem. The cognitive aid should be familiar to the person using it and as such should be incorporated into training. The use of cognitive aids improves technical performance in most studies; however, the effects on team dynamics and interpersonal communication, which are also important in crisis situations, are less clear.[29] The lack of uniform standards for simulators has also been a drawback in the advancement of common goals for training.[30]

In spite of increasing levels of fidelity in simulation environments, the majority of learning during residency training takes place in the operating room, critical care units, and procedural anesthetizing locations (e.g., in the endoscopy suite). The drawbacks of teaching in this setting include balancing patient safety with autonomy, impairment of nonverbal communication when masks must be worn, and the need for rapid action with little or no explanation during critical events. Techniques that facilitate learning in this environment include role modeling and thinking aloud while managing a crisis. Immediate debriefing after a critical event can help the learner to understand the thought process and the sequence of actions that occurred. For example, the Yale program makes use of different methods of learning for each level of Miller's pyramid[31] (Figure 12.3).

1. *Knows*: This level refers to the retention of factual information and is taught using podcasts in the *flipped classroom* model. These podcasts are assigned as prework for workshops, and assessments are multiple-choice questions at the end of the session.

2. *Knows how*: The interpretation and synthesis of knowledge. This is facilitated in the interactive sessions of the flipped classroom model and also case-based and problem-based discussions

3. *Shows how*: Demonstration of learning. Simulation sessions that follow the didactic sessions aim to facilitate this level of learning.

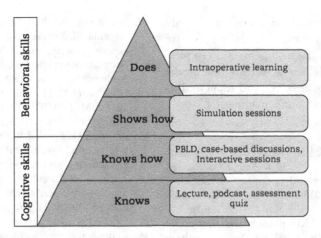

FIGURE 12.3: Integration of Miller's pyramid into anesthesia residency curriculum.

4. *Does*: Using information and knowledge in clinical practice. This level of understanding is assessed in the operating room. Ideally, topics that are discussed in the didactic sessions will be incorporated into patient care strategies.

THE LEARNER

Student engagement is used as a measure of the effectiveness of the lesson and depends on the presentation skills of the teacher as well as the learner's perceived value of the lesson content. Engagement seems to be the goal of all educational curricula and lesson plans. Are there particular factors that increase student engagement, and is it possible to use them to the advantage of the teacher and learner?

Survey instruments have been designed to measure student engagement. The National Survey of Student Engagement (NSSE) and the College Student Experiences Questionnaire (CSEQ) have recently been used to test institutional excellence.[32] Although the term *engagement* itself can be nebulous, the NSSE defines it as a part of student behavior and as such is something that can be observed. *Engagement* has three described areas: behavioral, emotional, and cognitive. Axelson defines *student engagement* as how "we engage (cognitively, behaviorally and emotionally) type X students most effectively in type Y learning processes/contexts so that they will attain knowledge,

skill or disposition Z."[32] Both the learner and the institution help to determine the level of student engagement. Institutions must create an inviting learning environment, while learners must demonstrate a commitment to learn and make an effort to use the resources at hand.

The meta-cognition of receiving feedback has also received much attention recently with respect to learner attributes. Douglas Stone and Sheila Heen describe the importance of meta-cognition when receiving feedback in their book *Thanks for the Feedback: The Science and Art of Receiving Feedback Well*. They identify a number of factors that prevent the learner from constructively using feedback. These factors include the truth trigger (set off by the content of the feedback), the relationship trigger (set off by the person giving the feedback), and the identity trigger (feedback threatening our image of ourselves).[33] Identifying these triggers will allow the learner to move past emotional blocks and improve performance.

CONCLUSIONS

It is possible to implement evidence-based practices in medical education, but they present the same difficulties as those encountered in clinical practice. It is now necessary to keep abreast of the the latest publications on educational science, to constantly evaluate training programs, and to make changes as necessary to ensure that "learning" takes place. Education must be a priority in residency departments, and innovation should be encouraged. Only then will it be possible to deliver on the promise to society to "train the next generation of physicians" who can deliver healthcare in a model that we as yet do not envision, and adapt to situations that as yet cannot be imagined.

REFERENCES

1. Bould MD, Naik VN, Hamstra SJ. Review article: new directions in medical education related to anesthesiology and perioperative medicine. *Can J Anaesth*. 2012;59(2):136–150. doi: 10.1007/s12630-011-9633-0. PubMed PMID: 22161241.

2. Kirkpatrick DL, Kirkpatrick JD. *Evaluating Training Programs*. 3rd ed. San Francisco: Berrett-Koehler; 1998.

3. Buchel TL, Edwards FD. Characteristics of effective clinical teachers. *Fam Med*. 2005;37(1):30–35. PubMed PMID: 15619153.

4. McMillan WJ. "Then you get a teacher": guidelines for excellence in teaching. *Med Teach*. 2007;29(8):e209–218. doi: 10.1080/01421590701478264. PubMed PMID: 18236265.

5. Kilminster S, Jolly B, van der Vleuten CP. A framework for effective training for supervisors. *Med Teach*. 2002;24(4):385–389. Epub 2002/08/24. doi: 10.1080/0142159021000000834. PubMed PMID: 12193321.

6. Cottrell D, Kilminster S, Jolly B, Grant J. What is effective supervision and how does it happen? A critical incident study. *Med Educ*. 2002;36(11):1042–1049. Epub 2002/10/31. PubMed PMID: 12406264.

7. Kilminster S, Cottrell D, Grant J, Jolly B. AMEE Guide No. 27: Effective educational and clinical supervision. *Med Teach*. 2007;29(1):2–19. Epub 2007/06/01. doi: 10.1080/01421590701210907. PubMed PMID: 17538823.

8. Gennis VM, Gennis MA. Supervision in the outpatient clinic: effects on teaching and patient care. *J Gen Intern Med*. 1993;8(7):378–380. Epub 1993/07/01. PubMed PMID: 8192744.

9. Roff S, McAleer S. What is educational climate? *Med Teach*. 2001;23(4):333–334. doi: 10.1080/01421590120063312. PubMed PMID: 12098377.

10. Menachery EP, Wright SM, Howell EE, Knight AM. Physician-teacher characteristics associated with learner-centered teaching skills. *Med Teach*. 2008;30(5):e137–144. doi: 10.1080/01421590801942094. PubMed PMID: 18576184.

11. Singh S, Pai DR, Sinha NK, Kaur A, Soe HH, Barua A. Qualities of an effective teacher: what do medical teachers think? *BMC Med Educ*. 2013;13:128. doi: 10.1186/1472-6920-13-128. PubMed PMID: 24044727; PubMed Central PMCID: PMCPMC3848658.

12. van Roermund TC, Tromp F, Scherpbier AJ, Bottema BJ, Bueving HJ. Teachers' ideas versus experts' descriptions of "the good teacher" in postgraduate medical education: implications for implementation. A qualitative study. *BMC Med Educ*. 2011;11:42. doi: 10.1186/1472-6920-11-42. PubMed PMID: 21711507; PubMed Central PMCID: PMCPMC3163623.

13. Branch WT, Frankel R, Gracey CF, Haidet PM, Weissmann PF, Cantey P, et al. A good clinician and a caring person: longitudinal faculty development and the enhancement of the human dimensions of care. *Acad Med*. 2009;84(1):117–125. doi: 10.1097/ACM.0b013e3181900f8a. PubMed PMID: 19116489.

14. Kannan J, Kurup V. Blended learning in anesthesia education: current state and future model. *Curr Opin Anaesthesiol*. 2012;25(6):692–698. doi: 10.1097/ACO.0b013e32835a1c2a. PubMed PMID: 23147669.

15. Nasca TJ, Day SH, Amis ES, Force ADHT. The new recommendations on duty hours from the ACGME Task Force. *N Engl J Med*. 2010;363(2):e3. doi: NEJMsb1005800 [pii] 10.1056/NEJMsb1005800. PubMed PMID: 20573917.

16. Kurup V, Hersey D. The changing landscape of anesthesia education: is Flipped Classroom the answer? *Curr Opin Anaesthesiol*. 2013;26(6):726–731. Epub 2013/10/16. doi: 10.1097/aco.0000000000000004. PubMed PMID: 24126692.

17. Prober CG, Khan S. Medical education reimagined: a call to action. *Acad Med*. 2013;88(10):1407–1410. doi: 10.1097/ACM.0b013e3182a368bd. PubMed PMID: 23969367.

18. Prunuske AJ, Batzli J, Howell E, Miller S. Using online lectures to make time for active learning. *Genetics*. 2012;192(1):67–72; quiz 1Sl-3SL. Epub 2012/06/21. doi: 10.1534/genetics.112.141754. PubMed PMID: 22714412; PubMed Central PMCID: PMCPmc-3430546.

19. Haller G, Myles PS, Taffé P, Perneger TV, Wu CL. Rate of undesirable events at beginning of academic year: retrospective cohort study. *BMJ*. 2009;339:b3974. PubMed PMID: 19826176; PubMed Central PMCID: PMCPMC2762036.

20. Hall RE, Plant JR, Bands CJ, Wall AR, Kang J, Hall CA. Human patient simulation is effective for teaching paramedic students endotracheal intubation. *Acad Emerg Med*. 2005;12(9):850–855. doi: 10.1197/j.aem.2005.04.007. PubMed PMID: 16141019.

21. Reznick RK, MacRae H. Teaching surgical skills: changes in the wind. *N Engl J Med*. 2006;355(25):2664–2669. doi: 10.1056/NEJMra-054785. PubMed PMID: 17182991.

22. Castanelli DJ. The rise of simulation in technical skills teaching and the implications for training

novices in anaesthesia. *Anaesth Intens Care.* 2009;37(6):903–910. PubMed PMID: 20014595.

23. Bose RR, Matyal R, Warraich HJ, Summers J, Subramaniam B, Mitchell J, et al. Utility of a transesophageal echocardiographic simulator as a teaching tool. *J Cardiothorac Vasc Anesth.* 2011;25(2):212–215. Epub 2010/10/27. doi: 10.1053/j.jvca.2010.08.014. PubMed PMID: 20974542.

24. Ericsson KA. Deliberate practice and the acquisition and maintenance of expert performance in medicine and related domains. *Acad Med.* 2004;79(10 Suppl):S70–81. PubMed PMID: 15383395.

25. Gallagher AG, Ritter EM, Champion H, Higgins G, Fried MP, Moses G, et al. Virtual reality simulation for the operating room: proficiency-based training as a paradigm shift in surgical skills training. *Ann Surg.* 2005;241(2):364–372. PubMed PMID: 15650649; PubMed Central PMCID: PMCPMC1356924.

26. Arriaga AF, Bader AM, Wong JM, Lipsitz SR, Berry WR, Ziewacz JE, et al. Simulation-based trial of surgical-crisis checklists. *N Engl J Med.* 2013;368(3):246–253. Epub 2013/01/18. doi: 10.1056/NEJMsa1204720. PubMed PMID: 23323901.

27. Gaba DM. Perioperative cognitive aids in anesthesia: what, who, how, and why bother? *Anesth Analg.* 2013;117:1033–1036.

28. Goldhaber-Fiebert SN, Howard SK. Implementing emergency manuals: can cognitive aids help translate best practices for patient care during acute events? *Anesth Analg.* 2013;117(5):1149–1161. Epub 2013/10/11. doi: 10.1213/ANE.0b013e318298867a. PubMed PMID: 24108251.

29. Marshall S. The use of cognitive aids during emergencies in anesthesia: a review of the literature. *Anesth Analg.* 2013;117(5):1162–1171. Epub 2013/09/14. doi: 10.1213/ANE.0b013e31829c397b. PubMed PMID: 24029855.

30. Cumin D, Weller JM, Henderson K, Merry AF. Standards for simulation in anaesthesia: creating confidence in the tools. *BJ Anaesth.* 2010;105(1):45–51. doi: 10.1093/bja/aeq095.

31. Miller GE. The assessment of clinical skills/competence/performance. *Acad Med.* 1990;65(9 Suppl):S63–67. PubMed PMID: 2400509.

32. Axelson R. Defining student engagement. *Change (New Rochelle, NY).* 2011;43(1):38–43.

33. Stone D, Heen. *Thanks for the Feedback: The Science and Art of Receiving Feedback Well.* New York: Penguin Group; 2014.

13

Regulating Quality

ROBERT S. LAGASSE

BACKGROUND

The healthcare industry is part of the free market economy of the United States and is, therefore, subject to the laws of supply and demand. Because the demand for healthcare services remains high, and is continuing to rise as technology advancement leads to the availability of new services, prices are increasing out of proportion to inflation. National healthcare expenditures reached $2.9 trillion in 2013, or $9,255 per person, and accounted for 17.4% of gross domestic product (GDP).[1] Health insurance in the United States has historically provided financial protection against the high costs associated with medical treatment, desensitizing individual consumers to the value of healthcare services. This cost is frequently borne by employers, who often provide health insurance as part of employee compensation in the United States. The government is the second major payer for healthcare in the United States. Federal, state, and local governments pay almost half of the national healthcare expenditure through Medicare, Medicaid, the Children's Health Insurance Program, and other programs.

In 2009, the Executive Office of the President's Council of Economic Advisers (CEA) provided an overview of the economic impacts of healthcare in the United States.[2] The CEA suggested that, if healthcare costs continued to grow at historical rates, its share of GDP would reach 34% by 2040. For households with employer-sponsored health insurance, this implies that a progressively smaller fraction of employee compensation would be in the form of take-home pay, while a significantly larger fraction would be in the form of health insurance, because health insurance premiums are growing more rapidly than employee compensation. Between 1996 and 2006, the average annual premium for family coverage obtained through an employer grew from $6,462 to $11,941.[2] Rising healthcare costs may also reduce the profitability and competitiveness of many US industries. To put this into perspective, General Motors spent $5.2 billion on employee health benefits in 2004,[3] which was more than their annual expenditure for steel. Perhaps most compelling, the 2009 CEA report projected that the current trend in Medicare and Medicaid spending would lead to an unsustainable rise in the federal deficit. This impact is even greater at the state level, where rising Medicaid costs for low-income populations compete with legislative requirements to balance state budgets.

The CEA also addressed the unacceptably high number of uninsured consumers of healthcare. For example, 45.7 million Americans did not have health insurance in 2007.[4] The increase in healthcare costs and the associated increase in insurance premiums are deterring an increasing number of employers from offering health insurance as part of workers' total compensation, and out-of-pocket premium requirements are becoming less affordable. The rising number of uninsured Americans leads to an increase in uncompensated healthcare costs, which include costs incurred by hospitals and physicians for the charity care that they provide, as well as bad debt that must be written off. Both the federal government and state governments use tax revenues to pay healthcare providers for a portion of these uncompensated costs through Disproportionate Share Hospital (DSH) payments, grants to Community Health Centers, and other mechanisms. In 2008, total government spending to reimburse uncompensated care costs incurred by medical providers was approximately $42.9 billion.[5]

Although the United States devotes a far larger share of GDP to healthcare than other developed countries, it does not achieve better health outcomes.[6] According to the Organization for Economic Co-operation and Development (OECD), the United States spent 16.9% of its GDP on healthcare in 2013. The next highest country was France, with 11.6%, while many high-income countries spent less than 10%.[6] Despite this level of expenditure, life expectancy in the United States is one of the lowest among developed countries. In 2010, life expectancy for all live births in the United States was 78.6 years, which was lower than that of 22 other developed countries. In fact, 18 countries had life expectancies of more than 80 years.[6] Infant mortality rate in the United States is also substantially above that of other developed countries. In 2010, there were 6.1 deaths for every 1000 live births in the United States, which was higher than the rates of 25 other developed countries. In the top-ranked countries, like Finland and Japan, the infant mortality rate was less than half the rate in the United States, at 2.3 deaths per 1000 live births.[7] Many factors other than healthcare costs affect life expectancy and infant mortality rates, but life expectancy has risen less in the United States than in other countries since 1970, when US healthcare costs were closer to those of other high-income countries.[8] These data strongly suggest that there are inefficiencies in the current US healthcare system.

The idea that healthcare quality is not optimal in the United States is certainly not a new concept. Since the late 1970s, John Wennberg has written about variations in clinical practice.[9-22] He examined factors such as surgery rates, drug use, and lab test ordering, which showed significant differences between industrialized countries. Eventually, he demonstrated that these same differences existed when comparing clinical practices from state to state, town to town, even between neighboring hospitals in the same town within the United States. More recently, Wennberg and colleagues, associated with the Dartmouth Atlas of Health Care, have shown that per capita Medicare spending varies as much as twofold by geographic region within the United States, and, in many cases, these variations are not associated with any substantial differences in health outcomes.[23] Because US states have fewer potential confounding variables than do independent countries, this comparison is even more compelling than the global comparison offered by the OECD.

In 1999, the Institute of Medicine (IOM), through its Quality of Healthcare in America Project, published a sentinel report, *To Err Is Human: Building a Safer Health System*. It reported that 44,000 to 98,000 Americans die each year as a result of medical errors. Even when using the lower estimate, deaths caused by medical errors exceeded the number attributable to the eighth leading cause of death in the United States at that time. According to the IOM, more people died in a given year as a result of medical errors than from motor vehicle accidents (43,458), breast cancer (42,297), or AIDS (16,516). Medication errors alone, occurring either in or out of the hospital, accounted for an estimated 7000 deaths annually. That is more than the estimated 6000 Americans who die each year as a result of workplace injuries. Translating quality into cost, the IOM estimated that preventable adverse outcomes increased healthcare spending by $17 billion to $20 billion annually.[24] This observation led the IOM, in a second report from the Quality of Healthcare in America Project, entitled *Crossing the Quality Chasm: A New Health System for the 21st Century*, to recommend that the US healthcare system be redesigned. According to this report, the healthcare system should focus on applying evidence to healthcare delivery, using information technology, aligning payment policies with quality improvement, and preparing the healthcare workforce for the necessary changes.[25]

Interest in improving healthcare quality while decreasing cost has increased significantly in recent years, but this concept has existed for decades. In 1983, for example, unit pricing based on diagnostically related groups (DRGs) shifted Medicare hospital payments from a retrospective, cost-based system to a prospective, condition-based system. With DRGs, Medicare paid hospitals a fixed amount to treat a patient with a specific condition, regardless of how long the treatment took or the resources expended in doing so. This new prospective payment system removed incentives for keeping patients hospitalized because longer stays did not result in additional reimbursements. DRGs resulted in lasting reductions in length of stay and services used in hospitals across the United States (Figure 13.1).[26] Unfortunately, however, overall healthcare spending was not significantly affected because the bulk of patient care merely shifted from inpatient to outpatient settings. This early experiment in the reform of healthcare financing did, however, demonstrate that payment incentives could modify the behavior of healthcare providers.

The delivery of healthcare and health insurance coverage are subject to an increasing amount of legislation that is created under the authority of several regulatory agencies. The Department of Health and Human Services (HHS) is the US government's principal regulatory agency for healthcare and is responsible for almost one-quarter of all federal spending.

HHS administers more grant money than all other federal agencies combined. HHS has implemented a variety of programs and initiatives that support its mission and cover a wide spectrum of activities that impact healthcare at every stage of life. Eleven operating divisions, including eight agencies in the US Public Health Service and three human services agencies, administer HHS's programs. HHS is required by the Government Performance and Results Act (GPRA) of 1993[27] and the GPRA Modernization Act of 2010[28] to update its strategic plan every 4 years. The strategic plan defines HHS's mission, its goals, and the means by which it will measure its progress in addressing specific healthcare issues over a 4-year period. The HHS Strategic Plan for 2014–2018[29] describes the Department's efforts within the context of four broad strategic goals:

1. Strengthen healthcare;
2. Advance scientific knowledge and innovation;
3. Advance the health, safety, and well-being of the American people;
4. Ensure the efficiency, transparency, accountability, and effectiveness of HHS's programs.

Multiple agencies within HHS, and several high-profile regulations, are targeting these strategic goals.

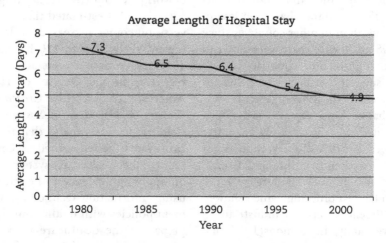

FIGURE 13.1: Effect of implementation of DRGs on average length of hospital stay.

The Patient Protection and Affordable Care Act and the Health Care and Education Reconciliation Act, collectively referred to as the Affordable Care Act (ACA), were signed into law in 2010.[30] The ACA makes healthcare more accessible by increasing the availability of health insurance, improving the value of Medicare, and encouraging states to expand access to Medicaid under federal subsidy. The ACA requires everyone in the United States to have health insurance and offers financial assistance through tax credits and cost-sharing reductions, protection against medical bankruptcy, and penalties for insurers discriminating because of a pre-existing patient condition. The Health Insurance Marketplace created by the ACA (also known as *Health Insurance Exchanges*) allows consumers to compare their insurance options based on price, benefits, and quality. The ACA additionally seeks to develop high-value healthcare by promoting efficiency, ensuring accountability, and improving quality outcomes by emphasizing prevention and safety across healthcare settings. HHS is responsible for implementing many of the provisions included in the Affordable Care Act as a means of achieving its first strategic goal. Among the many HHS agencies working to improve the value of healthcare are the Centers for Medicare and Medicaid Services (CMS).[31] CMS oversees Medicare, Medicaid, the Children's Health Insurance Program (CHIP), the Health Insurance Portability and Accountability Act (HIPAA), the Health Information Technology for Economic and Clinical Health (HITECH) Act,[32] and Clinical Laboratory Improvement Amendments (CLIA), among other services, all of which have a regulatory affect on anesthesia and perioperative care.

HHS is expanding its scientific understanding of how to advance healthcare, public health, human services, biomedical research, and the availability of safe medical and food products. HHS has been focusing on using technology to improve collaboration, modernizing the regulatory approval process, and expanding behavioral research. HHS is also promoting service integration and delivery through community-based approaches and collaboration with the private sector. Among the HHS agencies working to advance scientific knowledge and innovation are the Agency for Healthcare Research and Quality (AHRQ),[33] the Centers for Disease Control and Prevention (CDC),[34] and the National Institutes of Health (NIH).[35] All of these agencies affect the scientific basis of anesthesiology, as well as the delivery of perioperative care.

HHS advances their third goal by addressing the unique needs of vulnerable populations through program coordination within HHS, policy development, promotion of evidence-based practice, and research. Threats to population health include poverty, family problems, substance abuse, mental illness, limited health literacy, violence, trauma, an aging US population, and naturally occurring and man-made disasters. Protecting public health in the United States also requires international cooperation to promote the safety of imported medical products and lessen the impact of global outbreaks of disease. The Agency for Healthcare Research and Quality (AHRQ), Centers for Medicare and Medicaid Services (CMS), Centers for Disease Control and Prevention (CDC), Food and Drug Administration (FDA),[36] Health Resources and Services Administration (HRSA),[37] Indian Health Service (IHS),[38] and National Institutes of Health (NIH) work under the auspices of HHS, with other federal departments, to improve health, safety, and well-being. Anesthesiologists in the United States are affected by the regulatory efforts aimed at this goal on a daily basis through the CMS conditions of participation (COP). These regulations govern the delivery of healthcare to elderly and impoverished patients. Additionally, standards of care developed by private accrediting agencies with deeming authority, like the Joint Commission[39] and others,[40-44] enforce HHS agency recommendations and regulatory efforts. Moreover, if an institution is engaged in human subjects research, it must comply with the HHS regulations for the protection of human subjects.

The fourth goal is all-encompassing in its efforts to define the efficiency, transparency, accountability, and effectiveness of HHS programs. To improve performance and ensure the responsible stewardship of more than $900 billion in public investments, HHS continues to strengthen and integrate financial, performance, and risk management systems. HHS's risk management efforts focus on fraud, waste, and abuse. The Affordable Care Act and the Improper Payments Elimination and Recovery Act[27] provide for state-of-the-art fraud detection technology to prevent, reduce, and recover improper payments in the Medicare and Medicaid programs. In order to increase government transparency, HHS has made information easily accessible online through Web-based tools like HealthData.gov,[36] the CMS Data Navigator,[45] the Health Information Technology Dashboard,[46] and FDA-TRACK.[47] HHS has also focused on increasing the transparency of financial data by creating the Tracking Accountability in Government Grants System (TAGGS).[48] Regulations require departments and agencies to safeguard information technology systems containing certain categories of sensitive information such as personally identifiable information, proprietary information, and classified national security information. Anesthesiologists are most affected in their clinical practice by the HIPAA Standards for Privacy of Individually Identifiable Health Information (the Privacy Rule) and the CMS Conditions of Participation[31] that regulate billing and eliminate fraudulent claims in the Medicare and Medicaid programs.

Many of the regulations that are designed to accomplish the strategic goals of HHS affect the daily workflow of anesthesiologists and other perioperative healthcare professionals. The remainder of this chapter focuses on specific mandates regulating the quality of perioperative care, including those issued by private agencies granted authority by CMS to act on their behalf.

THE AFFORDABLE CARE ACT

On March 23, 2010, the Patient Protection and Affordable Care Act was signed into law.[49] The Affordable Care Act (ACA) is perhaps the most controversial healthcare legislation in a generation, and also carries the most influence on how healthcare is delivered. In addition to codified quality improvement and value-based purchasing initiatives, the ACA compels all Americans to buy health insurance or pay a penalty. The individual mandate was necessary to make health insurance more accessible to all Americans. The ACA makes health insurance more accessible by "mandatory issue" that prevents health plans from denying coverage to people with pre-existing conditions, and "community rating" that limits the premiums that health plans may charge based on pre-existing conditions. Without the individual mandate, insurance companies would fall victim to the phenomenon of "adverse selection" in which individuals only buy health insurance when they need it. This phenomenon would prevent insurers from spreading the economic risk among a large pool of insured that includes healthy people who do not use significant healthcare resources. Thus, the mandatory issue and community rating provisions were interdependent upon the individual mandate.

One of the primary goals of the ACA is to make health insurance more accessible for individuals with incomes at or below 133% of the federal poverty level. This is made possible by a new Medicaid category that is expected to expand coverage in the United States by 11.2 million adults. Most of the costs of this Medicaid expansion are covered by a federal subsidy. Average state spending is expected to increase by less than 3%, while federal Medicaid spending will increase by 26%.[50] The proportion of Medicaid patients in most anesthesiology and pain practices has been increasing since enactment of the ACA, while lower Medicaid reimbursement rates are becoming more prevalent in the healthcare market.

Some studies suggest that newly insured individuals will seek more medical care. For example, Massachusetts instituted healthcare reform in 2006 that achieved near-universal coverage by 2009. This increase in the numbers of insured was accompanied by a 30% growth in healthcare expenditure, or $418 billion, between pre-reform 2006 and post-reform 2009.[51,52] Non-obstetrical inpatient procedures were among the services showing the largest increase after reform. Newly insured people may be expected to consume more healthcare than they did prior to gaining coverage, and a new demand for surgical services may translate into a significant increase in the need for perioperative care by anesthesia professionals.

VALUE-BASED PURCHASING

The ACA is intended to reduce federal healthcare expenditure by rewarding high-value healthcare, not the volume of care. It requires HHS to adopt value-based payment methods for Medicare reimbursements for both physicians and hospitals, and to move away from the traditional fee-for-service system. In 2013, an estimated $850 million was distributed to approximately 3200 hospitals, for discharges occurring on or after October 1, 2012. These payments were based on a set of clinical process measures believed to improve quality of care and patient satisfaction. Evaluation of hospital performance is based on Clinical Process of Care measures (70%) and Patient Experience of Care (30%) measures as determined by completed Hospital Consumer Assessment of Healthcare Providers and Systems (HCAHPS) surveys. Hospitals receive points for achievement and improvement, for each measure in the two domains, with the greater set of points counting toward the domain total. The funds for these quality bonuses were made available by reducing total DRG payments to all participating hospitals by 1%. The size of the fund will gradually increase over time, through progressive DRG reductions, resulting in a shift from payments based on volume to payments based on performance.

There are currently 12 measures in the Clinical Process of Care domain, and eight HCAHPS "dimensions" in the Patient Experience of Care domain, but these measures are rapidly evolving. Within the current Clinical Process of Care domain are several measures for which anesthesia professionals can take or share responsibility; these are marked by an asterisk in Box 13.1. Anesthesia personnel can also contribute to the hospital's performance on all the dimensions of the Patient Experience of Care domain.

The Hospital Value-Based Purchasing (HVBP) program uses the hospital quality data-reporting infrastructure developed for the hospital Inpatient Quality Reporting (IQR) Program, which was part of the Medicare Prescription Drug, Improvement, and Modernization Act of 2003. Hospitals participating in the HVBP program began receiving incentive payments for providing high-quality care or improving care after October 1, 2012, based on a hospital's performance during the period from July 1, 2011, to March 31, 2012. In order to be eligible, each hospital was required to report on at least four HVBP measures during the performance period, with a minimum of 10 cases per measure (see Box 13.1). CMS chose this number to balance the need for statistically reliable scores, with their goal of including as many hospitals as possible in HVBP. The RAND corporation estimated that a hospital would need to report the results of at least 100 HCAHPS surveys to meet eligibility requirements for the Patient Experience of Care domain. For a list of measures and how data are collected, hospital administrators may visit the "For Professionals" section of the Hospital Compare website.[48]

VALUE-BASED MODIFIER

The Affordable Care Act also mandated that CMS apply a *value-based modifier* to the Medicare Physician Fee Schedule (MPFS) by 2015. Both cost and quality data are to be included in calculating payments for physicians. Group practices of 100 or more eligible professionals (EPs) who submit claims to Medicare under a single tax identification number (TIN) were subject to the value-based modifier beginning in 2015, based on their performance in calendar year 2013. Physicians in group practices of 10 or more EPs who participate in Fee-For-Service Medicare under a single TIN are subject to the value-based modifier beginning in 2016, based on their performance in calendar year 2014. For the years 2015 and 2016, the value-based modifier does not apply to groups of physicians who participate in the Medicare Shared Savings Program, Pioneer ACOs, or the Comprehensive Primary Care Initiative, as described in the following section. Beginning

---

BOX 13.1   CLINICAL PROCESS OF CARE DOMAIN

CLINICAL PROCESS OF CARE MEASURES

- AMI-7a fibrinolytic therapy received within 30 minutes of hospital arrival
- AMI-8 primary PCI received within 90 minutes of hospital arrival
- HF-1 discharge instructions
- PN-3b blood cultures performed in the ED prior to initial antibiotic received in hospital
- PN-6 initial antibiotic selection for CAP in immunocompetent patient
- SCIP-Inf-1 prophylactic antibiotic received within 1 hour prior to surgical incision*
- SCIP-Inf-2 prophylactic antibiotic selection for surgical patients
- SCIP-Inf-3 prophylactic antibiotics discontinued within 24 hours after surgery
- SCIP-Inf-4 cardiac surgery patients with controlled 6AM postoperative serum glucose*
- SCIP-Card-2 surgery patients on a β-blocker prior to arrival that received a β-blocker* during the perioperative period
- SCIP-VTE-1 surgery patients with recommended venous thromboembolism prophylaxis ordered
- SCIP-VTE-2 surgery patients who received appropriate venous thromboembolism prophylaxis* within 24 hours

DIMENSIONS OF PATIENT EXPERIENCE OF CARE*

- Nurse communication
- Doctor communication
- Hospital staff responsiveness
- Pain management
- Medicine communication
- Hospital cleanliness and quietness
- Discharge information
- Overall hospital rating

Measures for which anesthesia professionals can take or share responsibility.

---

in 2017, this value-based modifier affects all physicians who participate in Fee-For-Service Medicare.[30]

MEDICARE SHARED SAVINGS PROGRAM

The Medicare Shared Savings Program, created by the ACA, established Accountable Care Organizations (ACOs), which are responsible for the quality, cost, and overall care of a minimum of 5000 Medicare fee-for-service beneficiaries for at least 3 years. Medicare fee-for-service beneficiaries are assigned to an ACO based on those beneficiaries' primary care physicians participating in the ACO, thus emphasizing the "medical home" model. Because of the way the system is designed, primary

care physicians have a relationship with only one ACO. But because they account for the participating beneficiaries, primary care physicians will confer substantial influence within their respective ACOs. In contrast, anesthesiologists and other specialists have more flexibility and can belong to multiple ACOs, but exert less influence within an individual ACO. The American Society of Anesthesiologists has proposed a "perioperative surgical home" with anesthesiologists as the physicians determining beneficiary participation, but this model has not yet been accepted by CMS.

An ACO that meets specific quality performance standards set by the Secretary of HHS is eligible to receive Medicare shared savings to be distributed among the participating healthcare providers. Shared savings payments are in addition to the otherwise available Medicare reimbursement. The ACO physicians and other participating professionals will continue to receive payments under Part A and Part B of the Medicare fee-for-service program. ACOs will not receive monetary penalties if quality benchmarks are not attained. The Secretary will, however, have the ability to terminate ACOs that do not satisfy such quality standards. ACOs are prohibited from taking steps to avoid at-risk patients who are likely to negatively impact their success. In order to submit information necessary to determine their quality of care, each ACO will need a technology infrastructure, including an electronic health record (EHR), that is capable of maintaining, retrieving, and sharing relevant data.

CENTER FOR MEDICARE AND MEDICAID INNOVATION

The ACA also established mechanisms for the development of future regulation. A new Center for Medicare and Medicaid Innovation was established to research, develop, test, and expand innovative payment and delivery models. The Affordable Care Act will invest $10 billion in this center by 2020. Its three focus areas for Medicare, Medicaid, and CHIP beneficiaries include (1) improving care by exploring specific innovations, such as using bundled payments as opposed to fee-for-service billing; (2) developing new models that enable physicians in different care settings to work collaboratively; and (3) testing care and payment models that emphasize preventive medicine initiatives that alleviate public health issues such as smoking and obesity. Additionally, the ACA established the Independent Payment Advisory Board (IPAB) to study and present recommendations on private sector health spending and Medicare. IPAB submits annual recommendations to Congress, outlining methods to reduce Medicare expenditures when Medicare's spending grows faster than the Consumer Price Index and medical price growth as a whole. If Congress does not accept these recommendations, it must then enact policies that achieve equivalent cost reductions.[40] Although IPAB is projected to reduce Medicare costs by almost $24 billion by 2019, there was no applicable savings target for 2015 because the projected 5-year Medicare per capita growth rate did not exceed the Medicare per capita target growth rate set by the Consumer Price Index.[53]

The Pioneer ACO Model is another CMS Innovation Center initiative that is designed to test the impact of different payment models on an ACO's ability to provide quality patient care and reduce Medicare costs. This model allows providers that are already experienced in coordinating patient care across different settings to move from a shared savings payment model to a population-based payment model more quickly. These Pioneer ACOs begin using shared savings payment models, with generally higher levels of shared savings and risk than levels currently applied to the Medicare Shared Savings Program, for 2 years. In year 3, Pioneer ACOs that have demonstrated a specified level of savings will be eligible to move a substantial portion of their payments to a population-based model. Although this model is similar to the Medicare Shared Services Program in its efforts to improve quality and health outcomes across the ACO, it is designed to work in coordination with private payers as well.[1]

The Comprehensive Primary Care (CPC) initiative is an additional CMS Innovation Center initiative that is designed to strengthen the role of primary care. Since October 2012, CMS has collaborated with commercial and state health insurance plans in seven US regions to offer population-based care management fees and shared savings opportunities to participating primary care practices to support the provision of a core set of five primary care functions. These five "Comprehensive" functions include (1) Risk-Stratified Care Management; (2) Access and Continuity; (3) Planned Care for Chronic Conditions and Preventive Care; (4) Patient and Caregiver Engagement; and (5) Coordination of Care across the Medical Neighborhood. As with Pioneer ACOs, the purpose of this initiative is to determine whether multi-payer payment reform, data-driven performance improvement, and "meaningful use" of health information technology can improve care and lower costs.[1]

HEALTH INFORMATION TECHNOLOGY: MEANINGFUL USE

The Medicare and Medicaid Electronic Health Record (EHR) Incentive Programs provide financial incentives to eligible professionals and hospitals as they adopt, implement, upgrade, or demonstrate meaningful use (MU) of certified EHR technology. Anesthesiologists are automatically exempt, based on their Provider, Enrollment, Chain and Ownership System (PECOS) specialty designation, but may still choose to participate. Of note, this exemption does not apply to anesthesiologists who have enrolled in PECOS with pain medicine codes as their primary specialty designation, unless they are primarily hospital-based. Nonexempt physicians faced a 1% decrease in reimbursement for covered professional services under the Medicare Physician Fee Schedule in 2015 if they could not meet the MU objectives in each of three stages. This penalty increases to 2% in 2016 and 3% in 2017, for eligible providers who cannot meet the MU objectives in each of three stages. The difference between the stages lies in the number of MU objectives[31] and clinical quality measures[31] that must be reported.

HEALTH INFORMATION PORTABILITY AND ACCOUNTABILITY ACT (HIPAA)

The Health Insurance Portability and Accountability Act of 1996 (HIPAA)[54] required HHS to adopt national standards for electronic healthcare transactions and code sets, unique health identifiers, and security in order to improve the efficiency and effectiveness of the healthcare system. Under the Administrative Simplification provisions of HIPAA, all covered entities that submit electronic claims for services, including anesthesia and pain medicine services, are required

to do so via a common set of standards. Electronic data interchange (EDI) is an electronic communication system that provides standards for exchanging data through electronic means. At the same time, Congress recognized that advances in electronic technology could threaten the privacy of health information and mandated the adoption of federal privacy protections for individually identifiable health information as a key part of HIPAA. The finalized HIPAA regulations on Breach Notification impose responsibilities for securing "protected health information" (PHI) and financial penalties for privacy breaches resulting from unsecured PHI. Compliance with the Security Rule has been required since April 20, 2005. The Health Information Technology for Economic and Clinical Health Act (HITECH)[55] provides HHS with the authority to develop a nationwide health information technology infrastructure. HITECH also contains specific incentives designed to accelerate providers' adoption of electronic health record systems, and expands the scope of HIPAA while increasing the potential legal liability and penalties for noncompliance.

HUMAN RESEARCH PROTECTIONS

Institutions that are engaged in human subjects research must have an Institutional Review Board (IRB) that ensures compliance with the HHS regulations for the protection of human subjects. These regulations have been in place since 1991 and are often referred to as the *Common Rule*. In 2011, HHS made substantial changes to the regulations related to the ethics, safety, and oversight of human research.[54] These changes included the following:

1. Specific data security protections for IRB-reviewed research;
2. Consent requirements for research using existing biospecimens that do not have identifiers (e.g., from prior research);
3. Expanding the scope of the regulations to apply to all studies conducted by US

institutions that receive some federal funding for human subjects research;

4. Required reporting of research-related adverse events to a central repository;

5. Greater specificity for the requirements of informed consent, with a focus on key elements;

6. Requirements for a single IRB of record for studies that are conducted at multiple sites in the United States, although multiple IRBs may review a single study;

7. Uniform interpretation of the regulations across federal agencies using the Common Rule;

8. Higher levels of scrutiny by an IRB for higher-risk studies;

9. No need for an annual review after completion of study interventions because the risks are limited to privacy and confidentiality concerns, which would be dealt with by the new uniform protections;

10. Basing the risks imposed by various research activities on appropriate data, rather than a list approved by the HHS Secretary;

11. No longer requiring continuing review of low-risk studies that are approved by expedited review unless the reviewer, at the time of initial review, determines that the level of risk may change;

12. Limiting expedited review to research activities that are included in the HHS-approved list and, therefore, are assumed to involve minimal risk;

13. Allowing different approval criteria for expedited review and full IRB review;

14. Requiring reasonable data security protections for research subjects;

15. Specific criteria for determining whether a study is exempt;

16. No longer requiring administrative review before a study is determined to be exempt;

17. Allowing research to be exempt, even if subject information is recorded in an identifiable way, because the data are deemed secure.

CENTERS FOR MEDICARE AND MEDICAID SERVICES

CMS develops Conditions of Participation (CoPs) that healthcare organizations must meet in order to receive payment for services to Medicare and Medicaid beneficiaries. On January 14, 2011, the Centers for Medicare and Medicaid Services (CMS) issued revised Interpretive Guidelines (IGs) pertaining to the CoPs that changed the requirements for hospitals that provide any degree of anesthesia services.[56] According to these IGs, *anesthesia services* include general anesthesia, regional anesthesia, deep sedation or analgesia, and monitored anesthesia care, but do not include local or topical anesthesia, minimal sedation, and moderate sedation or analgesia (conscious sedation). Anesthesia services, as defined here, may only be administered by qualified anesthesia professionals, including anesthesiologists, non-anesthesiologist physicians, dentists, oral surgeons, or podiatrists qualified under state law. Nurse anesthetists (CRNAs) and anesthesiologist's assistants (AAs) are also considered qualified anesthesia professionals and, unless exempted under state law, work under the supervision of the operating practitioner or an anesthesiologist.

The CoPs require all anesthesia services provided in a hospital to be organized under the direction of a qualified physician, in accordance with state law and the hospital's governing body. A single anesthesia director must be responsible for planning, directing, and supervising all anesthesia services throughout the hospital including all departments on all campuses and off-site locations where anesthesia services are provided.[56] The director is also responsible for monitoring the quality of anesthesia care as incorporated into the hospital-wide Quality Assurance and Performance Improvement Program. Anesthesia services must be organized and staffed in a manner that emphasizes safety for all patients.

Each hospital must establish policies and procedures, based on nationally recognized guidelines, in order to determine whether specific clinical situations involve "anesthesia" and how the anesthetic care must be conducted.

These policies must include, at a minimum, the qualifications, responsibilities, and supervision required of all personnel who administer anesthesia; informed anesthesia consent; infection control measures; safety practices in all anesthetizing areas; protocols for emergency life support; reporting requirements; documentation requirements; and equipment requirements. A qualified anesthesia provider must perform a pre-anesthesia evaluation within 48 hours of inpatient or outpatient surgery. This evaluation must include a risk assessment; drug and allergy history; potential anesthesia problems anticipated; and the patient's condition prior to induction of anesthesia. The anesthesia professional must maintain an intraoperative anesthesia record that includes patient identifiers; anesthesia provider(s); drugs and anesthesia agents; intravenous fluids; blood or blood products, if applicable; oxygen flow rate; continuous recordings of blood pressure, and heart and respiratory rate. Any complications or problems occurring during anesthesia must be included, as well as the patient's response to treatment. A post-anesthesia follow-up must also be written within 48 hours after surgery by an individual qualified to administer anesthesia in accordance with state law and hospital policy. At a minimum, the post-anesthesia follow-up report documents must include cardiopulmonary status; level of consciousness; follow-up care required; and any complications occurring during post-anesthesia recovery. A similar post-anesthesia evaluation must be documented in the medical record of outpatients for proper anesthesia recovery, performed in accordance with policies and procedures approved by the medical staff.

The CoPs target quality, but CMS is also governed by regulations that are designed to control costs. The Sustainable Growth Rate (SGR)[57] was a method used by CMS to control the cost of physician services, and was established by the Balanced Budget Act of 1997 to ensure that the yearly increase in the cost per Medicare beneficiary did not exceed the annual growth in GDP. Every year, CMS set a conversion factor for physician fees in order to match the target expenditures. If the

expenditures for the previous year exceeded the target expenditures, then the conversion factor decreased payments for the following year. If the expenditures were less than expected, the conversion factor increased payments to physicians. The implementation of the physician fee schedule update to meet the target SGR could be suspended or adjusted by Congress, and has been done so regularly in the past decade. In April 2015, Congress passed the Medicare Access and CHIP Reauthorization Act of 2015 (MACRA), a bipartisan bill that replaced the SGR formula. Included in this legislation were provisions that physicians would receive a 0.5% update for the initial 5 years of the law, while a new system, known as the Merit-Based Incentive Payment System (MIPS),[58] was implemented.

Physician anesthesiologists, certified anesthesiologist assistants, and nurse anesthetists who opt to participate in MIPS will receive payments that will be subject to positive or negative performance adjustments. These payment adjustments will replace the incentives previously supplied to these eligible professionals (EPs) through the Physicians Quality Reporting System, the value modifier, and meaningful use. MIPS will measure EP performance in four categories to derive a "MIPS score" (0 to 100), which can significantly change an EP's Medicare payment in each payment year. The performance categories are as follows: Physician Quality Reporting System (PQRS) measured quality (up to 30 points); Value-Based Modifier (VBM) measured resource use (30 points); Meaningful Use (MU) (25 points); and a new category named Clinical Practice Improvement Activities (CPIA) (15 points). The MIPS score's maximum negative impact on payment increases from −4% for the 2019 payment year to −9% for the 2022 and subsequent payment years. Additionally, MIPS scores will be publicly reported on Physician Compare with ranges and benchmarks.[58]

The Medicare Access and CHIP Reauthorization Act (MACRA) provides a bonus payment to physicians who are participating in alternative payment models (APMs), and it exempts them from participating in

MIPS. Eligible professionals receiving a substantial portion of their revenue from APMs will receive an annual lump-sum payment equal to 5% of their Medicare physician fees from 2019 to 2024. Eligible APMs, such as Medicare Shared Savings Program Accountable Care Organizations or The Health Care Quality Demonstration Programs, must require that participants use certified EHR technology, pay based on quality measures comparable to those used in the MIPS quality category, and place material financial risk on EPs.

ACCREDITATION ORGANIZATIONS

The CMS CoPs are the foundation for improving quality and protecting the health and safety of Medicare beneficiaries. Because of this, CMS requires that the standards of accrediting organizations, which are recognized by CMS through a process called *deeming*, meet or exceed the Medicare standards set forth in the CoPs. Under the Social Security Act, CMS may recognize national accreditation organizations as having *deeming authority* if they demonstrate that their health and safety standards, and their survey and oversight processes, meet or exceed those used by CMS for the CoPs. In other words, hospitals accredited by these recognized organizations are "deemed" to have met most of the requirements set forth in the CoPs for participation in Medicare. Deeming authority was granted to the Joint Commission in 1965 through the Social Security Act.[59] Other organizations were permitted to apply for deeming authority, and the American Osteopathic Association has done so since 1966 with its Health Facilities Accreditation Program (HFAP).[41] Statutory deeming authority under the Social Security Act was removed in 2010, so the Joint Commission now applies for deeming authority granted by the federal government, just like all other accreditation programs. Det Norske Veritas (DNV)[40] received deeming authority for hospitals in 2008, and the Center for Improvement in Healthcare Quality (CIHQ)[42] received deeming authority for hospitals in 2013.

Hospital accreditation, though voluntary, offers several advantages beyond deemed status.

Some insurers and third-party payers require accreditation in order to participate in managed care plans or to bid on contracts. Some liability insurers also offer a discount to organizations that are accredited. Accreditation may also fulfill some regulatory requirements in select states. In Georgia, for example, a healthcare facility must be accredited in order to be certified by the state as a cancer treatment center. In Alabama, accredited hospitals may not need to undergo state licensing surveys. In Ohio, accreditation may be beneficial to help defend against negligent credentialing suits. Despite its voluntary nature, an estimated 88% of hospitals in the United States are accredited or seeking accreditation.[60] Because the Joint Commission had statutory deeming authority and minimal competition for over 40 years, it accredits more than 80% of the hospitals in the United States.

Accrediting organizations with deeming authority have similar accreditation requirements because of the need to meet, or exceed, the CoPs, but there are subtle differences. The Joint Commission, for example, has additional healthcare standards, sentinel event alerts, and national patient safety goals that are developed in cooperation with healthcare professionals, the public, and other key stakeholders. HFAP standards include other nationally recognized standards, as well as evidenced-based best practice and selected patient safety initiatives from organizations such as AHRQ and the Institute for Healthcare Improvement. The National Integrated Accreditation for Healthcare Organizations (NIAHO)[61] is DNV's hospital accreditation program. The NIAHO standards integrate requirements based on the CMS CoPs with the internationally recognized ISO 9001 Standards.[61] ISO 9001 is an infrastructure for quality management systems that enable organizations to reach maximum effectiveness and efficiency in processes that should lead to improved outcomes, both clinically and financially. CIHQ has some standards that cover gaps in the CoPs in the areas of patient safety and quality care (e.g., temporary privileges, fair hearing processes, physician health, and telemedicine).[62] Like the CoPs, these additional accreditation requirements are based on the healthcare facilities patient population and services provided.

CONCLUSIONS

Because of the high demand for healthcare in our free market economy, the costs exceed 17% of US GDP, and that number may double by 2040. Because federal, state, and local governments assume nearly half of our national healthcare costs, governmental regulation has made several attempts to increase the value of healthcare by lowering costs and improving quality. In the 1980s, this took the form of unit pricing based on DRGs that shifted Medicare hospital payments from a retrospective, cost-based system to a prospective, condition-based system that paid hospitals fixed amounts for hospitalizations associated with specific conditions, regardless of the resources expended in treating those conditions. More recently, the Affordable Care Act codified value-based purchasing initiatives, and compelled all Americans to buy health insurance or pay a penalty. Value-based purchasing initiatives are being funded through progressive reductions in DRG payments, resulting in a shift from payments based on volume to payments based on performance. Hospital performance is currently based on Clinical Process of Care measures and Patient Experience of Care measures. The ACA also established Accountable Care Organizations through the Medicare Shared Savings Program. ACOs must be willing to be accountable for the quality, cost, and overall care of a minimum of 5000 Medicare fee-for-service beneficiaries. Medicare beneficiaries will be assigned to an ACO based on those beneficiaries' primary care physicians in a "medical home" model. Although the American Society of Anesthesiologists has proposed a "perioperative surgical home" model with anesthesiologists as the physicians determining beneficiary participation, this model has not yet been accepted by CMS. On the physician side, Congress passed a bill that replaced the Sustainable Growth Rate formula in April 2015. Included in this legislation was implementation of a new system, known as the Merit-Based Incentive Payment System

(MIPS) for physicians, but the details remain uncertain. The legislation also provides for physician participation in Alternative Payments Models, such as the Shared Savings Program. With an emphasis on effectiveness and efficiency in processes that should lead to improved outcomes, hospital accreditation is beginning to require the application of quality management systems used in other industries, such as ISO 9001. The effect of regulation on cost and quality in healthcare may be uncertain, but further regulatory changes seem inevitable.

REFERENCES

1. Centers for Medicare and Medicaid Services. http://innovation.cms.gov/initiatives/Pioneer-ACO-Model/. Accessed June 2015.
2. Council of Economic Advisors. The economic case for health care reform. 2009. https://www.whitehouse.gov/administration/eop/cea/TheEconomicCaseforHealthCareReform/. Accessed June 2015.
3. Hirsh S. GM plant a sign of decline. The Baltimore Sun. May 9, 2005. http://articles.baltimoresun.com/2005-05-09/news/0505090070_1_general-motors-gm-baltimore-workers. Accessed April 2016.
4. DeNavas-Walt C, Proctor BD, Smith JC. Income, poverty, and health insurance coverage in the United States: 2007. US Census Bureau. Washington, DC: US Government Printing Office; 2008.
5. Hadley J, Holahan J, Coughlin T, Miller D. Covering the uninsured in 2008: current costs, sources of payment, and incremental costs. Health Aff (Millwood). 2008;27(5):399–415.
6. Organisation for Economic Co-operation and Development. https://data.oecd.org/searchresults/?hf=20&b=0&r=%2Bf%2Fdata_portal_v2_topics_en%2Fhealth&l=en&s=score. Accessed June 2015.
7. Rettner R. US ranks behind 25 other countries in infant mortality. Accessed June 2015.
8. Garber AM, Skinner J. Is American health care uniquely inefficient? J Econ Perspect. Fall 2008;22(4):27–50.
9. McPherson K, Wennberg JE, Hovind OB, Clifford P. Small-area variations in the use of common surgical procedures: an international comparison of New England, England, and Norway. N Engl J Med. Nov 18 1982;307(21):1310–1314.
10. Wennberg J, Gittelsohn. Small area variations in health care delivery. Science. Dec 14 1973;182(4117):1102–1108.

11. Wennberg J, Gittelsohn A. Variations in medical care among small areas. *Scientific American.* Apr 1982;246(4):120–134.

12. Wennberg JE. Dealing with medical practice variations: a proposal for action. *Health Aff (Millwood).* Summer 1984;3(2):6–32.

13. Wennberg JE. Variations in medical practice and hospital costs. *Conn Med.* Jul 1985;49(7):444–453.

14. Wennberg JE. Practice variations: why all the fuss? *Internist.* Apr 1985;26(4):6–8.

15. Wennberg JE. Unwanted variations in the rules of practice. *JAMA.* Mar 13 1991;265(10):1306–1307.

16. Wennberg JE. Future directions for small area variations. *Med Care.* May 1993;31(5 Suppl):YS75–80.

17. Wennberg JE. Practice variations and the challenge to leadership. *Spine (Phila Pa 1976).* Jun 15 1996;21(12):1472–1478.

18. Wennberg JE. On the appropriateness of small-area analysis for cost containment. *Health Aff (Millwood).* Winter 1996;15(4):164–167.

19. Wennberg JE. Understanding geographic variations in health care delivery. *N Engl J Med.* Jan 7 1999;340(1):52–53.

20. Wennberg JE. Unwarranted variations in healthcare delivery: implications for academic medical centres. *BMJ.* Oct 26 2002;325(7370):961–964.

21. Wennberg JE. Practice variation: implications for our health care system. *Managed care.* Sep 2004;13(9 Suppl):3–7.

22. Wennberg JE. Practice variations and health care reform: connecting the dots. *Health Aff (Millwood).* 2004;Suppl Variation:VAR140–144.

23. Wennberg JE, Fisher ES, Skinner JS. Geography and the debate over Medicare reform. *Health Aff (Millwood).* Jul–Dec 2002;Suppl Web Exclusives:W96–114.

24. Kohn L, Corrigan J, M. D, eds. *To Err Is Human: Building a Safer Health Care System.* Washington, DC: National Academy Press; 1999.

25. Committee on Quality Health Care in America. *Crossing the Quality Chasm: A New Health System for the 21st Century.* Washington, DC: 2001.

26. Kozak LJ, DeFrances CJ, Hall MJ. National hospital discharge survey: 2004 annual summary with detailed diagnosis and procedure data. *Vital and Health Statistics. Series 13, Data from the National Health Survey.* Oct 2006(162): 1–209.

27. The White House PBO. https://www.whitehouse.gov/omb/mgmt-gpra/gplaw2m. Accessed March 2015.

28. GPRA Modernization Act of 2010. 2010.

29. US Department of Health and Human Services. OIG Strategic Plan 2014-2018. 2013.

30. The Patient Protection and Affordable Care Act. 2010.

31. Centers for Medicare and Medicaid Services. http://www.cms.gov/Regulations-and-Guidance/ Legislation/EHRIncentivePrograms/Meaningful_Use.html. Accessed March 2015.

32. Office of the National Coordinator for Health Information Technology. http://www.healthit.gov/policy-researchers-implementers/health-it-legislation-and-regulations Accessed March 2015.

33. Agency for Healthcare Research and Quality. http://www.ahrq.gov/. Accessed March 2015.

34. Centers for Disease Control. http://www.cdc.gov/ . Accessed March 2015.

35. National Institute of Health. http://nih.gov/. Accessed March 2015.

36. Food and Drug Administration. http://www.fda.gov/. Accessed March 2015.

37. Health Resources and Services Administration. http://www.hrsa.gov/index.html. Accessed March 2015.

38. Indian Health Services. http://www.ihs.gov/. Accessed March 2015.

39. The Joint Commission. http://www.jointcommission.org. Accessed March 2015.

40. Det Norske Veritas. http://dnvglhealthcare.com/ Accessed March 2015.

41. Health Facilities Accreditation Program. http://www.hfap.org/. Accessed March 2015.

42. Center for Improvement in Healthcare Quality. http://www.cihq.org/. Accessed March 2015.

43. Accreditation Association for Ambulatory Health Care. http://www.aaahc.org/. Accessed March 2015.

44. American Association for Accreditation of Ambulatory Surgical Facilities. http://www.aaaasf.org/. Accessed March 2015.

45. Centers for Medicare and Medicaid Services. http://dnav.cms.gov. Accessed June 2015.

46. Office of the National Coordinator for Health Information Technology. http://dashboard.healthit.gov/index.php. Accessed March 2015.

47. Food and Drug Administration. http://www.fda.gov/AboutFDA/Transparency/track/default.htm. Accessed June 2015.

48. Health and Human Services. http://www.hospitalcompare.hhs.gov/staticpages/for-professionals/poc/data-collection.aspx/ Accessed March 2015.

49. Mira T. http://www.beckersasc.com/anesthesia/the-affordable-care-act-the-supreme-court-and-anesthesiologists-just-the-facts-please.html. Accessed March 2015.

50. Kaiser Family Foundation. http://kff.org/medicaid/press-release/report-finds-state-costs-of-implementing-the/. Accessed March 2015.

51. Long SK, Stockley K. The impacts of state health reform initiatives on adults in New York and Massachusetts. *Health Serv Res.* Feb 2011;46(1 Pt2): 365–387.

52. Kolstad JT, Kowalski AE. The impact of health care reform on hospital and preventive care:

evidence from Massachusetts. *J Public Econ.* Dec 1 2012;96(11–12):909–929.

53. Kliff S. As health-care costs slow, IPAB's launch is delayed. http://www.washingtonpost.com/blogs/wonkblog/wp/2013/05/03/as-health-care-costs-slow-ipabs-launch-is-delayed/. Accessed March 2010.

54. Health and Human Services. http://www.hhs.gov/ocr/privacy/hipaa/administrative/index.html. Accessed June 2015.

55. Office of the National Coordinator for Health Information Technology. http://www.healthit.gov/policy-researchers-implementers/select-portions-hitech-act-and-relationship-onc-work. Accessed June 2015.

56. CMS Manual System. Department of Health & Human Services (DHHS) Pub. 100-07 State Operations Provider Certification Centers for Medicare & Medicaid Services (CMS). December 2, 2011; Transmittal 74:1-11.

57. American College of Physicians. http://www.acponline.org/advocacy/state_health_policy/hottopics/sgr.pdf. Accessed June 2015.

58. Medicare Access and CHIP Reauthorization Act of 2015. *H.R. 22015.*

59. Association SS. Compilation of the Social Security Laws. http://www.ssa.gov/OP_Home/ssact/title18/1865.htm. Accessed June 2015.

60. The Joint Commission. http://www.jointcommission.org/facts_about_hospital_accreditation/. Accessed June 2015.

61. Det Norske Veritas. http://www.dnvusa.com/Binaries/NIAHO. Accreditation Requirements-Rev 307-8 0_tcm153-347543.pdf. Accessed June 2015.

62. Center for Improvement in Healthcare Quality. http://cihq.org/hospital_accreditation_division.asp. Accessed April 2016.

14

Creating a Quality Management Program

RICHARD P. DUTTON

INTRODUCTION

Every anesthesia department and practice requires a robust quality management (QM) program. The QM program enables good management of the operating room, response to patient and surgeon complaints, and submission of public performance measures to the Centers for Medicare and Medicaid Services (CMS). A robust QM program supports the professional obligation of anesthesiologists to continually improve the safety and efficiency of patient care. The QM program creates the measuring stick for improving outcomes over time, both for the group as a whole and for individual members. Collection and analysis of adverse events allow every professional to learn from the experience of any provider, and create the substrate for improving systems of care within a "safety culture" of open and honest discussion protected from legal discovery or public embarrassment.

This chapter reviews the steps involved in the creation and support of an anesthesia department QM program, including suggestions for data collection, incident reporting, and analysis. The goal is a department in which every member participates in continuous quality improvement (CQI) as an expected and valued activity.[1]

INSTITUTIONAL SUPPORT

The QM program begins with a firm commitment from senior leadership. In an era when quality and performance data are required by the hospital organization to meet its regulatory requirements, the department QM program offers a competitive advantage: groups that understand their own performance are best positioned to improve it, and can use this understanding to win and maintain their service contracts. Department chairs and practice governing committees are more willing to make the necessary investment in QM than in years past, but more than money and time are required. Senior leaders of the group and facility must make it clear by their attitude and actions that participation in QM activities is important. Leaders must be willing to acknowledge their own mistakes and adverse outcomes, and must model both compliance with changes in practice and the processes that create them. Not every member of the group has to take time out of clinical practice to attend hospital meetings or review adverse outcomes, but those who do must be respected by their peers who stay in the OR. Members of the group must recognize the contribution of QM activities to the success of the practice.

LEADERSHIP AND ORGANIZATION

At the head of every successful QM program is a clinical leader: the department's QM officer. Most often this is a mid- to late-career anesthesiologist, but enthusiasm and motivation for the work are more important than seniority. The QM officer should be supported by senior leadership, with positional authority established at the outset. While actual influence will be based more on persuasion than coercion, every member of the practice and all external stakeholders should know who the QM officer is and what his or her role will be.

The QM officer serves as the contact point for all members of the group with safety or quality concerns, and is the department's primary representative to the facility's QM program. The role of the QM officer is to gather data from everywhere in the clinical universe, synthesize it, and report on it to all stakeholders. He or she defines data collection, analysis, and reporting for the department, and works with peers in other departments and divisions of the hospital to frame interdisciplinary process improvement activities. The QM officer is responsible to the chair for understanding the group's performance, both in structured metrics and in reaction to complaints from patients and other stakeholders.

A good QM program does not consist of just one individual. The first activity of the QM officer should be to recruit and organize a department QM committee. This group will define performance metrics, launch focused reviews, and form the first layer of peer review for adverse and sentinel events. Diversity of clinical perspective is the most important criteria for forming the QM committee: the officer should seek representatives from established senior partners and new recruits, and from the ranks of physicians, nurse anesthetists, anesthesiologist assistants, nurses, and trainees. Participation of the practice business manager is desirable, because of the overlap between regulatory requirements and billing compliance. Both the committee and the QM officer should have the support of information technologists within the department and institution.

TOP-DOWN PERFORMANCE MEASUREMENT

Anesthesia department quality management can be thought of as two interlocking mechanisms: top-down aggregation of routine data, and bottom-up analysis of sentinel events and unusual cases. The QM officer must build infrastructure to accomplish each of these goals. Top-down performance measurement is often perceived as a daunting task, requiring masses of information recorded by already overworked clinicians, but in practice this need not be the case. In the Information Age, hospitals and anesthesia practices have access to extensive digital data. The efficient QM officer will pursue this information using a three-step approach: *acquire, collaborate,* and *create*.

Acquisition, Collaboration, and Creation

Top-down data collection begins with an inventory of data already available within the anesthesia practice, with an emphasis on data that are in digital form and thus easy to copy and transmit. All anesthesia billing information falls into this category, because most payment for anesthesia in the United States requires electronic transmission of individual case data to an insurance company. Rare exceptions to this rule occur in government programs such as the Department of Defense and the Veterans Administration and in pure health maintenance organizations (HMOs) such as Kaiser Permanente, but even in these settings, where anesthesia services are not billed independently, similar digital records are necessary for internal cost accounting. In all other settings, practice billing data are the critical first link in the performance measurement chain.

Billing records document every activity of the department and every patient who receives care, and include information about the surgical and anesthetic procedure; the date, time, and location of the case; the providers involved; and the patient's age, sex, and ASA Physical Status.[2] Although this is not the primary goal of QM—these data rarely include any information on the outcome of the procedure—they are essential for defining the work of the practice. Procedure codes, in particular, are used to create the denominator for the outcome measures that the QM program will define. Anesthesia and surgical procedures are coded using the Current Procedural Terminology™ (CPT) of the American Medical Association or the International Classification of Diseases (ICD) system. The QM officer should have some familiarity with each system and how they interact. Procedures can be coded in either system and "crosswalked" from one to the other; diagnostic codes are only found in ICD (i.e., the reason for the procedure and the patient's comorbidities). There are also ICD codes for "not present on admission" disorders, many of which represent complications of care.

Other data readily available for "harvest" by the QM program include hospital performance measures that are gathered by the QM department, registry information for surgical or procedural services, and reports generated for financial management. A quick walk through the executive suite will reveal reams of information generated by all elements of the facility, much of which reflects the work of the anesthesia department. Hospital administrators, including QM nurses, are usually more than willing to share copies of standing reports if asked politely, especially if the data are being requested and used in the spirit of improved patient care. Both hospitals and surgery centers are required to collect and report performance measures to state and federal agencies. Many of these reports are of relevance to procedural care, and can be useful to an anesthesia QM program. Although agencies' performance measures evolve and change, some examples include the Surgical Care Improvement Project (SCIP)[3] measures and the Consumer Assessment of Healthcare Providers and Systems (CAHPS)[4] of the CMS Hospital Compare program. These programs are currently undergoing significant changes, and not all of these measures apply to anesthesiologists, but it is important for the QM officer to be aware of the reports' contents, so as to avoid being blindsided when a performance problem is identified.

Most large healthcare institutions participate in multiple national registry and benchmarking projects, including the University Hospital Consortium,[5] the National Trauma Data Bank,[6] the National Cardiovascular Data Registry,[7] the National Surgical Quality Improvement Project,[8] and the Society for Thoracic Surgeons Cardiac Surgery Registry.[9] These registries offer a dual opportunity to acquire data for the anesthesia QM officer, by accessing both the report that is sent to the registry and participating in a review of the benchmarking that is returned to the institution. Working with the primary medical or surgical services to improve their position in the registry reports is a good way for the anesthesia department to demonstrate value; a surprising number of measures for other specialists can be influenced by changes in operative anesthesia, pain management, or preoperative assessment. A recent study of outcomes from cardiac surgery in New York State, for example, demonstrated similar variability in mortality based on the primary surgeon *or* the primary anesthesiologist.[10]

After existing data have been made available to the anesthesia program, the QM officer should consider *collaborating* to create new information. The institution's QM office is a good place to start because it is likely to have more resources for chart review and data collection than would an individual department. The institution has its own requirements for reporting performance in procedural care, and may be willing to devote resources to joint projects. For example, it is not unusual for nurses in the PACU to contact patients who have been discharged after surgery; the QM officer can collaborate in this process both by suggesting questions to ask and by helping to interpret and respond to the results.

Finally, and only after more efficient methods have been exhausted, the QM committee should consider gathering new information. This usually leads to the creation of an outcomes capture form that is completed after every anesthetic. A sample form is shown in Figure 14.1. This form—either electronic or on paper—will capture outcomes specific to anesthesia, including the occurrence of events such as postoperative nausea and vomiting, inadequate pain management, dental injuries, medication errors and reactions, difficult airway management, respiratory complications, hemodynamic instability, intraoperative cardiac arrest, and perioperative mortality. A core set of measures and recommended definitions can be found on the Anesthesia Quality Institute website at www.aqihq.org/quality.aspx, with the understanding that these are suggested templates that every practice will want to customize to match their own patient population, common surgeries, and issues of concern.

Anesthesia Quality Improvement PACU Discharge

Case Info		Anesthesia type	
Date		Provider ID	
MR #		CRNA ID	
ASA Class		Additional provider	

	Yes	No
Patient is awake and able to contribute to assessment		

Patient Physical Exam:	Yes	No	Pain Score (10-point VAS scale):	
Mental Status at baseline (Y/N)			on PACU admission	
Vital Signs at baseline (Y/N)			Highest pain score	
Airway patency at baseline (Y/N)			Pain score at time of assessment	

Nausea or vomiting requiring treatment		Any occurrence of vomiting	

Did the patient experience an unexpected event during perioperative care?

				Yes	No
Unplanned ICU admission		Anaphylaxis			
Unplanned hospital admission		Other medication reaction			
Intraoperative awareness		Delayed emergence			
Epidural hematoma		Respiratory arrest			
Peripheral neurologic deficit		Reintubation			
Corneal abrasion		Dental trauma			
Agitation requiring treatment		Aspiration			
Seizure		Cardiac arrest			
Uncontrolled blood sugar (high or low)		Hypotension requiring treatment			
Subcutaneous emphysema		Unplanned transfusion			
Vascular access complication		Unplanned return to OR			
Pulmonary Edema		Death			
Prolonged PACU stay—patient condition		Prolonged PACU stay—unrelated to patient condition			
New PVC's, bradycardia, arterial fibrillation, or other dysrhythmias requiring treatment		Use of sedation/narcotic reversal agent			
If other, please specify:					

This is a template. Please modify for local conditions.

The definitions for each measure can be found on the AQI website   Not Part of Patient's chart

FIGURE 14.1: A sample quality capture form, to be filled out at the time the patient is discharged from anesthesia care.

Anesthesia Quality Improvement PACU Discharge/2015, reprinted with permission from the American Society of Anesthesiologists. A copy of the full text can be obtained from ASA, 1061 American Lane, Schaumburg, IL 60173-4973 or online at www.asahq.org.

Creating and deploying an anesthesia-specific outcome capture form requires a relatively advanced patient safety culture, in which members of the department recognize the value of the data captured and are willing to take the time to report honestly and completely. If it is deployed too early in the development of the QM program, the form may be ignored or misused, creating mistrust or cynicism. Cynicism arises because this kind of self-reported data is inherently limited; it depends on fallible human consistency of purpose and it is subject to "gaming." In the long run, the QM officer should strive to capture most anesthesia outcomes from electronic data rather than self-reports. For example, it is more sensible to derive "hemodynamic instability" from the objective record of vital signs (e.g., a deviation exceeding a certain percentage of the patient's baseline) or medications (e.g., the use of pressors) than to require a practitioner to subjectively report it.

Data Analysis

After information has been found and aggregated, the next step is to determine how best to analyze and report the data. As with other aspects of the program, the most effective approach is one that starts with simple reports and delivers more complex reports over time. In some cases (e.g., data harvested from other systems), copying the native report will suffice. Billing and economic data may already contain hospital "key performance indicator" reports that show current demographics and changes over time.[11] In more sophisticated environments, these reports already include some benchmarking information, expressed as a desired target value or rate.

The simplest way to present data gathered within the anesthesia practice is just a count: how many patients received care or how many complications occurred, for example. Because case numbers and case mix will vary from month to month, however, it is usually desirable to take the next simple step and express key data as rates: a number of occurrences divided by a number of opportunities (e.g., the number of dural puncture headaches

[numerator] resulting from the combined number of spinals and epidurals performed [denominator]). This step normalizes the data for different sizes of denominators, and allows comparisons over time, across facilities, and between individual providers.

The first time QM data are analyzed and converted to rates, the committee will be limited in its ability to interpret the results. But the second time, a month or quarter later, value will begin to accrue. Presenting rates in a time series, showing the change from one period to the next, offers information about which processes are improving and which are not. When looking at short time series it can be hard to know whether the changes are occurring due to random chance or actually reflect a real shift in outcomes. As the series gets longer, however, more complex statistical methods can be brought to bear. A full explanation of statistical process control charts is beyond the scope of this chapter, but Figure 14.2 illustrates such a presentation, and there is good literature to demonstrate how this technique might be applied to anesthesia QM data.[12]

Data Reporting

Reporting from the QM database is a sensitive topic, and should be carefully considered.[13] Actionable data (e.g., patient satisfaction, adequacy of pain management, on-time starts, completion of QM outcome forms) should be reported at the level of the individual provider. If possible, this should be presented confidentially, allowing for "self-reflection," and should include benchmark data either from national norms or from the aggregate performance of the practice. Maintaining the confidentiality of personal performance information is critical to encouraging active participation in the QM program and to development of a culture of safety. Figure 14.3 illustrates this with quarterly presentation of the rate of PONV, with each provider seeing his or her own performance and that of all other providers in the group, but without specific identification of the peers. Creating and presenting this kind of performance scorecard may be all that is necessary to motivate improvement. Physicians in general are inherently competitive

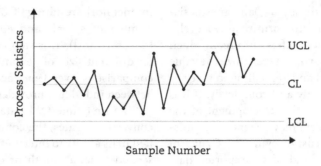

FIGURE 14.2: A sample statistical process control chart. Data are plotted as a series over time, on a graph that shows the upper and lower "control limits" (typically 2 standard deviations above and below the mean) to allow differentiation of random variation from systematic variation due to real changes in practice.

Reprinted with permission from the ProcessMA Excel Add-in by Process Excellence. http://www.processma.com/resource/spc.php.

individuals, and will strive to improve when presented with clear metrics.

Some QM data is not suitable for presentation at the individual level. This includes outcomes that happen so rarely that no individual provider will have enough occurrences for trend data to be statistically significant (e.g., perioperative mortality, cardiac arrest, anaphylaxis, malignant hyperthermia, myocardial infarction, stroke, postoperative visual loss). Other data (e.g., hospital length of stay, 30-day mortality) are unsuitable because the responsibility for improvement cannot be clearly attributed to any individual provider. In both of these cases, QM results are best presented at an aggregate level, for the facility, the practice, the hospital system, or even nationally.

Every member of the team shares responsibility for these shared accountability measures. Figure 14.4 shows the aggregate national rate of mortality in the immediate perioperative period from the National Anesthesia Clinical Outcomes Registry. With a mean rate of 3 per 10,000, this event is so rare that even facility-to-facility comparisons may lack the statistical power to demonstrate meaningful differences between groups.

Emerging requirements for public performance reporting are distorting the ability to keep QM data "within the family," because many of these programs require that data be made public at the level of individual physicians.[14] Selecting individual performance measures to share with the hospital (i.e., for Joint

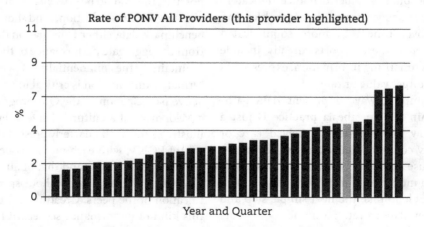

FIGURE 14.3: A typical confidential QM report for an individual provider, showing the rate of postoperative nausea and vomiting compared to all anesthesiologists in the group.

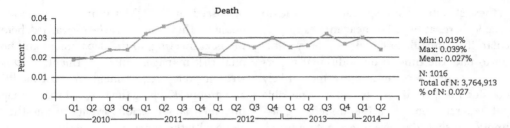

FIGURE 14.4: Mortality in the OR or PACU by quarter from the National Anesthesia Clinical Outcomes Registry. With a mean occurrence of 0.03% of cases, this outcome is too rare to enable statistically meaningful comparisons at the individual or even small-group level.

Commission purposes) or Medicare (for the Physician Quality Reporting System) is an important task of the QM officer. The desire to show good results in public is in direct conflict with the core purpose of the QM program to identify opportunities for performance improvement. Further, the use of measures for public reporting that are "safe," but not meaningful to providers or patients, undermines the credibility of the program and increases the cynicism of providers. For example, the timely administration of antibiotics at the start of a surgical case is a long-standing measure in the PQRS program. This is an important activity to reduce the risk of surgical site infection, but is not among the core concerns of anesthesiologists. Overemphasis on a collateral activity such as this may waste valuable time and attention in the QM program. The goal of the QM officer should be to align the measures that are publicly reported with measures that best demonstrate performance of the department. This may, however, require a substantial culture shift to convince the department that publicly reporting less-than-perfect performance will not have negative personal or financial consequences.

Public reporting may also demand that the data be risk adjusted, in order to account for differences in patient population, case mix, geographic region, and other factors outside the control of the anesthesiologist. For internal reporting, most of these variables will be identical for all members of the group, making risk adjustment unnecessary, but adjustment will be required for high-stakes external reporting in order to preserve confidence in the credibility of the results. Most variance in anesthesia outcomes can be controlled with adjustment for ASA Physical Status, age and the type of procedure, but this is still a mathematically cumbersome process. Increasing the risk adjustment's precision will require data that may not be readily available, such as detailed patient comorbidities. Even when carefully performed, risk adjustment is complicated enough that methodological issues can always be raised.[15] The QM officer must be aware of these concerns and their implications, so as to select the right degree of adjustment for the specific reporting purpose.

GROUND-LEVEL QUALITY MANAGEMENT

Collection of data for evidence-based decisions is important, but the management of unusual cases, adverse events, and serious patient injuries is another, equally important, role of the QM officer. Indeed, these anecdotal occurrences can have a much stronger role in driving hospital policy than rational analysis of data, partly because humans are naturally driven by stories instead of numbers, and partly because adverse events in anesthesia can be catastrophic. The goal of the QM officer in this area is to build a reporting network—both formal and informal—that ensures that every anesthesia-related adverse event is reported. Formal capture systems, often known as incident reports, may use either paper or digital forms to capture information about events. Most healthcare institutions and anesthesia departments have policies about the occurrences and near misses that are to be reported, but these structured systems catch only the tip of the iceberg, at best. For near misses in particular, it is difficult to convince a busy clinician to take the time to do additional paperwork. Actual adverse events are more likely to be documented, if only to mitigate possible legal repercussions, but the underlying assumption is that some events are not reported. An informal reporting system is therefore equally important. A network can be created simply by visiting various locations around the institution and talking to people both inside the department and out. Nurses, technicians, and residents all spend time at the bedside, and often know more than anyone else about what is really going on. They will be willing to share with the QM officer if approached in a collegial manner, especially if the information provided produces visible results.

After an adverse event collection and alerting system has been developed, the next step is to sort and triage the events. Many incident reports, both formal and informal, are relatively low-level or repeated events. Anesthesia-related examples include dental injuries or post-dural puncture headaches. These should be recorded, but not individually reviewed unless there is a cluster of events or an increase in rate. More serious occurrences, such as neurologic injuries, corneal abrasions, unplanned readmissions, and intraoperative cardiac arrests, should be brought to the QM committee for discussion. Members of the committee can take turns reviewing the medical records of assigned cases before each month's meeting, and can be responsible for presenting the clinical details and initial assessment to the committee. Discussion should focus on whether the event is isolated or part of a pattern, whether it was preventable through changes in practice, and whether it should be presented at a departmental Morbidity and Mortality (M & M) conference. These events, and the discussion that follows, are a critical tool for ongoing professional education; a well-run M & M conference is one of the most visible and educational features of the QM program.

Serious events, especially those that cause permanent patient harm or death, should be discussed in the QM Committee as soon as possible. They should also be forwarded, before the next meeting, to the department and hospital risk management department. This is a written policy requirement in most facilities and groups. Keeping the hospital risk manager informed about serious events in anesthesia, along with the expert review of the committee, will improve both communications and credibility for the anesthesia QM program. This is an important conduit for the QM officer to cultivate; occasionally the institutional QM or risk management officer will inform the anesthesia department about something that they should know. No matter how good the communications network, there will always be embarrassing events—especially patient complaints from out of the blue—that do not come directly to the anesthesia QM officer. Working with the institution's professionals is one more component of the desired communications network.

Certain serious events, such as wrong-site surgery, major blood or medication errors, and unexpected deaths, will initiate mandatory reporting to external agencies such as state regulators or the Joint Commission.[16] These "sentinel events" require a rapid and specific response, typically including a formal root cause analysis (RCA).[17] The RCA is a tool that can be used at many levels of the QM process, and if done well it can be a powerful way to effect change. The analysis begins with creation of a clear timeline of facts related to the case, often developed by serial, one-on-one interviews with all participants and witnesses. The QM officer should assemble this timeline and then schedule a meeting with key stakeholders to review it in detail and to solicit opinions about what went wrong and what could be improved. Multidisciplinary participation in the RCA is critical to its success. The purpose of the RCA is to look beyond the obvious desire to have individuals make better decisions—something that can never be fully attained—and to seek opportunities to improve systems and practices to make subsequent errors less likely. The RCA should not be a "blame and shame" event, nor should it attempt to gloss over critical faults. Instead, it should be an honest attempt to review the policies and practices that might be improved. An RCA is typically followed by an educational presentation at the M & M conference, during which the insights gained are shared with the entire department.

One useful technique for RCA discussions is the idea of the "Five Whys." The facilitator for a sentinel event discussion should ask "Why did this occur?" and should keep asking "why?" until an appropriate level of understanding is achieved. Box 14.1 shows an example of this process (that actually runs to seven "whys"). Any event can be infinitely dissected, of course, but the Five Whys are a good way to ensure that system variables predisposing to error are discovered before premature closure of thinking about the event.

The M & M conference is an important tool for the QM officer. Not only can it serve as a forum for case-based teaching and for presentation of aggregate statistics for the department, it can also serve an important role in advancing the desired safety culture. Within-the-family discussion of difficult cases and human errors creates an opportunity to detect legitimate interprovider differences in practice (e.g., the individual threshold for canceling a case), and can point out the need for systematic discussion of policy and protocol. Further, transparency in identifying and admitting error makes it safe for others to do the same. This is a situation in which the QM officer (or even the department chair) may need to lead from the front, by being the first to openly admit an error and discuss how it might have been prevented. As long as no ill effect is seen to result for this individual, such an activity will make it safer for others to self-report and will increase participation in the QM process.

DRIVING CHANGES IN PRACTICE

The final major step in departmental quality management is to react to the information gathered. Whether through quantitative analysis of electronic data or simple aggregation of adverse events, the QM officer will inevitably find ways in which practice can be improved. Turning this knowledge into action will improve outcomes over time, but can be a major challenge. There are many methods of doing this, including some name-brand systems reviewed in this section, but the process itself is deceptively simple. Find a problem, quantify it, gather experts, consider solutions, implement changes, and keep measuring. Small steps taken incrementally work better than grand solutions, and most groups will be more receptive to a small change in practice that is first implemented as a pilot or short-term experiment. Do this often enough, and continual improvement becomes a normal expectation. Keep it up long enough, and substantial change will occur.

Six Sigma is one methodology for change management, based on achieving an error rate lower than one case in a million (6 standard deviations on a normal distribution curve).[18]

BOX 14.1   AN ILLUSTRATION OF THE "FIVE WHYS" APPROACH TO ROOT CAUSE ANALYSIS

Questions are asked and answered until all facets of the adverse event are fully explored. At least 5 layers of explanation should be sought.

- Why did this patient die? Answer: He bled to death.
- Why did hemorrhage occur? Answer: A laparoscopic trocar injured the inferior vena cava.
- Why wasn't this noticed? Answer: The injury occurred in the retroperitoneum and the surgeons were operating in the abdomen.
- Why did the trocar hit the IVC? Answer: It was longer than the surgeons were used to.
- Why were the trocars changed? Answer: The hospital changed suppliers.
- Why wasn't this communicated? Answer: The OR manager was on vacation that week.
- Why didn't someone else communicate this? Answer: No one was assigned this task.

The terminology comes from the manufacturing world as a desirable goal for manufacturing processes, and the application of this method to industry was historically responsible for improvement in the Japanese economy after World War II. Of course humans are not objects, and there is far more variability present in similar patients having the same operation than there is on the average assembly line. The QM professional will therefore temper the Six Sigma quest for standardized processes and procedures—often derided as "cookbook medicine" by detractors—with flexible application to particular patients and situations. Done correctly, Six Sigma asks practitioners to follow mutually agreed-upon guidelines and standards, but allows for variation when needed. When enabled by templated electronic records, this approach will improve routine patient care and may even reduce the burden of clinical documentation.

Six Sigma is often conflated with Lean methodology[19] and the Toyota Production System, which are other terms for the same basic approach of systems-level thinking, focused and iterative change, and ongoing measurement. A specific discussion of these and other systems for managing change goes beyond the dimensions of this chapter, and will provide diminishing returns in any case. The terminology most important to the QM officer will be that adhered to by his or her own counterparts in leadership within the facility. The QM officer should take any opportunity that presents to learn about the local system for change management, and should actively participate in available courses and projects. These courses are also a good way to network with key external stakeholders.

CONCLUSION

The final task of the QM officer, really a summation of all the steps described, is to create a culture of continuous quality improvement in the anesthesia practice. This includes the expectation that performance will be measured, reported, and discussed; that emphasis will be placed on system function over individual results; that adverse events will be deconstructed

within the group; and that incremental change will be an ongoing expectation. The result will be a happy, harmonious department, confident in the delivery of the best possible patient care in the present and into the future.

REFERENCES

1. Dutton RP. Why have a quality management program? *Int Anesthesiol Clin.* 2013;51(4):1–9
2. Dutton RP, Dukatz A. Quality improvement using automated data sources: the anesthesia quality institute. *Anesthesiol Clin.* 2011;29:439–454.
3. Munday GS, Deveaux P, Roberts H, Fry DE, Polk HC. Impact of implementation of the Surgical Care Improvement Project and future strategies for improving quality in surgery. *Am J Surg.* 2014;208:835–840.
4. Crofton C, Lubalin JS, Darby C. Consumer Assessment of Health Plans Study (CAHPS). Foreword. *Med Care.* 1999;37(3 Suppl):MS1–9.
5. Simorov A, Bills N, Shostrom V, Boilesen E, Oleynikov D. Can surgical performance benchmarking be generalized across multiple outcomes databases: a comparison of University Health System Consortium and National Surgical Quality Improvement Program. *Am J Surg.* 2014;208(6): 942–948.
6. Haider AH, Saleem T, Leow JJ, Villegas CV, Kisat M, Schneider EB, Haut ER, Stevens KA, Cornwell EE3rd, MacKenzie EJ, Efron DT. Influence of the National Trauma Data Bank on the study of trauma outcomes: is it time to set research best practices to further enhance its impact? *J Am Coll Surg.* 2012;214:756–768.
7. Masoudi FA, Ponirakis A, Yeh RW, Maddox TM, Beachy J, Casale PN, Curtis JP, De Lemos J, Fonarow G, Heidenreich P, Koutras C, Kremers M, Messenger J, Moussa I, Oetgen WJ, Roe MT, Rosenfield K, Shields TPJr, Spertus JA, Wei J, White C, Young CH, Rumsfeld JS. Cardiovascular care facts: a report from the national cardiovascular data registry: 2011. *J Am Coll Cardiol.* 2013;62:1931–1947.
8. Ingraham AM, Richards KE, Hall BL, Ko CY. Quality improvement in surgery: the American College of Surgeons National Surgical Quality Improvement Program approach. *Adv Surg.* 2010;44:251–267.
9. Aronson S, Mathew JP, Cheung AT, Shore-Lesserson L, Troianos CA, Reeves S. The rationale and development of an adult cardiac anesthesia module to supplement the society of thoracic surgeons national database: using data to drive quality. *Anesth Analg.* 2014;118:925–932.
10. Glance LG, Dick A, Kellerman A, Hannan EL, Fleisher L, Eaton M, Lustik S, Li Y, Dutton RP. Impact of anesthesiologists on CABG mortality. *Anesth Analg.* 2015 Mar;120(3):526–533.

11. Granata RL, Hamilton K. Exploring the effect of at-risk case management compensation on hospital pay-for-performance outcomes: tools for change. *Prof Case Manag.* 2015;20:14–27.

12. Seim A, Andersen B, Sandberg WS. Statistical process control as a tool for monitoring nonoperative time. *Anesthesiology.* 2006;105:370–380.

13. Petschonek S, Burlison J, Cross C, Martin K, Laver J, Landis RS, Hoffman JM. Development of the just culture assessment tool: measuring the perceptions of health-care professionals in hospitals. *J Patient Saf.* 2013;9:190–197.

14. Rodrigues R, Trigg L, Schmidt AE, Leichsenring K. The public gets what the public wants: experiences of public reporting in long-term care in Europe. *Health Policy.* 2014;116:84–94.

15. Iezzoni LI. The risks of risk adjustment. *JAMA.* 1997;278:1600–1607.

16. [No authors listed] Sentinel events statistics for 2011. *Jt Comm Perspect.* 2012;32:5.

17. Williams PM. Techniques for root cause analysis. *Proc (Bayl Univ Med Cent).* 2001;14:154–157.

18. JL, Wang Z, McCaughey D, Langabeer JR2nd, DelliFraine2nd, Erwin CO. The use of Six Sigma in health care management: are we using it to its full potential? *Qual Manag Health Care.* 2014

19. Ahmed S, Manaf NH, Islam R. Effects of Lean Six Sigma application in healthcare services: a literature review. *Rev Environ Health.* 2013;28:189–194.

15

Health Information Technology Use for Quality Assurance and Improvement

CHRISTINE A. DOYLE

INTRODUCTION

Health information technology (HIT) has become an important part of patient care, and can provide useful solutions for a quality assurance and improvement (QA&I) program by illustrating current quality and demonstrating gaps in quality that can be targeted for improvement. Like any other information technology (IT) project, however, HIT solutions can give misleading results if the wrong information is selected for review, or if there are systematic errors in data handling. Although many health information systems are sometimes maligned as a glorified statistical tool or billing document, well-designed and implemented anesthesia information management systems (AIMS), perioperative electronic health records (EHR), and other software solutions can provide an excellent vehicle for use in quality programs. For the purposes of this chapter, the term EHR includes both an electronic health record and an anesthesia information management system.

When planning the implementation of a major HIT project, it is usually best to start at the "end"—the desired workflow and goals of the project—and then work backward. Properly determining goals and objectives will define the project requirements. This in turn will determine the data points that are necessary to meet these goals, and ensure that they are built into the record so that the data are captured. These selected data points should be reviewed on a regular basis and added to, subtracted from, or altered as the project progresses and the needs of the institution change.[1-4]

EHRs can easily be used for both automated and ad hoc event identification, standardized and custom reporting, and individual case review. Analytics capabilities may be incorporated into the EHR, or may be an add-on module or program. Such programs often include standard reports (typical queries) along with the ability to create custom reports. Some programs require additional work to create custom reports, while others can create reports with little additional effort and without making changes to the underlying software. It is therefore important to understand the capabilities of each analytics system.

The small number of publications that describe the use of EHRs for QA&I or patient outcomes is rapidly growing, including several ongoing projects that use the capabilities of EHRs to facilitate data mining (e.g., the Anesthesia Quality Institute and the Multicenter Perioperative Outcomes Group).[5-9] Moreover, the traditional role of a QA&I committee has increased in scope as outside quality initiatives have been promulgated by groups such as the Institute for Healthcare Improvement (IHI) and the Agency for Healthcare Research and Quality (AHRQ).

REPORTS VERSUS ANALYTICS

Although the terms are often used interchangeably, *reporting* and *analytics* are different tasks. *Reports* are static snapshots of a specific situation at a given point in time and are most often formulated as routine and periodic views of data. Reports may include scorecards (a statistical record used to measure progress toward a goal), dashboards (a visualization tool that displays metrics for the entire enterprise), and alerts. Reports may be reviewed annually, quarterly, or daily, depending on their content. They should answer questions such as "Is the institution meeting its goals?" and use gap analysis to generate questions such as "Where can performance be improved?" *Analytics* refers to a real-time and relational view of data that is then used to drive decisions in both the near and long term. Analytics should generate insight and answer questions generated by reports while also raising additional questions. Analytics typically answers the "why" and "how" questions, producing ideas that can lead to improvement. Reporting and analytics are often collectively referred to as *business intelligence* (BI).

> Example: The OR director was concerned with on-time starts at the beginning of the day. Several surgeons were routinely late. An attempt to specify a time by which everyone was in the OR and ready to go produced mixed results. Surgeons claimed that the "preoperative nurses" or "anesthesia" or something else was responsible for delaying the schedule. A First-Case On-Time report

was created. A case was defined as "late" if the patient was brought into the operating room more than 15 minutes after the scheduled start time. It was found that late starts had a variety of causes, including delays in the preoperative holding area, surgeons not being on time, and less common causes, including equipment or staff unavailability. The Pre-Op admission process was reviewed and streamlined. Surgeons who displayed a pattern of late arrivals were counseled by the department chairman, while those who were consistently on time were listed on a "wall of praise." Follow-up analysis after implementation of these processes demonstrated that the number of cases that started late fell significantly (Figure 15.1).

EVENT IDENTIFICATION

Most anesthesia departments use specific events to trigger QA&I reviews, ranging from case delays to episodes of cardiac arrest. QI programs typically rely on self-reporting of adverse events or identify complications from post-discharge claims coding. This can lead to significant delays in review and decrease opportunities to prevent harm in future patient

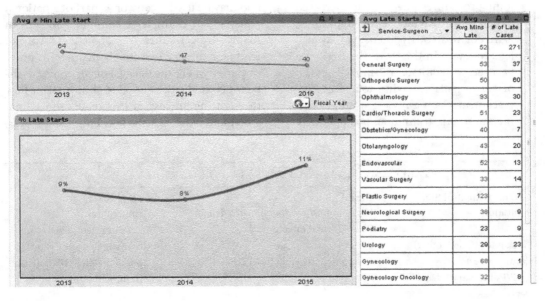

FIGURE 15.1: On-time starts.

care events. Each department or organization selects criteria that are required by regulatory agencies such as the US Centers for Medicare and Medicaid Services (CMS) and may also add criteria that are appropriate for their own facility. Review of these standard criteria should occur on a regular basis, at least annually, and routine reports should be run at least monthly. Typical criteria are seen in Table 15.1.

Single reports on a specific topic are often required for questions related to patient care or developing trends. For example, a report might be generated for a specific disease process (e.g., pseudocholinesterase deficiency) in order to determine whether the group has cared for such a patient before. A report might also be generated about a specific physician, for example, a surgeon whose cases seem to be delayed or canceled more frequently than others. Lastly, a report can help to determine whether there should be a concern about something happening outside the operating room ("There seems to be an increase in the incidence of postoperative falls. Could this be related to the anesthetic technique?").

Consider, for example, a hypothetical situation in which a group of orthopedic surgeons did not want regional anesthesia in patients undergoing total joint procedures "because it increased patient falls." An alternative hypothesis is that orthostatic hypotension may also lead to a fall. In this case, the EHR can be used to facilitate a 3-month review of all patients receiving total joint replacement. Such a review would examine anesthetic technique, postoperative transfusions, hypotension, and falls or near falls. Such a review might show that the incidence of falls was not increased in patients who received regional anesthesia, but that patients who were hypotensive or who required postoperative transfusion were at risk for falling. This would then suggest that postoperative management strategies be changed. The next step would then be to implement those changes and monitor the results generated by this report for a decreased incidence of postoperative falls.

REPORTS, DASHBOARDS, AND EXTRACTS

The EHR can be used to generate reports for a variety of purposes other than event identification and quality management. For example, reports about case and procedure volume for individuals may be part of the departmental Ongoing Professional Practice Evaluation (OPPE) process. Typical reports should include extracts for the reporting required by the US Centers for Medicare and Medicaid. Additional reports may include registry reporting to the Anesthesia Quality Institute (AQI) and the Society of Thoracic Surgeons (STS). Standard reports should be generated based on the data and identification schema set by the facility, and may be used locally or as part of a national registry. For example, a common problem in many surgical suites is that patients are not ready for surgery in a timely manner. In order to clarify where the delay(s) occur, a new dashboard could be developed to show patient flow through the process. If this report shows that sicker and older patients take longer to process,

TABLE 15.1. TYPICAL CRITERIA FOR QA&I REVIEW

Adverse Drug Reaction	Dental Injury	PTX p/ CVP
Aspiration	Nerve injury/peripheral neuro deficit	Reintubation
	PDPH (spinal or epidural)	Stroke or other neuro event
Block issue (failed, other)	PONV	Unanticipated admission
Cardiac arrest	Postop hypothermia (not planned)	Unanticipated ICU admission
CHF/Pulmonary Edema	Postop MI	Vision/ocular injury
Death		

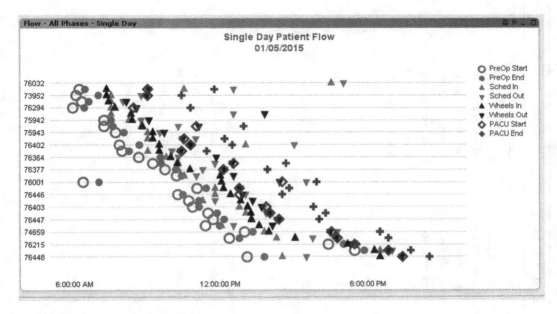

FIGURE 15.2. Patient throughput.

it might then be possible to develop criteria that would allow sicker patients to be seen in a preoperative clinic and then brought to the hospital earlier. This could potentially yield a significant improvement in on-time patient readiness, as well as patient satisfaction (Figure 15.2).

PERFORMANCE IMPROVEMENT AND QI TOOLS

The ultimate goal of quality management is to improve overall and provider-specific performance. Several schemata can be used to view the insights provided by information contained in the EHR and apply this knowledge to performance improvement. The most commonly used techniques include Failure Mode Effects Analysis (FMEA), Root Cause Analysis (RCA), and Plan Study Do Act (PSDA).[10–15]

FMEA is a tool designed to *anticipate* what might go wrong with a process or product, to identify the potential causes of failure, and to propose potential solutions that can be implemented in order to prevent an adverse event. FMEA is best used at the beginning of a project. A complete discussion of FMEA is beyond the scope of this chapter, but there are two primary phases: identifying every step in a given process along with potential errors

or issues, and then assigning and calculating risk. Evaluating the severity of an event, the risk of its occurrence, and the probability of its detection requires information that can be generated by a good HIT system. Levels of risk are then calculated using these three numbers, and the priority of a given corrective action is determined by the highest combined risk. Re-evaluation after action has been taken is often done to ensure that risks have been reduced. Table 15.2 provides an example of an FMEA template that was developed at a facility during the transition from paper to electronic physician order entry.

RCA is used to identify precipitating factors and areas for preventive changes in existing process *after* an event or near miss. Although a complete discussion of an RCA is beyond the scope of this chapter, its goal is to identify and eliminate factors that ultimately led to an event. In this analysis, a *root cause* is defined as a factor that, when removed from the sequence, prevents the final undesirable event from occurring; *causal factors* affect the event's outcome, but their removal does not prevent it from occurring. Root causes usually fall into one of three categories: *physical, human,* and *organizational.*

TABLE 15.2. FAILURE MODES AND EFFECTS ANALYSIS (FMEA)

Process Step	Potential Failure Mode	Potential Causes	Potential Failure Effects	SEV	OCC	Current Process Controls	DET	RPN
		What causes the step to go wrong? (i.e., How could the failure mode occur?)				*What are the existing controls that either prevent the failure mode from occurring or detect it or should it occur?*		
MD Writes new order	1) Wrong chart; 2) Physician writing in the order using the wrong patient label; 3) MD writes wrong date and time; 4) Once the order is written, it is modified by MD.	Wrong label, wrong chart	Delay in treatment, incorrect patient received the treatment/medication	9	4		3	108
Chart flagged to identify order has been written (red/stat; green/routine)	1) Not flagged after the order is written by MD; 2) Wrong color flagged by the MD; 3) No communication between MD and RN after the order is written.	No flags in the chart (missing flags); missing one or two flags from the chart.	Delay in treatment	9	7	Nurses not checking the charts in a timely manner. Holding nurses accountable for not doing the chart checks. Chart audits will help identify nurses who are not following the policy	6	378
Chart placed back in chart rack	1) Not flagged and placed the chart in chart rack; 2) Chart not placed back in the chart rack after MD order is written by MD.	Physician busy and left the chart on a back counter; physician called away without placing the chart back in the rack; interruption	Delay in treatment	9	8		1	72

Process step	Causes	Failure mode	Effect	Severity	Occurrence	Detection	RPN
Chart with orders identified by RN/ unit secretary	1) Delay in RN looking orders; 2) One unit secretary for 6 pods; 3) No light on the pod indicating orders are written; 4) Communication issue.	RN doesn't push the light for secretary indicating orders are written; light not working; RN/secretary not communicating	Delay in treatment	9	5	8	360
Order scanned/faxed to pharmacy	1) Distraction; 2) Communication issue; 3) Machines not working.	Scanner not working; wrong fax number entered to fax the order; scanned the orders twice; orders not scanned to pharmacy	Orders scanned twice to pharmacy, creating double work for pharmacist. No paper in the fax machine adds up queue in pharmacy, potential for confusion causes wrong treatment or delayed treatment.	10	6	7	420
Pharmacy reviews scanned orders and processed in order received—orders with stat box checked will be processed first.	1) Communication issue; 2) All orders marked as stat.	Orders marked stat when they are not stat; all entries are stat when noted using the approved format of order enter sheet.	Delays pharmacy due to overuse of stat orders; overuse of stat creates alert fatigue	10	8	1	80
Pharmacy validates medication order and enters meds into EHR MAR	1) Human error; 2) Distraction; 3) Staffing issue.	Human error while transcribing the orders; multiple screens opened by pharmacist to enter multiple orders creates confusion; incomplete order clarification.	Pharmacist overwhelmed by the orders if staffing issues; over-ride alerts; prescribing physician not available.	10	6	6	360

(continued)

TABLE 15.2. CONTINUED

Process Step	Potential Failure Mode	Potential Causes	Potential Failure Effects	SEV	OCC	Current Process Controls	DET	RPN
Unit secretary/ RN enters order in EHR for non-pharmacy items	1) Human error; 2) Distraction; 3) Performance issue.	Orders entered in a wrong patient; wrong selection of the lab from the drop-down menu; wrong time entered; incomplete orders; too many orders and trying to keep the fast pace; entering the wrong orders; no unit secretary during the shift; busy shift, alert fatigue.	Delay in treatment	7	4		7	196
Chart flagged (yellow) indicating orders needed to be checked by RN	1) Chart not being flagged by unit secretary; 2) RN too busy to note the orders; 3)Hard to see the charts with flag; 4) Communication issue.	RNs too busy to see the new orders	Delay in treatment	10	9		4	360

New orders identified in EHR "in" box	1) Performance issue of RNs; 2) Technology issue.	RNs ignore the "in" box with orders; RNs creating shortcuts to check the orders; busy shift with too many admissions and discharges; overwhelm; technological challenges	Delay in treatment	10	By having the "Check all" box in EHR for nurses to sign off all the medication orders at once.	9	Following are the five steps in place to prevent the failure mode. 1) Pharmacy check; 2) RN checking the EMAR against physician orders; 3) 8-hour chart check; 4) 24-hour chart check; 5) Handover between shifts.	8	720
Primary RN validates paper MD orders to those viewed in the EHR "in" box	1) Not following the policies	Charts not available for RNs to review the orders; too many orders; time management issue; lack of prioritization; effectiveness of training; standardization of training; too busy.	Delay in treatment	10	By having the "Check all" box in EHR for nurses to sign off all the medication orders at once. RNs are held accountable by department managers and directors and progressive disciplinary action is taken by them.	10	Following are the five steps in place to prevent the failure mode. 1) Pharmacy check; 2) RN checking the EMAR against physician orders; 3) 8-hour chart check; 4) 24-hour chart check; 5) Handover between shifts.	8	800
If medication order incorrect, primary RN completes and scans Medication Communication Form to the Pharmacy	1) Inventory stock too low of the MCF; 2) Distraction; 3) Forms not in place.	No standard forms for the MCF and forms being out of stock; different forms in different units due to photocopying of the forms.	Delay in communication to pharmacy and due to which delay in giving the medication to patients on right time.	6		6		3	108

(continued)

TABLE 15.2. CONTINUED

Process Step	Potential Failure Mode	Potential Causes	Potential Failure Effects	SEV	OCC	Current Process Controls	DET	RPN
Primary RN on night shift reviews all orders in past 24 hours by comparing original order against electronic/written evidence of order transcription	1) Not following the policies	Too busy to do the 24-hour chart check; quick turnover of the patients; performance issues; distraction; cultural issues.	Delay in treatment	10	8	Following are the five steps in place to prevent the failure mode. 1) Pharmacy check; 2) RN checking the EMAR against physician orders; 3) 8-hour chart check; 4) 24-hour chart check; 5) Handover between shifts.	9	720

By having the "Check all" box in EHR for nurses to sign off all the medication orders at once. night shift nurses not doing the 24-hour chart check and therefore not following the policy.

SEV = How severe is the effect on the customer? (higher numbers mean more impact)
OCC = How frequent is the cause likely to occur? (higher numbers mean more often)
DET = How probable is detection of the cause? (lower number means more likely)
RPN = Risk Priority Number, SEV x OCC x DET (higher numbers mean higher risk)
EMAR, MAR = Electronic Medication Administration Record
MCF = Medication Communication Form

Organizational causes are usually at the core of the problem, and correcting them usually offers the best opportunity to prevent future recurrences; they may not be easily addressable, however. Physical causes are associated with a specific piece of equipment or part of the operational environment (e.g., a physiologic monitor that allows alarms to be permanently silenced and causes a life-threatening arrhythmia to go unnoticed). Human causes include mistakes and violations, and are usually the most difficult to correct. As with FMEA, the first step is to identify every step of the process. The EHR can be used to collect this information, assuming that the necessary data are being collected. This underscores the need for thoughtful analysis of current and future needs when designing the system, and for continual reassessment of the system. Data collection and reports should also be designed to be in a usable format (i.e., related data points should be viewable together).

Both FMEA and RCA are often seen as costly, time-consuming processes, but they are also parts of *agile* and *rapid-cycle change* QI strategies. The Plan-Do-Study-Act (PDSA) process is a specific rapid-cycle change tool initially developed by W. Edwards Deming. Under PDSA, the first step is to establish objects and the processes that are necessary to achieve specific goals. These processes are then implemented, and the actual results are compared to the expected results. This information is then used to modify the processes that were put in place. PDSA is intended to test for change (i.e., whether the process worked), and is best used to evaluate a pilot project before a large-scale implementation effort. Multiple cycles may run sequentially with incremental changes, or several cycles may run in parallel and then be combined. Using the EHR to collect the data needed for PDSA can simplify each of these steps if the data are available, but this may necessitate changing the EHR or its data architecture, which might be difficult to do quickly in response to changing data requirements.

COMPLIANCE

Healthcare professionals and institutions must now demonstrate compliance with a constantly expanding and changing set of regulations and guidelines. HIT solutions can automate much of this process, simplifying assessment while improving efficiency and timely completion of the necessary elements. As with all information technology development and implementation, it is critical to understand the rules as well as their exceptions. Consider, for example, a facility that routinely fails to document compliance with Surgical Care Improvement Project (SCIP) guidelines for antibiotic administration. Relying on an outside reviewer may delay the results of an audit for several months, which precludes any sort of rapid-cycle change. If an AIMS system is in use, a standard report can be created that allows daily review of antibiotic administration in the operating room. This in turn will reveal patterns (e.g., specific procedures, specific providers) that require attention. In this case, it is also necessary to apply rules for the appropriate use of addendum notes in the chart when antibiotics are not administered. Use of standard language comments, such as "patient infected, already on antibiotics," is preferred because it permits automated processing, although free text can still be used when necessary.

When designing the data-collection and reporting architecture, it is important to distinguish between hospital-based metrics and physician-based metrics, because in some cases designing around one may make it difficult to create reports for the other. Software should ideally be designed to collect the necessary data and provide reports for both simultaneously. For example, a hospital system using several different software applications (a "best-in-breed" schema, as opposed to an "enterprise" product) might be unable to import the home medications of its surgical patients into the system EHR because of a delay in the vendor's development of an interface. In this situation, the Chief Information Officer (CIO) might make a decision to enter all home medications entered into the EHR instead of the

AIMS, as this would ensure that the hospital would meet its Meaningful Use (MU) criteria. This could cause the data to no be longer available from within the AIMS. Although the CIO had envisioned a custom extract that would combine data from each system, this could not be created. The anesthesiologists would therefore have to manually re-enter the patients' home medications in order to extract them for reporting or they would lose the MU bonus.

UPDATES AND SECURITY

Updates and incremental changes are an inevitable part of any HIT system, and in many cases produce significant improvements in performance and security. Update cycles should be carefully tested and planned to ensure that upgrades do not "break" existing relationships or export capabilities. Even within enterprise systems, changing one section may cause problems with another; this is typically caused by IT staff who are unaware that there is an underlying linkage between subsystems in use and therefore fail to test that linkage. Such a problem might occur during the installation of one module of an EHR, when, for example, a new allergy category scheme is created without review of the existing categories in other parts of the EHR. This could cause a complete failure of data transfer between the modules. Extensive testing should be performed to ensure that implementing a new or updated program or module will not cause additional problems.

DATA INTEGRITY AND SECURITY

As with paper records, documentation must be retained after the care is provided in order to facilitate future care of the same patient as well as compliance audits, and to ensure that the chart is available should there be any legal action. Data integrity and data security are full-time concerns with any system. Distinguishing between integrity and security is important, as there may be some processes that favor one to the exclusion of the other. Many IT professionals now use the concept of CIA—confidentiality, integrity, and accessibility—when designing systems related to data integrity and security.

Separate from concerns related to the Health Insurance Portability and Accountability Act (HIPAA), the confidentiality and security of the medical record have always been a major goal. One disadvantage of electronic records is that a breach is likely to affect far more records than a breach of a paper chart collection. Vigilance must be ongoing: assessing for weak links, identifying breaks in procedures, and penetration testing are the keys for maintaining confidentiality and security. Conflicts between medical devices and interfaces are important to identify and mitigate. Anecdotal stories about a medication delivery device crashing due to a virus, a neuro-imaging device being affected with malware, and so on, are often told, although the actual frequency of such events is not clear.

Data integrity involves many things, ranging from concerns about mathematical accuracy of conversions (i.e., pounds to kilos), to copy/paste or cloning, to inability to delete erroneous data. Issues unique to an AIMS include direct and continuous data capture from the physiologic monitors, electrocautery interference, minimum/maximum values on invasive monitoring lines (before placed, when drawing ABG, etc.).

Accessibility should focus on real-time (or near real-time) ability to work with the chart—whether merely reviewing data or entering data. The use of virtual access and single sign on (SSO) software (i.e., VMWare) has facilitated this significantly for hospitals and other facilities, while simultaneously simplifying the IT workload with use of thin client desktops (where the software is on a central server). SSO functionality should be avoided for anesthesia workstations, however, because logging into another workstation at another location (e.g., in the pre-op area or break room) might unintentionally log out the workstation, causing loss of data. If SSO software is used for an anesthesia workstation, a policy should be created that the relieving professional will log out the current user and then log back in using his or her credentials. Before implementing this policy, the system should be tested to ensure that vital sign data are not lost during this process.

LIMITATIONS

Common pitfalls involving EHR are the same as in other areas of IT or software development. Poorly designed processes produce bad data, bad data are easily cloned, and removing erroneous data is nearly impossible. Data validation schemes may not identify such problems, as the form of the data may be valid even if the content is not. Placeholder data (for example, a case created to block a room from double-booking) may skew analytics if it is not accounted for; it may also be valuable data to analyze in and of itself. Drop-down lists may make it easy to select the wrong item on the list (a line too high or too low). Radio-button sets make it impossible to select multiple options.

CASE LAW AND CHART REVIEW

There are many occasions where chart review and verification may need to occur. Most are for the QI reasons listed earlier in the chapter. But legal action does take place and requires a slightly different view of the chart. Case law specific to EHRs is starting to appear.

Medical malpractice insurance carriers have noted that cases involving EHR issues have doubled in recent years. QA data may not be properly protected within the EHR, making it discoverable in the event of a lawsuit. Log files that allow review of chart access may be crucial in deciphering the timeline around a critical event—if they exist.

Discrepancies between screens for nurses and doctors and the printouts taken to court have led some judges and juries to discredit provider testimony.[16] It is currently unclear where this is going, but it will continue to be a concern as we gather more data into the electronic record.

SUMMARY

Use of electronic records can facilitate a robust QA&I process for a group, department, or hospital. It can contribute to both rapid-cycle and detailed analysis of patient care documentation. But like paper methods, it is subject to the limits of data accuracy. And, in the end, if something was not documented, it cannot be reviewed.

REFERENCES

1. Creating clear project requirements—differentiating "what" from "how." http://www.pmi.org/~/media/PDF/Publications/ADV06NA08.ashx. Accessed January 29, 2016.
2. Mede/Analytics, Analytics versus reporting: the salient differences. www.medeanalytics.com. Accessed April 13, 2012.
3. Benn J, Arnold G, Wei I, Riley C, Aleva F. Using quality indicators in anaesthesia: feeding back to improve care. *Br J Anaesth*. 2012;109(1):80–91.
4. Haller G, Stoelwinder J, Myles PS, McNeil J. Quality & safety indicators in anesthesia: a systematic review. *Anesthesiology*. 2009;110:1158–1175.
5. National Quality Measures Clearinghouse. Measure regarding normothermia. http://www.qualitymeasures.ahrq.gov/content.aspx?id=27987. Accessed January 20, 2015.
6. Bender SP, Paganelli WC, et al. Intraoperative lung-protection ventilation trends and practice patterns: a report from the multicenter perioperative outcomes group. *Anesth Analg*. 2015121(5): 1231–1239
7. Kheterpal S, Healy D, et al. Incidence, predictors, and outcomes of difficult mask ventilation combined with difficult laryngoscopy: a report from the Multicenter Perioperative Outcomes Group. *Anesthesiology*. 2013:119(6):1360–1369.
8. Whitlock EL, Feiner JR, Chen LL. Perioperative mortality, 2010 to 2014: a retrospective cohort study using the National Anesthesia Clinical Outcomes Registry. *Anesthesiology*. 2015; 123(6): 1312–1321
9. Cnattingius S, Ericson A, Gunnarskog J, Kallen B. A quality study of a medical birth registry. *Scand J Public Health*. 1990;18(2):143–148. http://sjp.sagepub.com/content/18/2/143.short.
10. Chang B, Kaye AD, et al. Complication of non-operating room procedures: outcomes from the National Anesthesia Clinical Outcomes Registry. *J Patient Saf*. 2015, http://journals.lww.com/journalpatientsafety/Abstract/publishahead/Complications_of_Non_Operating_Room_Procedures__.99676.aspx, Apr 7. Accessed May 31, 2016.

11. http://www.isixsigma.com/tools-templates/fmea/quick-guide-failure-mode-and-effects-analysis. Accessed January 20, 2015.

12. http://www.ihi.org/resources/Pages/Tools/PlanDoStudyActWorksheet.aspx. Accessed January 20, 2015.

13. http://asq.org/learn-about-quality/root-cause-analysis/overview/overview.html. Accessed January 20, 2015.

14. Root Cause Analysis: tracing a problem to its origins. http://www.mindtools.com/pages/article/newTMC_80.htm. Accessed January 20, 2015.

15. http://www.institute.nhs.uk/quality_and_service_improvement_tools/quality_and_service_improvement_tools/plan_do_study_act.html. Accessed January 20, 2015.

16. http://www.politico.com/story/2015/05/electronic-record-errors-growing-issue-in-lawsuits-117591. Accessed May 31, 2016.

16

Safety in Remote Locations

SAMUEL GRODOFSKY, MEGHAN LANE-FALL, AND MARK S. WEISS

INTRODUCTION

Non-operating room anesthesia (NORA) is an umbrella term that describes the anesthetic care of patients undergoing procedures outside the conventional operating room setting. These procedures include gastrointestinal endoscopy, endobronchial procedures, electrophysiologic procedures, and radiologic procedures (Table 16.1). The common thread connecting these procedures is that they occur outside the operating room in locations that were designed for the use of specialty equipment, including fluoroscopes, with anesthesia as a secondary consideration. Nurse-delivered moderate sedation and monitored anesthesia care are more common in these settings, enabling faster turnover and decreased patient length of stay.

At the authors' institution, for example, NORA case volume increased 300%, from 2400 cases in 2005 to 9600 cases in 2012. Although precise case volumes at a national level are unknown, this increase in the volume of NORA cases is emblematic of a larger trend, as was reported by Chang et al. in their analysis of the National Anesthesia Clinical Outcomes Registry from the Anesthesia Quality Institute.[1]

There are at least three reasons that NORA case volume has increased. First, the greater use of mild and moderate sedation and monitored anesthesia care increases throughput and decreases post-procedural length of stay. Second, technological advances have improved the ability of proceduralists' ability to diagnose and treat disease using minimally invasive techniques. A third and related factor is that the minimally invasive nature of techniques used in NORA settings has increased the safety profile of procedures that previously had a high complication rate. As a consequence, patients presenting for NORA cases span the gamut of health from ASA Physical Status 1 patients undergoing screening procedures to ASA 4 or ASA 5 patients who are too ill to withstand conventional surgery. Irrespective of the health status of patients undergoing procedures involving NORA, however, the provision of safe, high-quality care remains the shared goal of both the anesthesiologist and the proceduralist.

Each NORA location presents unique challenges imposed by the procedure to be done, its associated equipment, room setup and ergonomics, support staff, and patient comorbidities. This chapter will discuss the safety concerns associated with NORA care, including (1) structural and design factors, (2) pre-anesthesia checkout, (3) preoperative evaluation, (4) intra-procedural care, (5) post-procedural care, and (6) specialty-specific considerations. Finally, office-based anesthesia will be discussed, along with the common practice of sedation administration by non-anesthesia clinicians (e.g., proceduralists or registered nurses) occurring alongside NORA care. In addition to NORA, "remote" (i.e., non-operating room) services, such as airway management on hospital wards, are rendered by anesthesia personnel, but the scope of this chapter is limited to the NORA suite.

STRUCTURAL AND DESIGN FACTORS IN NORA CARE

Safety starts with design. In the operating room (OR), standard configurations of equipment such as the anesthesia machine, drug delivery

TABLE 16.1. EXAMPLES OF NORA PROCEDURES

Specialty	Example Case Types
Gastroenterology, general surgery	Upper and lower endoscopy; endoscopic retrograde cholangiopancreatography (ERCP); endoscopic ultrasound; percutaneous endoscopic gastrostomy (PEG)
Interventional cardiology	Atrial fibrillation ablation; cardioversion cardiac catheterization; lead extraction for pacemaker or implantable cardioverter defibrillator
Interventional pulmonology	Bronchoscopy tracheobronchial stenting; transbronchial biopsy
Radiology	Diagnostic imaging requiring sedation / anesthesia; cerebral aneurysm coiling; vascular access procedures
Urology	Extracorporeal shock wave lithotripsy (ESWL)

systems, and gas delivery and scavenging allow safety checks to be standardized and therefore streamlined. In locations away from the OR, the anesthetist's workflow may not have been incorporated into room design, but anesthesia staff must nevertheless ensure that all necessary equipment is present and functional. It may be prudent to use guidelines such as the American Society of Anesthesiologists' (ASA) 2008 modification of the US Food and Drug Administration's 1993 pre-anesthesia checkout procedures.[2] These guidelines address routine checks of anesthesia equipment, including the anesthesia gas machine, medical gases, suction, and airway equipment, as well as the availability of emergency medications.

The ASA has also released a statement that specifically addresses standards and practice parameters for NORA locations.[3] This 11-point statement discusses the availability of oxygen, suction, and waste gas scavenging, as well as emergency equipment such as self-inflating resuscitator bags. Specific attention is devoted to the adequacy of the physical space: "There should be in each location, sufficient space to accommodate necessary equipment and personnel and to allow expeditious access to the patient, anesthesia machine (when present) and monitoring equipment" (Item #7).

As the ASA statement on NORA implies, physical space is often at a premium in procedure suites. Especially in older facilities, these locations may not have been designed with the anesthetist's workflow in mind. In their consideration of workspace requirements, Lebak and colleagues submit that a minimum of 64 square feet of workspace is needed for the anesthesia professional.[4] There should also be 3–4 feet of space on at least three sides of the procedure table to allow access to the patient. Finally, each space should be outfitted with an anesthesia gas machine (where applicable) and a supply cart. Where space is limited, the desire to have anesthesia-related equipment close by must be balanced with the need to have other types of equipment and accessories available. Some consideration should be given to which equipment must be immediately accessible inside the NORA suite, and which equipment can be safely stored in a nearby location.

Human factors and ergonomics (HFE) is the scientific discipline focused on the interactions between humans and their environment, with a goal of optimizing overall system performance.[5] Ergonomic factors are also an important component of a safe clinical environment. There are numerous HFE considerations in the NORA suite that can affect the safety of anesthesia care:

- Lighting should be sufficient to allow for safe anesthesia care.
- Supplies should be easily accessible.
- Monitors should be easy to see and access.
- Noise levels must allow for monitor alarms to be heard and to allow for unfettered communication between staff members.
- Equipment should be positioned so as to avoid tripping hazards or injury from low-hanging equipment.

Failure to design procedural suites for these factors may increase the risk of harm. For example, an unreliable oxygen supply or oxygen concentration monitor increases the risk of hypoxia. The ASA Closed Claims database includes a number of adverse events related to inadequate oxygen delivery, and a disproportionate fraction of these oxygen-related claims occurred in NORA settings as compared to conventional ORs.[6,7] According to the Closed Claims database, the most common oxygen-related problems were attributed to oxygen delivery tubing (e.g., improper use or kinking) and gas supply tank mix-ups (e.g., connecting the patient to a carbon dioxide cylinder instead of an oxygen cylinder).[7] In order to avoid adverse events related to hypoxia, both a primary oxygen supply and a backup source of oxygen are essential. The primary supply ideally should come from a central location, accessible through wall outlets or specially configured booms, but reliable oxygen can also be supplied via "E" cylinders.[8] Oxygen cylinders offer several advantages in remote settings: They are portable, easy to use, and do not require electricity. The most important factors limiting the use of E cylinders include their weight and high inventory cost. Some sites have circumvented the problems associated with pressurized oxygen sources by using oxygen concentrators,[9] which use pressure swing adsorption technology to provide an oxygen-enriched gas mixture from ambient air. These devices usually require specialized training and a consistent supply of electrical power.

Electric hazards present an additional safety concern in NORA settings. Institutional standards are designed to prevent electrical shock through proper isolation, appropriate use of grounding, and, historically, conductive flooring material.[10] Steps that can be taken to minimize electrical hazards include proper placement of multi-outlet power strips and boxes, regular checks for electrical wire fraying, and checks for the contamination of electrical equipment by fluid spills (including bodily fluids). An electrical safety checklist should include a contingency plan in the event of a sudden power outage. This contingency plan should include provisions for battery-powered backup of the anesthesia machine, infusion pumps, lighting, electronic drug dispensing systems, and communication devices.

As the demand for NORA grows, new facilities will be built, which will offer opportunities for the anesthesiologist to become involved in the design process. The ASA statement on NORA standards and practice parameters[3] should be consulted during the design process. Considerations that should be addressed early in the planning process include room size, ergonomics for the procedural and anesthesia staff, pharmacy support, emergency planning, and post-anesthesia care needs. Also important are the availability of magnet-safe equipment in magnetic resonance imaging suites, maintaining the anesthesiologists' ability to access the patient throughout all room and equipment configurations, and computing and two-way communication resources to facilitate communication about patient care. Finally, there should be a plan in place for managing emergency situations that might include sudden loss of power, equipment malfunction, or patient emergencies, including anaphylaxis and cardiac arrest. Team-based simulation exercises facilitate training staff on emergency responses, identifying gaps in knowledge and resuscitative capacity, and improving communication between staff members.

PRE-ANESTHESIA CHECKOUT

A properly performed pre-anesthesia checkout can reduce the risk of adverse outcomes associated with anesthetic care. In the operating room, standardization of and familiarity with the OR environment allows a rapid and accurate assessment of a safe working environment.[11] In NORA locations that were not designed according to operating room standards, these checks may be even more important. The pre-anesthesia check in the NORA suite should pay special attention to life-critical issues such as the availability of supplemental oxygen, access to emergency medications and equipment, and a means of communication and escalation of care in the event that additional assistance is needed.

The pre-anesthesia check should confirm proper functioning of the primary oxygen source and circuit, as well as a backup oxygen supply and self-inflating ventilator device (e.g., Ambu™ bag). As part of the safety check, the clinician should confirm the presence of a standardized gas delivery system with functional tubing that is long enough to reach the patient. Inappropriate rigging of oxygen delivery systems, such as direct connection of the patient to a high-pressure oxygen system, has been associated with barotrauma and pneumothorax.[7]

Emergency medications and equipment must be available at all anesthetizing locations. Emergency medications include treatments for anaphylaxis, laryngospasm, malignant hyperthermia (in locations using inhaled anesthetic gases and/or succinylcholine), and cardiovascular emergencies such as cardiac arrest and atrial or ventricular tachyarrhythmias. A functioning cardiac defibrillator (ideally with transcutaneous pacing capability) must also be available. The responsibility for checking and maintaining emergency supplies is often shared among the anesthesia clinician, the procedural physicians, and the nursing staff. This shared responsibility presents a potential organizational challenge in settings that are shared by multiple procedural teams (e.g., interventional radiology and gastroenterology). Organizational policies should address this need to maintain a consistent ability to manage life-threatening emergencies despite team changes; these policies should be reassessed and updated on a regular basis.

Finally, before starting the procedure, the anesthesia and procedural staff should consider the possibility of unanticipated complications and develop a plan to transfer the patient to a higher level of care if needed. If the NORA setting is located in a hospital, this may simply require that the patient be transferred to the post-anesthesia care unit, emergency department, inpatient ward, or a traditional operating room. For freestanding surgery centers or office-based practices, an ambulance may be required to transport the patient to a hospital. Preoperative discussion of this process may avoid a delay in treatment if the patient deteriorates.

PREOPERATIVE EVALUATION

The preoperative evaluation is critically important, especially in the NORA setting. Even though procedures employing NORA are generally shorter and less invasive than surgery, there remains a risk of physiologic deterioration as a result of sedation, anesthesia, or procedural complications. A consensus standard of care places emphasis on the performance and documentation of a preoperative evaluation prior to establishing intraoperative care.[12] This evaluation is particularly important when working in areas with fewer material resources and alternative staffing arrangements, as is commonly the case in NORA settings. The key benefit of the preoperative evaluation lies in the identification of those patients for whom the "typical" anesthetic approach must be altered as a result of patient preference, comorbidity, or procedural details. The clinician must therefore exercise due diligence during the pre-anesthetic evaluation, when the majority of the practice consists of high patient volumes undergoing low-risk procedures. To encourage the safest possible practice, administrative leaders should encourage an institutional culture that upholds preoperative evaluation as a priority for patient safety.

It is common for patients undergoing non-OR procedures to be evaluated by an anesthesiologist on the day of the procedure. Indeed, proceduralists will often determine in advance which patients are likely to need anesthesia care instead of moderate sedation (also known as *conscious sedation*). When anesthesia care has been requested by a procedural team, it is important to understand why the patient requires the care of an anesthesiologist, or why the aspects of a given procedure require deep sedation or general anesthesia. Box 16.1 presents examples of reasons that a patient might be referred for anesthesia care in a NORA setting. Table 16.2 discusses preoperative considerations of particular interest to clinicians who practice in NORA settings.

Many procedures in remote settings tend to be short and cause minimal blood loss, so specific preoperative testing is often not indicated. As with any patient undergoing surgery, however, specific comorbidities, such as

---

BOX 16.1   REASONS THAT A PATIENT MIGHT BE REFERRED FOR ANESTHESIA CARE IN A NORA SETTING

Patient factors

- Patient request
- Obstructive sleep apnea
- Reactive airway disease
- Heart disease: congestive heart failure, coronary artery disease
- Chronic renal insufficiency
- Chronic opioid use
- Hemodynamic instability
- Ventilator-dependent respiratory failure
- ASA physical status > 2

Procedural factors

- Need for extreme stillness or paralysis: extracorporeal shock wave lithotripsy, atrial fibrillation ablation, cerebral aneurysm coiling

Other factors

- Use of propofol*

The use of propofol is currently sufficient Medicare justification for provision of monitored anesthesia care. However, some procedural specialties have advocated for proceduralist supervision of propofol administration by nurses.

---

cardiac disease, diabetes mellitus, and renal impairment, may justify preoperative laboratory testing. The American Heart Association preoperative testing guideline for patients with cardiovascular disease undergoing noncardiac surgery[13] is a useful reference, as is the ASA practice advisory for pre-anesthesia evaluation.[12] Fasting guidelines for patients undergoing a procedure in a remote location are the same as those for conventional surgery because it may be necessary to secure the patient's airway. Patients scheduled for colonoscopy procedures may, however, be dehydrated from bowel preparation. They should be encouraged to drink clear liquids until 2 hours before sedation is scheduled to start, unless otherwise contraindicated.

INTRA-PROCEDURAL CARE

Many procedures employing NORA are often short, sometimes fewer than 10 minutes in duration. It is, therefore, important for the anesthesia and procedural teams to discuss expectations prior to initiating patient care in order to ensure that appropriate procedural equipment and monitors are available and that the patient receives the appropriate level of sedation.

Monitoring standards for non-OR settings have been updated to essentially the same standards as those for OR procedures. ASA guidelines call for standard monitors that include blood pressure monitoring at least every 5 minutes, continuous ECG and pulse oximetry, temperature monitoring (when appropriate), and continual monitoring of the adequacy of ventilation, ideally with end-tidal carbon dioxide ($ETCO_2$) monitoring.[14] $ETCO_2$ monitoring has previously been considered optional, but it provides a faster and more sensitive indicator of hypoventilation than does pulse oximetry. It is, therefore, more strongly encouraged in the most recent ASA standards. Although quantitative carbon dioxide measuring is not strictly required, it has become a de facto standard for anesthetic care. In fact, analysis of the ASA Closed Claims database has revealed that the absence of capnographic

TABLE 16.2. KEY AREA FOR PREOPERATIVE EVALUATION IN NORA SETTINGS

Preoperative Concern	Examples of Comorbid Conditions
Does the patient have an **increased risk of developing apnea or obstruction** at lower than conventional sedation doses with an unprotected airway?	• Obesity • Age > 50 years • Obstructive sleep apnea • Chronic opioid use*
Does the patient have an **increased risk of cardiovascular collapse** with sedation?	• Hypovolemia • Decompensated heart failure • Unstable coronary artery disease • Valvular abnormalities • Autonomic instability • Uncontrolled hypertension
Does the patient have a **challenging airway** that in a remote location may prove problematic for ventilation or intubation?	• Obesity • Craniofacial abnormalities • Limited cervical spine mobility • Limited mouth opening • Tracheal stenosis
Does the patient have any medical conditions or take any medications that may **alter pharmacokinetics or pharmacodynamics?**	• Severe hepatic dysfunction • Severe renal dysfunction • Cytochrome P450 inducers • Cytochrome P450 inhibitors • Chronic opioid use • Chronic alcohol use
Does this patient have an **elevated aspiration risk?**	• Upper gastrointestinal pathology • Pregnancy • Diminished mental status • Dysphagia

*Chronic opioid use is associated with a higher risk of post-procedural apnea, likely related to higher requirements for procedural opioid dosing to achieve the desired level of sedation.

monitoring was the most common reason that care was designated as substandard.[6] It is important to note that while capnometry is a gold standard for ventilatory monitoring, there are specific settings or procedures in which accurate capnometry is difficult or impossible. This may be caused by problems with gas sampling (e.g., sampling line condensation, leaks, kinks); nasal cannula sampling devices have some sampling error, and patients may breathe through their mouth (which will lead to underestimation of ventilation). In procedures involving the airway, carbon dioxide measurement may be imperfect or inconsistent. Given the problems with capnometry, it is prudent to use a surrogate measure of respiration to supplement or replace capnometry. Chest wall movement can be detected from ECG electrodes, and this method has been proven to be valid for detecting obstructive sleep apnea in children.[15]

The sedation goal is determined for each patient and procedure by the anticipated level of pain and the invasiveness of the procedure, as well as the patient's comorbidities and perceived level of anxiety. The ASA has characterized levels of sedation as *mild, moderate, deep,* and *general anesthesia* (with or without a protected airway).[16] Over-sedation may lead to inadequate ventilation and oxygenation or blunting of the sympathetic response to hypovolemia, and may decrease patient throughput. On the other hand, inadequate sedation may lead to excessive autonomic responses like tachycardia or hypertension. Inadequate sedation may also lead to sudden patient movement during the procedure that may cause direct trauma, compromise of the sterile field, or termination of the procedure as a result of suboptimal conditions.

The difficulty in safely reaching and maintaining targeted levels of sedation prompted one author to rename MAC (monitored anesthesia care) as "maximum anesthesia caution."[17] Clinicians who provide anesthesia care must anticipate and respond promptly to changes in procedural stimulation that may lead to concomitant changes in the level of sedation. A calm, moderately sedated patient may rapidly awaken and become disinhibited in response to a painful stimulus or may become deeply sedated with hypopnea and inadequate oxygenation or ventilation during a pause in the procedure. Rescue airway equipment must be immediately available in case the patient requires ventilatory assistance. The ASA Closed Claims studies indicate that inadequate oxygenation and ventilation are at the root of most NORA-related claims, so procedure- and setting-specific approaches to airway management (with contingency plans) should be developed.

SPECIALTY-SPECIFIC INTRA-PROCEDURAL CONSIDERATIONS

Anesthetic care is conceptually similar in OR and non-OR settings, but specific procedures require special consideration:

Gastroenterology—endoscopic retrograde cholangiopancreatography (ERCP): This procedure may require lateral or prone positioning. The patient should be supported with padding to prevent pressure injury and to enable adequate diaphragmatic excursion. Patients with increased abdominal girth may be particularly difficult to position.

Interventional cardiology—atrial fibrillation ablation: Respiratory movement can interfere with mapping and ablation of electrical foci. For this reason, some centers have reported shorter procedural times and greater proceduralist satisfaction with the use of high-frequency jet ventilation (HFJV) to support oxygenation and ventilation while minimizing respiratory motion.[18]

Interventional cardiology—lead extraction (pacemaker or implantable cardioverter defibrillator): Intramyocardial lead extraction carries a risk of cardiac perforation, which may cause hemorrhage and cardiovascular collapse. Some institutions therefore require backup support from a cardiothoracic surgeon. Because of the risk of this life-threatening complication, the proceduralist and anesthesiologist must discuss the timing of lead extraction to facilitate rapid detection and treatment if it occurs.

Interventional pulmonology—bronchoscopy: The airway is shared by the anesthesia staff and the procedural staff during tracheobronchial procedures. It is therefore critical that the entire team communicate about anticipated procedural course, likely complications, and plan for maintaining the airway at all times. HFJV can be useful for ventilation during rigid bronchoscopy.

Urology—extracorporeal shock wave lithotripsy: As with atrial fibrillation ablation, HFJV decreases diaphragmatic excursion and may shorten procedural time.[18]

POST-PROCEDURAL CARE

Recovery after NORA is similar to that of outpatient surgical procedures conducted in an OR. Patients recovering from sedation and anesthesia should receive care in a dedicated area that meets ASA standards for post-anesthetic care. Skilled nursing staff must be available, and these nurses must be familiar with the unique requirements of patients who are recovering from sedation and anesthesia. Although patients who have not had general anesthesia generally meet discharge criteria more rapidly than those who have received general anesthesia, recovery staff should assess patients for late effects of sedation such as delayed hypoventilation. Provisions for transfer to a higher level of care (e.g., an acute care hospital) should be in place in the event that a patient experiences an unanticipated complication.

SPECIALTY-SPECIFIC SAFETY CONSIDERATIONS

Some NORA settings—radiology, gastrointestinal endoscopy, and cardiac electrophysiology—present specific safety challenges.

Radiology

Anesthesia professionals care for patients undergoing both diagnostic studies and therapeutic procedures in the radiology suite. Sedation is often required for diagnostic procedures in pediatric patients and patients who are unable to cooperate because of diminished cognitive abilities. Anesthesia care may be requested for therapeutic procedures in order to allay patient anxiety or to provide complete immobility for procedures that demand extreme precision (e.g., neurovascular procedures).

Anesthesia care in the radiology suite presents challenges that may not be encountered in a conventional OR. Physical distance from the patient is one of the most notable differences. It is often necessary for the anesthetist to monitor the patient from a control room adjacent to the imaging equipment. Visual contact is maintained through a window or with a live camera feed. This requires particular attention to monitors, cables, and tubing to ensure that no tension is placed on catheters, sensors, or equipment. Sufficient length should be maintained throughout the full range of motion of radiology tables, which may rotate or move back and forth to obtain images. It is also important to consider how positioning and procedure length may impact the sedation plan. For example, an obese patient with severe obstructive sleep apnea might be safely managed with MAC and a natural airway for a computed tomography scan, but might require general anesthesia with an endotracheal tube for a prolonged radiologic procedure.

Managing NORA patients involves risks to both patients and staff. Perhaps the most obvious risk is exposure to ionizing radiation. Computed tomography and fluoroscopy machines emit radiation from three sources: directly from the imaging beam, from the radiation source itself (i.e., a poorly shielded X-ray tube), and via scatter from the patient; this latter source may present the greatest risk to anesthesiologists. The organs most likely to be damaged by radiation include the eye, the thyroid gland, and the gonads.[19] The Sievert (Sv) is a derived unit of exposure to ionizing radiation that reflects the probability of developing cancer. Exposure to one Sievert carries a 5.5% risk of developing cancer. The maximal annual radiation dose recommended by the International Commission on Radiological Protection is 50 milliSieverts (mSv). The maximum recommended dose per lifetime is 10 mSv x age in years. For pregnant women, the maximum recommended monthly dose is 0.5 mSv.[20]

Protective measures for patients involves using the minimum dose of radiation to achieve the desired image and shielding those regions of the body that are not involved in the procedure. Modern fluoroscopy equipment also warns proceduralists about the fluoroscopy time accumulated in a given procedure.

Staff who are exposed to ionizing radiation should be protected as much as possible, and their exposure should be monitored with dosimetry devices. At a minimum, staff should wear leaded aprons (at least 0.5 mm thick for proceduralists, at least 0.25 mm thick for those on the periphery of the procedure room), thyroid shields, and glasses.[21] Ideally, staff are fitted for lead coverings appropriate to body size. These coverings should cover both the front and the back of the body to allow staff to move freely within the radiology suite. Additional protection is conferred by X-ray blocking curtains and transparent leaded panels. Staff who are consistently exposed to ionizing radiation should wear dosimeters that are queried monthly to determine their exposure. Pregnancy is not necessarily a contraindication to working with ionizing radiation, but extra care should be taken to ensure that protective wear completely covers the pregnant staff member, and the dosimeter should be worn at the waist level.[21] Some institutions have a policy of reassigning pregnant staff so that they are not frequently exposed to ionizing radiation.

Patients undergoing both interventional and diagnostic imaging are often administered intravenous iodinated contrast that absorbs X-rays. This contrast material has rare but potentially life-threatening side effects. These include glottic edema, bronchospasm, pulmonary edema, arrhythmias, seizures, cardiac arrest, and anaphylaxis. Mild side effects are much more common and include urticaria, pruritus, erythema, and upper respiratory effects such as nasal congestion, scratchy throat, or sneezing. Contrast nephropathy is another complication that may occur from contrast administration. The anesthesiologist may reduce this risk by expanding the circulating blood volume with isotonic crystalloid and avoiding other nephrotoxic drugs.[22] There is some limited evidence that isotonic sodium bicarbonate may further reduce the risk of contrast nephropathy in patients with mild preexisting renal dysfunction.[23]

The field of interventional neuroradiology (INR) is experiencing rapid growth as a result of improving technology and emerging evidence that procedures such as endovascular coiling aneurysms demonstrate better long-term results than surgical clipping for some patients.[24,25] INR comprises a spectrum of procedures that range from low-risk, elective procedures that may be performed under local anesthesia (e.g., cerebral angioplasty) to high-risk emergency care, such as management of ruptured intracranial aneurysms. In order to ensure safe and efficient completion of an INR procedure, anesthesiologists must work with the proceduralist to maintain mutually established target physiologic variables such as cerebral perfusion pressure goals, anticipating potential procedural complications and ensuring patient immobility for digital subtraction angiography. Anesthetic considerations for INR are similar to those for open neurosurgery, and include the use of pharmacologic and ventilatory techniques to avoid increases in intracranial pressure. Often, systemic arterial blood pressure monitoring is required to maintain optimal hemodynamic parameters and to withdraw blood samples for activated clotting time measurements and arterial blood gas testing. A key safety measure in the interventional radiology suite is maintaining access to resources similar to those available in centrally located ORs, such as a blood bank.

Magnetic resonance imaging (MRI) presents a different set of challenges for NORA care. MRI applies a strong static magnetic field (typically 1.5–3 Tesla) and a second magnetic field created by pulsed radiofrequency (RF) to a target tissue area. A subsequent RF signal is emitted from tissue and is detected by an RF coil, which is then used to construct an image. In order to obtain satisfactory imaging data, long scanning times, sometimes over an hour, may be required; this must be considered during anesthetic planning. Furthermore, emission of the pulsed RF signal creates a loud sound that may impair the anesthetist's ability to hear monitor tones or to communicate with radiology staff. For the patient, these sounds may prove bothersome or anxiety provoking, and may cause hearing loss. For this reason, ear protection should be provided to the patient.[26]

While there is little evidence that MRI technology poses direct tissue injury, severe patient harm and death have been caused by ferromagnetic objects being pulled into the strong magnetic field, and thermal burns have been caused by various equipment, including ECG electrodes and pulmonary artery catheters. [27–29,30] The room containing the MRI scanner should have clearly marked warning signs about the dangers of unsupervised entry. Anesthesia and radiology departments should collaborate on policies for the training required for entry into MRI areas, and there should be a strict screening protocol in place for all individuals entering strong magnetic fields.[31] This includes thorough questioning for the presence of implantable medical devices such as pacemakers, implantable cardiac defibrillators, programmable ventricular shunts, intracranial aneurysm clips, neurostimulators, and other devices, which are generally contraindicated in MRIs and require documentation as being MR-safe and MR-conditional. Patients should also be queried about drug delivery patches that may contain a metallic foil.[32]

Complications related to medication administration and positioning should be a concern for every anesthetic professional. The most common malpractice claims against anesthesiologists who have cared for a patient undergoing an MRI procedure occurred as a result of injuries related to over-sedation, burns from incompatible MRI equipment, and nerve damage from poor arm positioning in the scanner.[7] As part of the preparation for an MRI anesthetic, staff should confirm the availability of MR-safe and MR-compatible anesthesia equipment, including monitors (e.g., pulse oximeters, ECG electrodes), ventilators, gas-delivery systems, intravenous tubing, patient pumps, and warming devices. The FDA has instituted a standardized labeling system that identifies items as *MR-unsafe, MR-safe* (can be used within any static or gradient field), and *MR-conditional* (can be used only in static magnetic fields less than a given strength or defined gradient fields).[32] To reduce the risk of thermal injury, monitor wires should be free and as straight as possible, without loops. Equipment should be regularly inspected for worn or frayed wires.[33]

Management of critical events in the MRI setting requires some awareness of the logistical challenges at hand. If a cardiac arrest occurs, it is impossible to bring resuscitation equipment into the MRI room. The anesthesia team must therefore coordinate the transportation of the patient to a suitable area, while CPR is being performed, in order for a code team to work effectively. Additional emergency management includes the need to quench the magnet, which rapidly releases the cryogenic gas (usually liquid helium), which quickly dissipates the magnetic field. This can quickly create a hypoxic environment in the scanner room, and should only be considered if the patient or a staff member is trapped in the bore of the magnet by another piece of equipment, or if an injury will occur if a ferromagnetic object

is not retrieved from the room in a timely manner.[34]

Gastrointestinal Endoscopy

Gastrointestinal (GI) endoscopy suites produced the largest number of NORA claims in the ASA Closed Claims database, comprising 32% of claims.[7] Gastrointestinal endoscopic procedures, such as colonoscopies, upper endoscopies, and endoscopic retrograde cholangiopancreatography (ERCP), have created unique NORA challenges because endoscopy suites are often high-volume facilities that require high turnover of MAC cases. Although sedating healthy patients undergoing colonoscopy rarely leads to an adverse event, patients with multiple comorbidities frequently undergo procedures in these settings. Risk stratification during the pre-anesthetic evaluation is therefore critical, with additional consideration warranted for patients with the following comorbidities: morbid obesity and obstructive sleep apnea, full stomach, hypovolemia (particularly after bowel prep), chronic pain with high-dose opioid use, and hepatic or renal insufficiency (Box 16.1 and Table 16.2). The majority of GI endoscopy claims were attributed to over-sedation leading to respiratory depression. This most frequently occurred during upper GI endoscopy and ERCP procedures, with propofol as the most commonly attributed anesthetic agent (78% of cases).[7] Risk-reduction strategies to accommodate these common challenges include slow drug titration, the early use of a nasal airway with a breathing circuit, and close communication with proceduralists.

One of the most controversial safety-related issues in GI endoscopy involves the use of routine capnometry during moderate sedation. The ASA has provided clear language supporting its use; the clinical reasoning is that a change in carbon dioxide exhalation is an earlier and more sensitive indicator of ventilatory compromise than is oxygen desaturation. In contrast, the American Gastroenterology Association (AGA) released a statement questioning the evidence supporting the routine use of capnometry, and cites the increased cost and intrusion of false alarms as justification to avoid the routine monitoring of exhaled CO_2.[35] The anesthesia care team should have a low threshold for using $ETCO_2$ monitoring if factors related to the patient or procedure are present that prevent easy visual determination of chest rise or other signs of adequate respiratory effort.

Cardiac Electrophysiology

Interventional electrophysiology (EP) and cardiac catheterization are becoming increasingly common, and have fundamentally transformed care for patients with heart disease while decreasing the need for surgical intervention in select patients. Mapping of the coronary arteries and electrical pathways is achieved through a combination of fluoroscopy, MR, and ultrasound, allowing patients to undergo complex procedures through a minimally invasive approach. Anesthesia professionals are rarely required for cardiac catheterization procedures, but are sometimes called to assist in rescue scenarios. Anesthesia care is, however, more common for patients undergoing electrophysiology (EP) procedures. There are at least two major safety hazards in cardiac electrophysiology procedures: ionizing radiation, which was discussed earlier, and the requirement for both the anesthesiologist and the proceduralist to jointly manage the patient's hemodynamics.

Patients undergoing EP procedures typically have one or more significant comorbidities that may include severe systolic and diastolic dysfunction and malignant tachyarrhythmia. Unlike in the OR, the patient's hemodynamic status is managed by both the anesthetist (by administering medications) and the interventional cardiologist (by administration medications and through direct manipulation of the cardiac rhythm). The anesthetic plan for these patients should include special attention to using agents that minimize impairment of myocardial contractility. Perhaps more important, however, is direct and continuous communication between the anesthesia and procedural teams in the EP suite. Unless the two teams engage in a continuing discussion of the patient's status and the treatment plan, the anesthetist and cardiologist

may institute overlapping (e.g., both teams administer vasopressors) or contradicting therapies (e.g., one team administers a vasopressor while the other administers a vasodilator). Defibrillation, often necessary to terminate provoked arrhythmias, poses an additional risk to anesthesia team members, who may be subject to shock if they are not aware when defibrillation occurs. Communication may at times be difficult because of differences in training and expectations and the physical distance between proceduralists (who are located in a control room) and anesthesia staff (who are located near the patient). The use of pre-procedural briefings and two-way communication devices (e.g., "walkie-talkie" headsets) may decrease misunderstandings that can result in patient harm or provider dissatisfaction.

Office-Based Anesthesia (OBA)

Office-based surgery has increased in prevalence, and this growth has prompted an expansion of state and federal regulations related to OBA. It is difficult to assess the absolute risk of OBA because offices are decentralized, and compiling a meaningful database is therefore problematic. Centers that strictly adhere to accepted standards of care have been shown to produce excellent patient outcomes, and the low rates of hospital admissions are mainly related to surgical complications.[36,37] The ASA has created a set of broad outlines for OBA, with emphasis on ensuring the presence of the basic safety infrastructure found in hospital-based operating rooms.[38] The greatest obstacle may be tied to the decentralized nature of practice and less imposing bureaucracy than that found in the hospital setting; experts have expressed concern that this administrative structure may lead to a lapse in safety standards.[39] To help address safety concerns, anesthesiologists should participate in the administrative oversight of office-based surgical practices, and should encourage continuous quality improvement. Investments in accreditation, professional board certification, and proper credentialing of proceduralists may also improve patient outcomes. Safety culture should also be promoted; this includes the use of checklists and appropriate patient and procedure selection for the office setting.[40] An emergency transfer contingency plan with a clear protocol for managing an acutely ill patient is a critical measure to minimize risk if a complication that exhausts an office's resources should occur.

SEDATION BY NON-ANESTHESIA PRACTITIONERS

The parallel provision of sedation by both anesthesia professionals and sedation providers who are not trained in anesthesia is a major challenge facing anesthesiologists in the NORA setting. Given the sheer volume of NORA cases, it is unrealistic for anesthetists to care for all patients who undergo procedures outside the operating room. For this reason, non-anesthesia professionals (e.g., registered nurses, non-anesthesia physicians) are commonly credentialed to provide sedation.[41] Sedation is typically driven by a comprehensive administrative protocol that requires the proceduralist to supervise drug administration and typically limits providers to using shorter acting drugs such as midazolam and fentanyl.[42] Anesthesiologists have expert knowledge in this area and should therefore ensure that all sedative and analgesic drugs are delivered safely throughout the healthcare institution. This responsibility may include training of non-anesthesia practitioners and the development of policies and protocols for sedation and for referral of selected patients for anesthesia care. Examples of poor candidates for sedation care by non-anesthesia professionals include those with morbid obesity, severe OSA, decompensated cardiac function, anxiety, and chronic opioid use (Box 16.1).

Sedation protocols that rely on benzodiazepines and opioids may be problematic for at least two reasons: First, it may be difficult to create acceptable procedural conditions within a short time frame using these drugs. Second, high doses of fentanyl or midazolam may be required to keep patients still and comfortable, particularly in patients with tolerance to these drugs. These high doses may exceed protocol limits, necessitating anesthetist intervention, or may place patients at risk for post-procedural over-sedation that prolongs length of stay and/or requires airway support. Propofol offers a favorable sedation profile because it is potent and short-acting, but controversy exists as to whether non-anesthesia practitioners should administer this drug. There are data that support the administration of propofol by non-anesthesia professionals to patients who are designated with ASA physical status I and II for gastrointestinal endoscopy cases.[43,44] In higher-risk cases (ASA PS III and above), the evidence demonstrates that anesthesia professionals do in fact decrease the risk of complications in NORA cases when propofol is used. [45]

Anesthesia professionals have training and experience in a variety of situations that allow them to develop familiarity with benzodiazepines, opioids, propofol, ketamine, dexmedetomidine, and other sedating drugs. Non-anesthesia practitioners such as sedation nurses do not share this familiarity and experience. Off-label use of propofol via physician oversight, as with gastroenterologist-directed nurse administration, is a common practice.[44] Although the ASA guidelines for sedation and analgesia for non-anesthesiologists suggest that non-anesthesia practitioners use benzodiazepines for moderate sedation cases, the use of propofol requires preparation for deep sedation even if this is not the intended goal.[16]

One of the most comprehensive reports concerning NORA safety data comes from the Pediatric Sedation Research Consortium.[45] Pediatric sedation is commonly indicated for diagnostic radiology procedures (e.g., magnetic resonance imaging), which requires small children to be motionless for long periods of time. The Consortium's publication of almost 50,000 sedation cases from 37 institutions employing propofol offers insight into safe sedation practices. Their study reported no deaths and two events requiring cardiopulmonary resuscitation after sedation. Just one in 70 cases required airway management and controlled ventilation. Overall, the data demonstrate that propofol use by non-anesthesia professionals can be performed safely, but the persistence of adverse events suggests that there is still a role for anesthesiologists to optimize patient safety in NORA settings.

QUALITY IMPROVEMENT IN NORA SETTINGS

The rapid growth in procedures employing NORA, combined with the multidisciplinary, interprofessional nature of NORA care, creates opportunities for innovation in patient care. However, non-OR procedures may also cause unusual system stresses and communication difficulties. For this reason, it is important that anesthesia staff, procedure staff, and facility administrative staff maintain open lines of communication about patient care.[46] Regular meetings to discuss procedures, protocols, and adverse events are helpful, as is the presence of an anonymous event-reporting system. Even though there may be emphasis placed on efficiency and throughput, at least some staff should have dedicated non-clinical time to collect and analyze data about patient outcomes and productivity measures. Also, as mentioned earlier, simulation exercises may improve team communication and allow for prompt responses to rare clinical emergencies.

CONCLUSION

The ever-growing number of innovations in patient care technology permits noninvasive or minimally invasive diagnosis of treatment of an increasing number of diseases. As a result, non-operating room procedures have become commonplace. Anesthesiologists can facilitate high-quality patient care in NORA settings by helping design facilities for non-operating room procedures, by helping determine which patients need anesthesia care, and by participating in quality improvement initiatives to achieve and maintain care excellence.

REFERENCES

1. Chang B, Kaye AD, Diaz JH, Westlake B, Dutton RP, Urman RD. Complications of non-operating room procedures: outcomes from the National Anesthesia Clinical Outcomes Registry. *J Patient Safety.* 2015; epub ahead of print.
2. American Society of Anesthesiologists Committee on Equipment and Facilities. *Guidelines for Pre-Anesthesia Checkout Procedures.* 2008. http:// www.asahq.org/resources/clinical-information/ 2008-asa-recommendations-for-pre-anesthesia-checkout. Accessed 9 April, 2016.
3. American Society of Anesthesiologists Committee on Standards and Practice Parameters. *Statement on Nonoperating Room Anesthetizing Locations.* 2013. http://www.asahq.org/~/media/legacy/for% 20members/documents/standards%20guidelines%20stmts/nonoperating%20room%20anesthetizing%20locations.pdf. Accessed 9 April, 2016
4. Lebak K, Springman S, Lee J. designing safety and engineering standards for the non-operating room anesthesia procedure site. In: Weiss MS, Fleisher LA, eds. *Non-Operating Room Anesthesia.* Philadelphia: Elsevier Saunders; 2015:8–10.
5. Xie A, Carayon P. A systematic review of human factors and ergonomics (HFE)-based healthcare system redesign for quality of care and patient safety. *Ergonomics.* 2014;58(1):33–49.
6. Metzner J, Domino KB. Risks of anesthesia or sedation outside the operating room: the role of the anesthesia care provider. *Curr Opin Anaesthesiol.* 2010;23(4):523–531.
7. Metzner J, Posner KL, Domino KB. The risk and safety of anesthesia at remote locations: the US closed claims analysis. *Curr Opin Anaesthesiol.* 2009;22(4):502–508.
8. Love-Jones S, Magee P. Medical gases, their storage and delivery. *Anaesth Intensive Care Med.* 2007;8(1):2–6.
9. McCormick BA, Eltringham RJ. Anaesthesia equipment for resource-poor environments. *Anaesthesia.* 2007;62:54–60.
10. Helfman S. Electrical service. In: Block FE, Helfman S, eds. *Operating Room Design Manual.* American Society of Anesthesiologists; 2010:69–74.
11. Olympio MA, Goldstein MM, Mathes DD. Instructional review improves performance of anesthesia apparatus checkout procedures. *Anesth Analg.* 1996;83(3):618–622.
12. Practice advisory for preanesthesia evaluation: an updated report by the American Society of Anesthesiologists Task Force on Preanesthesia Evaluation. *Anesthesiology.* 2012;116(3):522–538.
13. Fleisher LA, Fleischmann KE, Auerbach AD, et al. 2014 ACC/AHA guideline on perioperative cardiovascular evaluation and management of patients undergoing noncardiac surgery: a report of the American College of Cardiology/American Heart Association task force on practice guidelines. *Circulation.* 2014;130(24):e278–e333.
14. American Society of Anesthesiologists Committee on Standards and Practice Parameters. *Standards for Basic Anesthetic Monitoring.* 2010. http:// www.asahq.org/~/media/sites/asahq/files/public/

resources/standards-guidelines/standards-for-basic-anesthetic-monitoring.pdf. Accessed 9 April, 2016.

15. Shouldice RB, O'Brien LM, O'Brien C, De Chazal P, Gozal D, Heneghan C. Detection of obstructive sleep apnea in pediatric subjects using surface lead electrocardiogram features. *Sleep.* 2004;27(4):784–792.

16. American Society of Anesthesiologists Task Force on Sedation and Analgesia by Non-Anesthesiologists. Practice guidelines for sedation and analgesia by non-anesthesiologists: an updated report by the American Society of Anesthesiologists task force on sedation and analgesia by non-anesthesiologists. *Anesthesiology.* 2002;96(4):1004–1017.

17. HugJr CC. MAC should stand for maximum anesthesia caution, not minimal anesthesiology care. *Anesthesiology.* 2006;104(2):221–223.

18. Raiten J, Elkassabany N, Mandel JE. The use of high-frequency jet ventilation for out of operating room anesthesia. *Curr Opin Anaesthesiol.* 2012;25(4):482–485.

19. McCollough CH, Primak AN, Braun N, Kofler J, Yu L, Christner J. Strategies for reducing radiation dose in CT. *Radiol Clin N Am.* 2009;47(1):27–40.

20. The 2007 recommendations of the International Commission on Radiological Protection. ICRP publication 103. *Annals of the ICRP.* 2007; 37(2–4):1–332.

21. Association of Surgical Technologists. AST Standards of Practice for Ionizing Radiation Exposure in the Perioperative Setting. 2010. http://www.ast.org/uploadedFiles/Main_Site/Content/About_Us/Standard%20Ionizing%20Radiation%20Exposure.pdf. Accessed 8 January, 2016.

22. Dickinson MC, Kam PC. Intravascular iodinated contrast media and the anaesthetist. *Anaesthesia.* 2008;63(6):626–634.

23. Ho KM, Morgan DJ. Use of isotonic sodium bicarbonate to prevent radiocontrast nephropathy in patients with mild pre-existing renal impairment: a meta-analysis. *Anaesth Intens Care.* 2008;36(5):646–653.

24. Molyneux AJ, Kerr RS, Yu LM, et al. International subarachnoid aneurysm trial (ISAT) of neurosurgical clipping versus endovascular coiling in 2143 patients with ruptured intracranial aneurysms: a randomised comparison of effects on survival, dependency, seizures, rebleeding, subgroups, and aneurysm occlusion. *Lancet.* 2005;366(9488):809–817.

25. Molyneux AJ, Kerr RS, Birks J, et al. Risk of recurrent subarachnoid haemorrhage, death, or dependence and standardised mortality ratios after clipping or coiling of an intracranial aneurysm in

the International Subarachnoid Aneurysm Trial (ISAT): long-term follow-up. *Lancet Neurology.* 2009;8(5):427–433.

26. Rubin D. Anesthesia for ambulatory diagnostic and therapeutic radiology procedures. *Anesth Clin.* 2014;32(2):371–380.

27. Dempsey MF, Condon B. Thermal injuries associated with MRI. *Clin Radiol.* 2001;56(6):457–465.

28. Colletti PM. Size "H" oxygen cylinder: accidental MR projectile at 1.5 Tesla. *J Magn Reson Imaging.* 2004;19(1):141–143.

29. Chaljub G, Kramer LA, Johnson RF, 3rd, Johnson RF, Jr., Singh H, Crow WN. Projectile cylinder accidents resulting from the presence of ferromagnetic nitrous oxide or oxygen tanks in the MR suite. *Am J Roentgenol.* 2001;177(1):27–30.

30. Levine GN, Gomes AS, Arai AE, et al. Safety of magnetic resonance imaging in patients with cardiovascular devices: an American Heart Association scientific statement from the Committee on Diagnostic and Interventional Cardiac Catheterization, Council on Clinical Cardiology, and the Council on Cardiovascular Radiology and Intervention: endorsed by the American College of Cardiology Foundation, the North American Society for Cardiac Imaging, and the Society for Cardiovascular Magnetic Resonance. *Circulation.* 2007;116(24): 2878–2891.

31. Practice advisory on anesthetic care for magnetic resonance imaging: a report by the Society of Anesthesiologists Task Force on Anesthetic Care for Magnetic Resonance Imaging. *Anesthesiology.* 2009;110(3):459–479.

32. Committee on Standards and Practice Parameters, Apfelbaum JL, et al. Practice advisory for preanesthesia evaluation: an updated report by the American Society of Anesthesiologists Task Force on Preanesthesia Evaluation. *Anesthesiology.* 2012;116(3):522–538.

33. Stensrud PE. Anesthesia at remote locations. In: Miller RD, ed. *Miller's Anesthesia.* Vol 2, 7th ed. Philadelphia: Churchill Livingstone Elsevier; 2010:2461–2484.

34. Expert Panel on MRS, Kanal E, Barkovich AJ, et al. ACR guidance document on MR safe practices: 2013. *J Magn Reson Imaging.* 2013;37(3): 501–530.

35. American Society of Gastrointestinal Endoscopy Statement. Universal adoption of capnography for moderate sedation in adults undergoing upper endoscopy and colonoscopy has not been shown to improve patient safety or clinical outcomes and significantly increases costs for moderate sedation. 2012. http://www.asge.org/assets/0/71542/71544/90dc9b63-593d-48a9-bec1-9f0ab3ce946a.pdf Accessed: 9 April 2016.

36. Shapiro FE, Punwani N, Rosenberg NM, Valedon A, Twersky R, Urman RD. Office-based anesthesia: safety and outcomes. *Anesth Analg.* 2014;119(2):276–285.

37. Blake DR. Office-based anesthesia: dispelling common myths. *Aesthet Plast Surg.* 2008;28(5):564–570; discussion 571–562.

38. American Society of Anesthesiologists Committee on Ambulatory Surgical Care. Guidlines for Office-Based Anesthesia. 2014. http://www.asahq.org/~/media/Sites/ASAHQ/Files/Public/Resources/standards-guidelines/guidelines-for-office-based-anesthesia.pdf. Accessed 9 April, 2016.

39. Bridenbaugh PO. Office-based anesthesia: requirements for patient safety. *Anesth Prog.* 2005;52(3):86–90.

40. Shapiro FE, Punwani N, Urman RD. Office-based surgery: embracing patient safety strategies. *J Med Pract Manage.* 2013;29(2):72–75.

41. Manickam P, Kanaan Z, Zakaria K. Conscious sedation: a dying practice? *World J Gastroenter.* 2013;19(28):4633–4634.

42. Fassoulaki A, Theodoraki K, Melemeni A. Pharmacology of sedation agents and reversal agents. *Digestion.* 2010;82(2):80–83.

43. Tohda G, Higashi S, Wakahara S, Morikawa M, Sakumoto H, Kane T. Propofol sedation during endoscopic procedures: safe and effective administration by registered nurses supervised by endoscopists. *Endoscopy.* 2006;38(4):360–367.

44. Rex DK, Heuss LT, Walker JA, Qi R. Trained registered nurses/endoscopy teams can administer propofol safely for endoscopy. *Gastroenterology.* 2005;129(5):1384–1391.

45. Cravero JP, Blike GT, Beach M, et al. Incidence and nature of adverse events during pediatric sedation/anesthesia for procedures outside the operating room: report from the Pediatric Sedation Research Consortium. *Pediatrics.* 2006;118(3):1087–1096.

46. Lane-Fall MB, Weiss MS. Engineering excellence in non-operating room anesthesia care. In: Weiss MS, Fleisher LA, eds. *Non-Operating Room Anesthesia.* Philadelphia: Elsevier Saunders; 2015:2–6.

17

Medication Safety

ALAN F. MERRY

INTRODUCTION

Medication safety is often thought of as achieving the "rights" of medication administration: the Joint Commission listed five of these "rights,"[1] and an accurate record of the administration is also important (Box 17.1).[2] It is not difficult to achieve these six "rights" for any single administration of a medication, but an anesthesiologist may administer medications perhaps a quarter of a million times during his or her career (e.g., on average 10 administrations per anesthetic, 5 anesthetics a day, 4 days a week, 45 weeks a year, for 30 years = 270,000); in this context, achieving all six every time is statistically improbable with current approaches to the administration of drugs in this specialty, particularly for intravenous (IV) drugs. In fact, failures to achieve these rights occur more often than one might expect (see Tables 17.1 and 17.2).

Such failures are often attributed to medication errors, which may be defined as "errors in the prescription, dispensing, or administration of a medication," [3] with an error defined in Chapter 3 ("Errors and Violations") of this volume as "the unintentional use of a wrong plan to achieve an aim, or failure to carry out a planned action as intended." Medication errors may be errors of commission or errors of omission.

The coupling between medication errors and their consequences is loose (see Chapter 3, "Errors and Violations").[4] It has been estimated that about 1% of medication errors result in an adverse drug event (ADE),[5] defined as "any injury arising from the use of a drug." Many medication errors are without consequence, and

it is even possible for a medication error to have a positive impact on patient outcome (Box 17.2). Furthermore, not all ADEs are caused by error—for example, anaphylactic and other allergic reactions to drugs are ADEs, but they may occur in the absence of medication errors. Some ADEs are preventable while others are not, because they reflect intrinsic properties of certain medications. These ADEs may be accepted as predictable and acceptable side effects of valuable therapies (e.g., hair loss after administration of chemotherapeutic agents), but they are still relevant to medication safety, because they may be reduced through drug development. Some intrinsic ADEs are partly preventable: for example, nausea and vomiting, or constipation, after the administration of opioids.

Anesthesiologists working in the operating room (OR) are unusual in that they prescribe, dispense, and administer many medications themselves, without any checks from pharmacists and nurses. This probably increases the risk of error, although errors may occur even with the benefit of such checks. In the wider context of perioperative medicine, errors and ADEs also occur preoperatively and postoperatively, in post-anesthetic care units (PACU),[6,7] intensive care units (ICU),[8,9] on wards,[10] or even at home after discharge from the hospital. Medications in these areas are often administered by nurses, and may be prescribed by various doctors, including anesthesiologists and surgeons, or surgical residents or interns (depending on the system prevailing in the particular country and institution).

Anesthesiologists' autonomous management of medications in the OR provides

1. The right drug
2. To the right patient
3. At the right time
4. In the right dose
5. By the right route
6. Recorded right (i.e., correctly)

*It can also be argued that one should be able to
demonstrate that the six rights have been achieved.*

unparalleled opportunity for abuse.[11] This is a
second important element of medication safety.
The abuse of drugs is an example of a *violation*
(see Chapter 3, "Errors and Violations"). The
potential impact of such abuse on anesthesiologists' cognition and performance creates an
additional risk to the safety of patients in their
care, and to the anesthesiologists themselves,
including a risk of death, either by deliberate
suicide or by accident.

Access to essential drugs of adequate quality is a third key element of perioperative medication safety.[12]

Thus failures in medication safety are
common in perioperative medicine, and varied
in nature. Many of these failures are influenced by factors in the system, and many are
underpinned by errors or violations. It follows
that an understanding of medication safety
depends on an understanding of errors, violations, and complex systems in general. The
relevant principles are discussed in detail in
Chapter 3 of this volume. In this chapter, specific aspects of medication safety are considered
in light of these generic principles.

MEASUREMENT AND MEDICATION SAFETY

Measurement is an important element in
improving safety: if one cannot quantify a
problem, it is difficult to evaluate the effectiveness of initiatives designed to address it.
Unfortunately, accurately quantifying failures
in medication safety is both difficult and resource intensive. Understandably, there seems
to have been a tendency for studies to focus on
individual parts of the patient pathway, rather
than the entire perioperative experience of a
patient from admission to hospital to discharge
home, let alone the days and weeks that follow
discharge.

Incident Reporting

Several early studies of medication errors in
the perioperative period have involved voluntary incident reporting.[6,13–16] Studies of this
type typically document the fact that medication errors occur and provide some insight
into their nature, but substantially underrate

TABLE 17.1. RATES OF MEDICATION ADMINISTRATION ERROR
PER ANESTHETIC REPORTED IN FIVE STUDIES USING FACILITATED
INCIDENT REPORTING

Country	NZ[24]	USA	RSA	USA	China
Number of anesthetics	10806	6709	30412	10574	24380
Rate as 1 drug error per n anesthetics	1/133	1/163	1/450	1/302	1/137

For consistency, near misses have been excluded and the denominator used in this table is the total number of anesthetics given,
not the number of forms returned (therefore some rates may be different from those cited in the source publications). The assistance of Craig Webster in preparing this table is gratefully acknowledged.

Sources:
Bowdle A, Kruger C, Grieve R, Emmens D, Merry A. Anesthesia drug administration errors in a university hospital. ASA Meeting
    Abstracts 2003:A–1358.
*Llewellyn RL, Gordon PC, Wheatcroft D, et al. Drug administration errors: a prospective survey from three South African teaching
    hospitals.* Anaesth Intensive Care. 2009;37(1):93–98.
*Cooper L, DiGiovanni N, Schultz L, Taylor AM, Nossaman B. Influences observed on incidence and reporting of medication errors
    in anesthesia. [Erratum appears in Can J Anaesth. 2012 Oct;59(10):1006]. Can J Anaesth. 2012;59(6):562–570.*
*Zhang Y, Dong YJ, Webster CS, et al. The frequency and nature of drug administration error during anaesthesia in a Chinese hospi-
    tal.* Acta Anaesthesiol Scand. 2013;57(2):158–164.

TABLE 17.2. RATES OF ERRORS IN ADMINISTERING AND RECORDING DRUGS IN 509 CASES MANAGED WITH CONVENTIONAL METHODS OF DRUG ADMINISTRATION DURING ANESTHESIA

Type of Error	Errors per 100 Drug Administrations	Rate as 1 Error per n Anesthetics
Administration errors	**0.32**	**1/31**
Substitution errors	0.18	1/56
Omission errors	0.14	1/71
Recording errors	**11.35**	**1/1**
Drug given, not recorded at all	3.50	1/3
Drug given, dose not recorded	0.67	1/15
Discrepancy between given and recorded dose	7.18	1/1

Errors were identified prospectively by multiple means (see text).

See Merry AF, Webster CS, Hannam J, et al. Multimodal system designed to reduce errors in recording and administration of drugs in anaesthesia: prospective randomised clinical evaluation. *BMJ.* 2011;343:d5543.

their frequency. Errors are by definition unintended, so it follows that at the point of making the error the practitioner does not realize that he or she is doing so. Whether the error is subsequently identified, and how soon, depends on several things, including its consequences and certain aspects of technique (discussed in the following sections). Often, a practitioner simply won't know that an error has been made. This obviously represents an important barrier to recording the error in the notes, or to filing an incident report. Even if a practitioner does detect an error, he or she may be alone in this knowledge. Ideally, one would expect an accurate record and immediate and open disclosure of the error, if only in the interests of mitigating its consequences. In a just culture this behavior should be seen as positive and appropriate, and genuine errors accepted as unintentional and blameless. It is failure to disclose that should be viewed as undesirable. Not all institutions have reached a point where practitioners feel

---

BOX 17.2   EXAMPLES OF THE RELATIONSHIP BETWEEN MEDICATION ERRORS AND ADVERSE DRUG EVENTS

The failure to give a prophylactic antibiotic at the right time during surgery (i.e., within 60 minutes prior to the incision—an example of an error of omission) illustrates the loose coupling (see Chapter 3 of this volume) that often exists between a medication error and an ADE. Overall, there is good evidence for the value of timely antibiotic prophylaxis in reducing surgical site infection, but on an individual basis it would be difficult to know whether such an infection should be attributed to a particular instance of this type of medication error, because other factors might also have contributed to the infection, and giving the antibiotic correctly might not have prevented it. Furthermore, the possible link between the event (which may manifest weeks later) and the error might not even be identified.

Some medication errors have no consequences (e.g., inadvertently using saline instead of sterile water to dilute a drug) and some may even have a positive influence on patient outcome (e.g., inadvertently administering a second dose of an anti-emetic—a "repetition error"—could decrease the risk of postoperative nausea and vomiting in some patients).

Conversely, the accidental administration of a potent vasoactive agent such as dopamine is likely to have immediate and dramatic harmful consequences[4]—in this case the coupling is tight.

confident in such a response. One way or another, it is clear that many errors go unreported.

Facilitated Incident Reporting

Facilitated incident reporting has been used in the OR (see Table 17.1). This involves asking anesthesiologists to complete a form at the end of *every* anesthetic, answering a single primary question: Did a medication error occur during this anesthetic or not? If the answer is "no," no further information is sought. If "yes," then more questions follow. This approach is predicated on the notion that many people will perceive a substantial difference between simply forgetting to fill in a form when an error occurs and deliberately falsifying an answer to a direct question. Furthermore, the initial effort required is the same either way, although the number of subsequent questions in the case of a "yes" answer should be limited in order to avoid creating a disincentive to answering at all. The studies listed in Table 17.1 have all used this approach and have consistently identified much higher rates of medication error during anesthesia than studies based on voluntary incident reporting alone.

Note Review

Studies of this type typically use trained researchers to review a large random sample of medical records from an institution or several institutions over a defined period of time. Interrater reliability is usually fairly low, and the method is very costly.

Note review does not seem to have been widely used in the context of perioperative error in particular, but medication errors have typically featured prominently in more general studies of iatrogenic harm associated with acute care hospital admissions, such as the Harvard Medical Practice Study.[17]

Trigger Tools

The use of triggers[18] is predicated on the idea that certain easily identifiable events may assist in the identification of failures in safe process. For example, the administration of naloxone suggests an overdose of an opioid and may be used as a trigger. With electronic record systems, it may be quite simple and cost effective to identify triggers. The identified notes can then be reviewed in more detail, or alternatively, with large data sets, the rates of selected triggers can be used without further analysis as high-level indicators of safety. The major drawback of using triggers to monitor medication safety is that the variety of failures that can occur is considerable, and even relying on several triggers will miss many of them.

Prospective Observation

The most reliable, but resource-intensive, method of identifying medication errors is by prospective observation, supplemented with various techniques to increase the rate of detection. In a recent prospective study of more than 1000 cases in the OR,[19] a full inventory of the contents of the drug drawer in the anesthesia cart was taken at the beginning and end of each case. Participating anesthesiologists were asked to retain all empty vials and ampoules (in a purpose-designed sharps container) and not to discard used syringes. At the end of each case, the remaining contents of the drug drawers were compared with the preoperative inventory, and the information was integrated with information from empty ampoules and vials, any residual drugs in syringes, and the drug administrations recorded on the final anesthetic record. This approach identified an even higher rate of failure in the processes of medication safety than facilitated incident reporting (Table 17.2), but it was very resource intensive. There is also the question of the effect of observation on performance, sometimes called the "Hawthorne Effect."[20]

Simulation

Observational studies may be seen as creating legal risk for participating clinicians by definitively identifying errors that may subsequently be linked to serious ADEs. One way of addressing this is through the use of high-fidelity simulation in which real medications are used. Simulation is controllable and the scenarios can be repeated.[21] Observation can be supported by video recording and debriefing. Much useful information can be obtained in this way, but realistic simulation of anesthesia is resource intensive, and it is not certain how findings in a simulated environment translate into clinical practice.[22]

The Denominator

There are different ways of reporting the rate of ADEs or medication errors. In the context of ward practice, ADEs are often reported per admission or per patient day. In anesthesia, a common approach has been to report the rate of medication errors or ADEs per anesthetic. However, there is substantial variation in case mix on wards, in the duration of anesthetics and in the number of medications given in any one anesthetic. For example, a child undergoing a myringotomy and tube insertion may receive only gases and vapors, and no IV drugs at all, whereas a complicated cardiac procedure may involve more than 100 boluses of IV medication in the OR, and a number of infusions, and many medications in the ICU and on the ward postoperatively.

It seems more logical to report rates of error or ADE per medication administration. This denominator may, however, be difficult to count. Moreover, the drug administrations of a particular anesthesiologist in a given case on a specific day are related to each other and different from those of another anesthesiologist on another day. Treating each administration of a drug as an independent event may give a false impression of precision (with respect to confidence limits or P values in between-group comparisons). One approach to dealing with this is to calculate the rate of error per administration for each case, and then use case as the unit of analysis. When measuring errors in the OR, it is also important to include the anesthesiologist as a factor in any between-group analyses.[19]

CLASSIFICATION OF PERIOPERATIVE MEDICATION ERRORS

There are various ways to classify failures in perioperative medication safety. The following approach is orientated toward facilitating the identification of possible solutions.

1. Failures relating directly to the drugs and their intrinsic properties;
2. Failures in access to essential medications of adequate quality;
3. Failures in the systems of distributing and presenting medications and the associated structural elements of a safer medication system within an institution;
4. Failures in the selection of drugs and doses;
5. Failures in the administration of drugs and doses once selected;
6. Deliberate sabotage (very rare, but included for completeness[23]).

Categories 4 and 5 can be subdivided by relating failures in the process of medication safety to the six rights[24] or to the cognitive processes involved in generating the error (see Chapter 3 of this volume)—a multidimensional matrix is often needed to fully characterize any individual failure.

Failures Relating Directly to the Drugs and Their Intrinsic Properties

Patients may suffer ADEs related to the intrinsic properties of drugs despite apparently acceptable contemporary practice at the time of the event (e.g., hepatitis after halothane,[25] nausea and vomiting after opioids[26] or nitrous oxide,[27] delayed hemorrhage associated with the postoperative use of nonsteroidal anti-inflammatory agents,[26] residual paralysis in PACU after muscle relaxants[28]). In general, the solution to this problem lies in the development of improved drugs (as in the case of halothane hepatitis, which has become exceedingly rare with the advent of newer volatile anesthetics), or in improved (often protocolized) approaches to minimizing the risk of the ADE (as in the case of routinely administering prophylactic antiemetics when using nitrous oxide[29]).

Failures in Access to Essential Medications of Adequate Quality

The Lancet Commission's recent report has placed the global crisis in surgery and anesthesia on the public health agenda.[30] Five billion patients do not have access to essential surgery with safe anesthesia. There are many reasons for this, but a lack of essential drugs for anesthesia and perioperative care is one important reason.[31,32] Even in high-income countries, the supply of some drugs has been unreliable in recent years and has occasionally affected the safety of anesthesia.[12,33,34] The quality of medications is also an important consideration— particularly in light of an emerging problem in relation to products intended for use in simulation only.[35] Adequate access to essential drugs, with confidence about adequate quality, is essential for medication safety.

Medications represent a substantial proportion of healthcare costs, and unnecessary expenditures constitute an opportunity cost in the face of limited resources. Attempts to control costs may, however, have unanticipated effects. For example, when hospitals change to a supplier that offers medications at a lower cost, changes in presentation and packaging are rarely taken into consideration; this may increase the risk of error by the practitioners who must then administer them. Those who create the latent factors that predispose to errors seldom share in the accountability for errors when they occur.

Failures in the Systems of Distributing and Presenting Medications and the Associated Structural Elements of a Safer Medication System Within an Institution

The standardization and integration of systems of distributing and presenting medications and supporting their use are very important. At the most basic level, it is valuable to involve pharmacists directly in units where medications are administered in order to support practitioners in their safe use.[36]

Failures in the Selection of Drugs and Doses

Failures in the selection of drugs or doses may involve decisions made with various combinations of Type I and Type II thinking, and

may reflect failures at several points in the process, illustrated in Figure 3.2 of Chapter 3 of this volume, and discussed in detail in that chapter. Among other things, these decisions require broadly based expert knowledge of medicine, pathology, physiology, and pharmacology. The careful application of this knowledge requires comprehensive assessment of patients, notably in relation to their medication history, including their history of allergies, and the accurate documentation and communication of key findings. To this end, much effort is invested in the training of anesthesiologists. Learning is a lifelong enterprise, however, and continuing medical education is also important. The recent series of case reports drawn from the Anesthesia Incident Reporting System (AIRS), a national incident reporting system established by the American Society of Anesthesiologists, is particularly effective in highlighting key safety messages, including messages about medication safety.[37,38] These reports are unusual in that they address *both* relevant aspects of expert knowledge *and* the various other ways in which the process of making decisions can go wrong. The education of nurses, technicians, and others who support anesthesiologists in and beyond the OR is also important—the contribution of these health professionals to checking and supporting the processes of medication management in anesthesia in the OR deserves greater emphasis than it has hitherto received.[39] Of course, in many countries, especially those with low and middle incomes, anesthetics are frequently managed by non-physicians. In the context of the global crisis in surgery and anesthesia, the Lancet Commission has emphasized the need for task *sharing*, with physician oversight, in surgery, obstetrics, and anesthesia.[30]

Failures in the Administration of the Drugs and Doses Once Selected

Many of these failures are slips or lapses (see Chapter 3). Many factors contribute to errors of this type (Box 17.3). They typically reflect distraction in the presence of latent conditions in the system, notably poor labeling and presentation of ampoules, syringes, and tubing. Interchangeable connectors are also a weakness in the defenses against error: it is all too easy to inject a drug intended for intravenous administration into an intrathecal or epidural catheter, or vice versa.[40,41] Errors have even involved injections into feeding tubes and intracranial catheters.

Workspace Organization

Anecdotal observation suggests that anesthesiologists tend to be idiosyncratic and variable in their approach to organizing the workspace on which they keep the ampoules, vials, and syringes that they use. Untidiness and poor design of drug drawers have the potential to increase the risk of error. More systematic approaches have been described.[19,36] This is an area where tidiness makes sense, and to the extent that anesthesiologists relieve each other or supervise residents or other practitioners, standardization also makes sense, at least within an institution.

Look-Alike Sound-Alike Drugs: Labels, Color and Tall Man Lettering

Errors attributable to the problem of so-called look-alike sound-alike (LASA) drugs have been reported repeatedly.[43] Ampoules of drugs for IV use often look very similar, and the names of the drugs they contain may sound similar as well—dopamine and doxapram being one example.[4] Labels are also often difficult to read, and are cluttered with information that is more important for regulatory purposes than for the safe administration of the drug to a patient. Similar considerations apply to the labeling of lines—clear labeling to distinguish between intravenous, intra-arterial, intrathecal and other lines has recently received strong emphasis.[44]

Legible labels, both for ampoules and for application to syringes,[44] are primary requirements. Nevertheless, people tend to see what they expect to see, even with highly readable labels. Words are read as a whole, rather than letter by letter. The use of two levels of nomenclature makes the word pictures more distinct (e.g. "inotrope dopamine" is easier to distinguish from "analeptic agent doxapram" than the single words "doxapram" and "dopamine").[36] Tall Man lettering is another useful way to create more distinctive word patterns[43]—not for all drugs, but for those drugs that are frequently associated with errors leading to ADEs.[45]

The role of color coding in the prevention or genesis of medication errors has not been definitively resolved, but there is support for color coding by class of drug for user-applied labels in anesthesia from the majority of authorities identified in a systematic review of strategies to reduce medication error[46] and from some empirical data.[47] This makes intuitive sense—a substitution error between drugs of the same class is less likely to cause a complication than a between-class error. Several different color codes were initially used for syringe labels, which could be very confusing for practitioners who move from one institution to another. Canada, the United States, the United Kingdom, Australia, and New Zealand have all adopted standardized color codes. Unfortunately, the color codes used in Australia for tubing labels partially overlap with color codes used for labeling syringes in anesthesia.[44]

SOME ASPECTS OF MEDICATION SAFETY THAT PRESENT PARTICULAR CHALLENGES

Sterile Fields

Administering drugs within a sterile field, by surgeons or for epidural or spinal injections, involves particular challenges. Syringes used in sterile fields should ideally be labeled,[44] which implies the availability of suitable labels, or pre-labeled syringes, which, anecdotally, is still very uncommon. This makes it possible to confuse different solutions (e.g., local anesthetic and chlorhexidine in unlabeled bowls), with tragic consequences.[48] It may be more practical to insist that all drugs for intrathecal or epidural injection should be double-checked when drawn up, and then administered without the syringe ever leaving the practitioner's hand. If an unlabeled syringe is put down, the risk of error increases substantially. Interventions might include labeling the syringe before putting it down or discarding it and starting the entire process again.

Children

Children are exposed to the same failures in medication safety as adults, but are typically more vulnerable to their consequences because of fundamental differences in their physiology.[2]

Dosage errors are common in children. Clearance of most drugs is immature at birth, matures progressively over the first few years of life, and has a nonlinear relationship to weight. There is a paucity of pharmacodynamics and integrated pharmacokinetic-pharmacodynamic (PKPD) research in children, notably in relation to total intravenous anesthetics. This, along with the difficulty inherent in monitoring the effects of anesthesia in infants, may predispose to an increased risk of awareness.

Infants cannot swallow pills, but liquid formulations with adequate information on hepatic extraction ratio and the effects of diluents used to improve palatability are often unavailable. Practitioners may therefore administer intravenous preparations orally, which decreases confidence about the dose actually given. Alternatively, adult formulations may be diluted, which also increases the risk of dosage error.[49] Some medication may be retained in the dead space of an intravenous administration set or syringe[50] when medications are given intravenously. This may mean that the desired effect is not obtained or that the retained drug is accidentally given later. Children are not always weighed, or an inaccurate weight is used, and practitioners' estimates of weight tend to be unreliable.[2]

Remote Locations

Anesthesia or sedation in outpatient locations, or during MRI or CT scanning, or cardiac catheterization, can be particularly challenging for many reasons.[51] Even institutions that have standardized anesthesia equipment in their ORs may use different, usually older, equipment in the remote location. Monitoring may also be less well supported, and observation of the effect of administered drugs may also be difficult. Assistance may not be readily available. These challenges are compounded with pediatric patients.

Intravenous Drugs and Surgical Site Infection

Surgical site infection (SSI) is a major problem in all countries.[52] There is a growing body of literature supported by progressively more data that suggests that the failures in the aseptic practices of anesthesia personnel may contribute to SSI.[53,60] In particular, the way in which anesthesiologists draw up, handle, and administer intravenous drugs may on occasion lead to the inadvertent injection of microorganisms into patients.[60] The care of ports used for injecting into intravenous lines is also relevant. The significance of these findings is still not completely clear, but there is clearly a need for meticulous asepsis in the handling of intravenous drugs.

STRATEGIES FOR IMPROVING PERIOPERATIVE MEDICATION SAFETY

Improving Medication Safety in the Operating Room

There has been considerable interest in improving medication safety in the OR, and the need for this is well established. Simple exhortation to practice more safely is unlikely to be successful (see Chapter 3). If anesthesia professionals continue to administer drugs in the same way that they have always done, they will continue to make errors at much the same rate as they always have. Systematic change is required. The Anesthesia Patient Safety Foundation (APSF) advocates a "new paradigm" (Box 17.4).[61] This paradigm is entirely consistent with the principles discussed in this chapter and Chapter 3, and aligns with previously identified principles that are supported by empirical and theoretical data, and by expert consensus (see Box 17.5).[19,45,61]

Most elements of the new paradigm are within reach of most, if not all, anesthesia professionals. The use of technology requires adequate financial resources. Two anesthesia information management systems that support key elements of the new paradigm have been described for use in the OR (the SAFERsleep System [Safer Sleep, LLC, Nashville, TN][19] and the DocuSys System [DocuSys, Inc., Mobile, AL]), and various technological solutions have emerged to support the administration of medications on wards, and these have been described in more detail elsewhere.[3] The integration of these systems with each other and with the overall patient record systems of the institution is an important aspect of providing technological support for medication safety.[63] In reality, the biggest challenge is that of culture. Providing technology is not enough—practitioners must embrace the underlying principles and then apply them in order to improve safety.[19] Arguably, failure to check a drug before administering it will often represent a blameless error attributable to distraction or other factors (see Chapter 3), but the persistent failure to engage in appropriate practices to improve patient safety is more properly categorized as violation.[64] A response is overdue to the numerous calls that have been made to improve medication safety in the OR.[65-68] A comprehensive perioperative medication safety program should be underpinned by ongoing education and should also address the risk of substance abuse by various practitioners.

BOX 17.4   THE NEW PARADIGM ADVOCATED BY THE ANESTHESIA PATIENT SAFETY FOUNDATION

- Standardization (drugs, concentrations, equipment)
- Technology (drug identification and delivery, automated information systems)
- Pharmacy (satellite pharmacy, premixed solutions, and prefilled syringes whenever possible)
- Culture (recognition and reporting of drug errors to reduce recurrences)

See Medication Safety in the Operating Room: Time for a New Paradigm. *Anesthesia Patient Safety Foundation; 2010.*

BOX 17.5   STRATEGIES FOR REDUCING THE RISK OF MEDICATION ERROR IN ANESTHESIA IDENTIFIED THROUGH A SYSTEMATIC REVIEW OF THE LITERATURE

1. Systematic countermeasures should be used to decrease the number of drug administration errors in anesthesia.
2. The label on any drug ampoule or syringe should be read carefully before a drug is drawn up or injected.
3. The legibility and contents of labels on ampoules and syringes should be optimized according to agreed-upon standards.
4. Syringes should always be labeled (or almost always: if, during the process of drawing up and administering a single medication, the syringe never leaves the practitioner's hands, a case can be made that a syringe label is not necessary, but it is probably safer simply to label all syringes).
5. Medication drawers and workspace should be formally organized, and potentially hazardous medications (e.g., epinephrine, halothane, bupivacaine) not used during routine and uneventful anesthetics should be separated from those that are (in another drawer, or outside the OR).
6. Labels should be checked with a second person or by means of a device (such as a bar code reader linked to a computer) before any medication is drawn up or administered.
7. Errors in intravenous drug administration during anesthesia should be reported and regularly reviewed.
8. Inventory management should focus on minimizing the risk of drug error: there is a strong case for designating a pharmacist to the operating theaters, and any changes in presentation should be notified ahead of time.
9. Similar packaging and presentation of medications should be avoided where possible.
10. Measurement of weight should be routine before the use of any medication in a child.
11. Satellite pharmacies should be involved with supporting medication safety at the level of the ward or the OR.

Modified from Jensen LS, Merry AF, Webster CS, Weller J, Larsson L. Evidence-based strategies for preventing drug administration errors during anaesthesia. Anaesthesia. *2004;59(5):493–504. See* [2,44,46,76,77].

Sources: Nott MR. Misidentification, in-filling and confirmation bias. Anaesthesia. *2001;56(9):906–924.*
Oldroyd K. Drug syringe labels. Anaesth Intensive Care. *1986;14(1):91–92.*

Ensuring Adequate Supply of Medications of Adequate Quality

The World Health Organization maintains a list of essential medications, which is primarily of value to low- and middle-income countries. In some high-income countries, notably the United States, much faith has been placed in the ability of the market to maintain competitive prices and standards. This approach has traditionally provided incentives to pharmaceutical companies to invest in relevant research and development, and the advent of many newer and safer drugs and agents in the decades following World War II may be attributed to this stimulus. Drug development for anesthesia seems to have slowed down recently. One or two countries, notably New Zealand, have established national purchasing agencies, which reduce cost and may, through long-term contracting, improve the security of supply as well. Whether such an approach could realistically be applied to larger economies is moot, but it seems likely that supply security will depend upon some form of coordinated national approach, perhaps through major societies and organizations, but probably in liaison with governments.

Improving Perioperative Medication Safety

Ideally, the wider picture of perioperative safety should be addressed, including all stages of the patient pathway, from admission to the hospital (when medication reconciliation ensures that pre-admission medications are appropriately managed), on the wards, in the OR, in the PACU, in the ICU, and on discharge (when medication reconciliation should occur again). This implies a more broadly based program, with integration between different areas. For example, labeling of infusions in cardiac ORs[69] should be aligned with subsequent practice in the ICU. This type of integration between different areas of practice probably requires the establishment of a multidisciplinary team within the institution to agree and coordinate common approaches to medication safety, and to align the purchase of technological solutions.[70, 71]

Measuring for Safety

Measurement is a key element of any program to improve medication safety. It may be difficult to identify appropriate and practical metrics for measuring perioperative medication, even in the context of research, let alone for routine use for quality assurance and improvement. One approach might be to adopt the well-known framework of *structure, process*, and *outcome*.[72] Depending on where an institution is in the evolution of its medication safety program for anesthesia, *structural* measures may include resources such as the presence of an agreed-upon perioperative safety program,[73] standardized layouts of drug drawers, color-coded labels for all drugs, facilities for barcode checking in the OR and on the wards and other technological solutions, trays for the orderly arrangement of syringes, and so forth (this list is illustrative, not comprehensive). *Process* measures might include the frequency of labeling of syringes, or of double-checking with a person or device, or of reconciling medications at the time of discharge from hospital and communicating with the primary healthcare team about the correct list, or of plausibly recording the correct time of all medications on an anesthetic record.

Outcome is typically the most difficult thing to measure. Error reporting is too prone to the vagaries of voluntary behavior to be of much value for monitoring or comparing levels of medication safety, and, furthermore, errors are not in themselves outcomes. ADEs, however, are, and should be reported. If this reporting used multiple sources (including patients, who could be surveyed regularly), it might prove fairly reliable and allow one to monitor changes in both the rate and the pattern of events (e.g., previously common catastrophic failures to administer oxygen—a medication—because of disconnections or misconnections of the circuit have virtually disappeared from incident reports, presumably because of various safety initiatives, including the introduction of pulse oximetry[74]).

Multisource ADE reporting could be combined with a selection of triggers, chosen to monitor at least the common outcomes attributable to failures in medication safety in anesthesia. These triggers might include the use of naloxone, supplementary doses of reversal agents in the PACU, re-intubation of the trachea, and the occurrence of postoperative surgical site infection. A proactive approach to identifying awareness under anesthesia (by routinely asking patients about this complication) might also be considered—awareness during anesthesia often reflects medication error.[75]

In such an approach to improving perioperative medication safety, one might start by thoroughly addressing the structural requirements for perioperative medication safety (after which there would be no need to continue measuring them). One might then monitor a suite of triggers such as those listed in this section and report on these on an ongoing basis. One might also measure and report key processes on an occasional basis, using observation in a purposive sample of cases, primarily to drive process improvement.

At an institutional level, the direct engagement of pharmacy with wards and ORs is key—and this is reflected in the New Paradigm of the APSF.

CONCLUSION

Perioperative medication safety depends on a complex interaction between the system in which patients are cared for and the practitioners who prescribe and administer drugs to them. Much attention has been paid to medication error in the OR, and this continues to be a prime area for attention. However, there is a strong case for integrating the management of medications across all parts of surgical patients' path, from admission through the ward, the OR, PACU, ICU, and other parts of the hospital. There is still considerable room for improvement in all of these areas.

REFERENCES

1. The Joint Commission. Accreditation essentials: tips for addressing the "rights" of medication administration. *Joint Commission Resources*. http://www.jcrinc.com/6840/. Accessed April 7, 2015.
2. Merry AF, Anderson BJ. Medication errors: new approaches to prevention. *Paediatr Anaesth*. 2011;21(7):743–753.
3. Cooper RL, Merry A. Medication management. In: Stonemetz J, Ruskin K, eds. *Anesthesia Informatics*. London: Springer; 2008:209–226.
4. Skegg PDG. Criminal prosecutions of negligent health professionals: the New Zealand experience. *Med Law Rev*. 1998;6:220–246.
5. Bates DW, Boyle DL, Vander Vliet MB, Schneider J, Leape L. Relationship between medication errors and adverse drug events. *J Gen Intern Med*. 1995;10(4):199–205.
6. Kluger MT, Bullock MF. Recovery room incidents: a review of 419 reports from the Anaesthetic Incident Monitoring Study (AIMS). *Anaesthesia*. 2002;57(11):1060–1066.
7. Hicks RW, Becker SC, Krenzischeck D, Beyea SC. Medication errors in the PACU: a secondary analysis of MEDMARX findings. *J Perianesth Nurs*. 2004;19(1):18–28.
8. Wheeler SJ, Wheeler DW. Medication errors in anaesthesia and critical care. *Anaesthesia*. 2005;60(3):257–273.
9. Flaatten H, Hevroy O. Errors in the intensive care unit (ICU): experiences with an anonymous registration. *Acta Anaesthesiol Scand*. 1999;43(6):614–617.
10. Charpiat B, Goutelle S, Schoeffler M, et al. Prescriptions analysis by clinical pharmacists in the post-operative period: a 4-year prospective study. *Acta Anaesthesiol Scand*. 2012;56(8):1047–1051.
11. Swanson SP, Roberts LJ, Chapman MD. Are anaesthetists prone to suicide? A review of rates and risk factors. *Anaesth Intensive Care*. 2003;31(4):434–445.
12. Dutton RP, Cohen JA. Medication shortages: are we the Iron Chefs or our own worst enemies? *Anesth Analg*. 2011;113(6):1298–1299.
13. Cooper JB, Newbower RS, Long CD, McPeek B. Preventable anesthesia mishaps: a study of human factors. *Anesthesiology*. 1978;49(6):399–406.
14. Cooper JB, Newbower RS, Kitz RJ. An analysis of major errors and equipment failures in anesthesia management: considerations for prevention and detection. *Anesthesiology*. 1984;60(1):34–42.
15. Currie M, Mackay P, Morgan C, et al. The "wrong drug" problem in anaesthesia: an analysis of 2000 incident reports. *Anaesth Intensive Care*. 1993;21(5):596–601.
16. Chopra V, Bovill JG, Spierdijk J. Accidents, near accidents and complications during anaesthesia. *Anaesthesia*. 1990;45:3–6.
17. Leape LL, Brennan TA, Laird N, et al. The nature of adverse events in hospitalized patients: results of the Harvard Medical Practice Study II. *N Engl J Med*. 1991;324(6):377–384.
18. Seddon ME, Jackson A, Cameron C, et al. The Adverse Drug Event Collaborative: a joint venture to measure medication-related patient harm. *N Z Med J*. 2013;126(1368):9–20.
19. Merry AF, Webster CS, Hannam J, et al. Multimodal system designed to reduce errors in recording and administration of drugs in anaesthesia: prospective randomised clinical evaluation. *BMJ*. 2011;343:d5543.
20. Parsons HM. What happened at Hawthorne? *Science*. 1974;183:922–932.
21. Merry AF, Weller JM, Robinson BJ, et al. A simulation design for research evaluating safety innovations in anaesthesia. *Anaesthesia*. 2008;63(12):1349–1357.
22. Weller J, Henderson R, Webster CS, et al. Building the evidence on simulation validity: comparison of anesthesiologists' communication patterns in real and simulated cases. *Anesthesiology*. 2014;120(1):142–148.
23. Dyer C. Public inquiry hears how Shipman killed patients with diamorphine. *BMJ*. 2001;322(7302):1566.
24. Webster CS, Merry AF, Larsson L, McGrath KA, Weller J. The frequency and nature of drug administration error during anaesthesia. *Anaesth Intensive Care*. 2001;29(5):494–500.
25. Ray DC, Drummond GB. Halothane hepatitis. *Br J Anaesth*. 1991;67(1):84–99.
26. Merry AF, Webster CS, Holland RL, et al. Clinical tolerability of perioperative tenoxicam in 1001 patients: a prospective, controlled, double-blind, multi-centre study. *Pain*. 2004;111(3):313–322.

27. Myles PS, Leslie K, Chan MT, et al. Avoidance of nitrous oxide for patients undergoing major surgery: a randomized controlled trial. *Anesthesiology.* 2007;107(2):221–231.

28. Yip PC, Hannam JA, Cameron AJ, Campbell D. Incidence of residual neuromuscular blockade in a post-anaesthetic care unit. *Anaesth Intensive Care.* 2010;38(1):91–95.

29. Myles PS, Leslie K, Chan MT, et al. The safety of addition of nitrous oxide to general anaesthesia in at-risk patients having major non-cardiac surgery (ENIGMA-II): a randomised, single-blind trial. *Lancet.* 2014;384(9952):1446–1454.

30. Meara JG, Leather AJ, Hagander L, et al. Global Surgery 2030: evidence and solutions for achieving health, welfare, and economic development. *Lancet.* 2015; 386:569–624.

31. Hodges SC, Mijumbi C, Okello M, McCormick BA, Walker IA, Wilson IH. Anaesthesia services in developing countries: defining the problems. *Anaesthesia.* 2007;62(1):4–11.

32. WHO Model Lists of Essential Medicines. 2013. http://www.who.int/medicines/publications/essentialmedicines/en/. Accessed March 15, 2015.

33. Ferguson K, Woodcock T. Ensuring a sustainable supply of drugs for anaesthesia and peri-operative care. *Anaesthesia.* 2012;67(12):1313–1316.

34. Hall R, Bryson GL, Flowerdew G, et al. Drug shortages in Canadian anesthesia: a national survey. *Can J Anaesth.* 2013;60(6):539–551.

35. US Food and Drug Administration. FDA's investigation into patients being injected with simulated IV fluids continues. 2015. http://www.fda.gov/Drugs/DrugSafety/ucm428431.htm. Accessed May 10, 2015.

36. Merry AF, Webster CS, Mathew DJ. A new, safety-oriented, integrated drug administration and automated anesthesia record system. *Anesth Analg.* 2001;93(2):385–390.

37. Dutton RP. Making a difference: the Anesthesia Quality Institute. *Anesth Analg.* 2015;120(3):507–509.

38. Learning from others: a case report from the anesthesia incident reporting system. *Anaesthesia Quality Institute.* 2015. https://www.aqihq.org/casereportsandcommittee.aspx. Accessed May 15, 2015.

39. Weller JM, Merry AF, Robinson BJ, Warman GR, Janssen A. The impact of trained assistance on error rates in anaesthesia: a simulation-based randomised controlled trial. *Anaesthesia.* 2009;64(2): 126–130.

40. Lanigan CJ. Safer epidural and spinal connectors. *Anaesthesia.* 2002;57:567–571.

41. Walker IA, Griffiths R, Wilson IH. Replacing Luer connectors: still work in progress. *Anaesthesia.* 2010;65(11):1059–1063.

42. Khan FA, Hoda MQ. A prospective survey of intra-operative critical incidents in a teaching hospital in a developing country. *Anaesthesia.* 2001;56(2):177–182.

43. Emmerton LM, Rizk MF. Look-alike and sound-alike medicines: risks and "solutions." *Int J Clin Pharm.* 2012;34(1):4–8.

44. Merry AF, Shipp DH, Lowinger JS. The contribution of labelling to safe medication administration in anaesthetic practice. *Best Pract Res Clin Anaesthesiol.* 2011;25(2):145–159.

45. Emmerton L, Rizk MF, Bedford G, Lalor D. Systematic derivation of an Australian standard for Tall Man lettering to distinguish similar drug names. *J Eval Clin Pract.* 2015;21(1):85–90.

46. Jensen LS, Merry AF, Webster CS, Weller J, Larsson L. Evidence-based strategies for preventing drug administration errors during anaesthesia. *Anaesthesia.* 2004;59(5):493–504.

47. Cheeseman JF, Webster CS, Pawley MDM, Francis MA, Warman GR, Merry AF. Use of a new task-relevant test to assess the effects of shift work and drug labelling formats on anesthesia trainees' drug recognition and confirmation. *Can J Anaesth.* 2011;58(1):38–47.

48. Clinical Safety Quality and Governance Branch. Safety Notice 010/10. Correct identification of medication and solutions for epidural anaesthesia and analgesia. NSW Department of Health; 2010.

49. Koren G, Barzilay Z, Greenwald M. Tenfold errors in administration of drug doses: a neglected iatrogenic disease in pediatrics. *Pediatrics.* 1986;77(6):848–849.

50. Bowman S, Raghavan K, Walker IA. Residual anaesthesia drugs in intravenous lines: a silent threat? *Anaesthesia.* 2013;68(6):557–561.

51. Webster CS, Anderson BJ, Stabile MJ, Merry AF. Improving the safety of pediatric sedation: human error, technology and clinical microsystems. In: Mason KP, ed. *Pediatric Sedation Outside of the Operating Room: A Multispecialty International Collaboration.* New York: Springer Science; 2015:587–612.

52. *Report on the Burden of Endemic Health-Care Associated Infection Worldwide: A Systematic Review of the Literature.* Geneva: World Health Organization; 2011.

53. Loftus RW, Patel HM, Huysman BC, et al. Prevention of intravenous bacterial injection from health care provider hands: the importance of catheter design and handling. *Anesth Analg.* 2012;115(5):1109–1119.

54. Loftus RW, Brown JR, Koff MD, et al. Multiple reservoirs contribute to intraoperative bacterial transmission. *Anesth Analg.* 2012;114(6): 1236–1248.

55. Loftus RW, Brindeiro BS, Kispert DP, et al. Reduction in intraoperative bacterial contamination of peripheral intravenous tubing through the use of a passive catheter care system. *Anesth Analg.* 2012;115(6):1315–1323.

56. Loftus RW, Muffly MK, Brown JR, et al. Hand contamination of anesthesia providers is an important risk factor for intraoperative bacterial transmission. *Anesth Analg.* 2011;112(1):98–105.

57. Koff MD, Corwin HL, Beach ML, Surgenor SD, Loftus RW. Reduction in ventilator associated pneumonia in a mixed intensive care unit after initiation of a novel hand hygiene program. *J Crit Care.* 2011;26(5):489–495.

58. Koff MD, Loftus RW, Burchman CC, et al. Reduction in intraoperative bacterial contamination of peripheral intravenous tubing through the use of a novel device. *Anesthesiology.* 2009; 110(5):978–985.

59. Loftus RW, Koff MD, Burchman CC, et al. Transmission of pathogenic bacterial organisms in the anesthesia work area. *Anesthesiology.* 2008;109(3):399–407.

60. Gargiulo DA, Sheridan J, Webster CS, et al. Anaesthetic drug administration as a potential contributor to healthcare-associated infections: a prospective simulation-based evaluation of aseptic techniques in the administration of anaesthetic drugs. *BMJ Qual Saf.* 2012;21(10): 826–834.

61. *Medication Safety in the Operating Room: Time for a New Paradigm.* Anesthesia Patient Safety Foundation; 2010.

62. Webster CS, Larsson L, Frampton CM, et al. Clinical assessment of a new anaesthetic drug administration system: a prospective, controlled, longitudinal incident monitoring study. *Anaesthesia.* 2010;65(5):490–499.

63. Pronovost PJ, Bo-Linn GW, Sapirstein A. From heroism to safe design: leveraging technology. *Anesthesiology.* 2014;120(3):526–529.

64. Weller JM, Merry AF. I. Best practice and patient safety in anaesthesia. *Br J Anaesth.* 2013;110(5): 671–673.

65. Merry AF, Anderson BJ. Medication errors: time for a national audit? *Paediatr Anaesth.* 2011;21(11): 1169–1170.

66. Llewellyn RL, Gordon PC, Reed AR. Drug administration errors: time for national action. *S Afr Med J.* 2011;101(5):319–320.

67. Merry AF, Webster CS. Medication error in New Zealand:time to act. *N Z Med. J.* 2008;121(1272): 6–9.

68. Orser BA. Medication safety in anesthetic practice: first do no harm. *Can J Anaesth.* 2000;47(11): 1051–1052.

69. Merry AF, Webster CS, Connell H. A new infusion syringe label system designed to reduce task complexity during drug preparation. *Anaesthesia.* 2007;62(5):486–491.

70. Merry AF, Weller J, Mitchell SJ. Improving the quality and safety of patient care in cardiac anesthesia. *J Cardiothorac Vasc Anesth.* 2014;28(5): 1341–1351.

71. Leslie K, Merry AF. Cardiac surgery: all for one and one for all. *Anesth Analg.* 2015;120(3): 504–506.

72. Donabedian A. *An Introduction to Quality Assurance in Health Care.* New York: Oxford University Press; 2003.

73. Stratman RC, Wall MH. Implementation of a comprehensive drug safety program in the perioperative setting. *Int Anesthesiol Clin.* 2013;51(1):13–30.

74. Runciman WB. Iatrogenic harm and anaesthesia in Australia. *Anaesth Intensive Care.* 2005;33(3):297–300.

75. Abeysekera A, Bergman IJ, Kluger MT, Short TG. Drug error in anaesthetic practice: a review of 896 reports from the Australian Incident Monitoring Study database. *Anaesthesia.* 2005;60(3):220–227.

76. Eichhorn J. APSF hosts medication safety conference: consensus group defines challenges and opportunities for improved practice. *APSF Newsletter* 2010;25(1):1–7.

77. Australian and New Zealand College of Anaesthetists. *Guidelines for the Safe Administration of Injectable Drugs in Anaesthesia.* Policy Document PS 51. Melbourne: The College; 2009.

18

Operating Room Fires and Electrical Safety

STEPHAN COHN AND P. ALLAN KLOCK, JR.

INTRODUCTION

Operating rooms and other anesthetizing locations contain dangerous electrical elements that can seriously injure patients or healthcare professionals with electrical injury, burns, or fires. Modern equipment, hospital infrastructure, and care practices have improved patient safety, but anesthesia professionals should appreciate the latent hazards of electrical equipment and the oxygen-enriched environment. Understanding modern electrical systems and the fundamentals of fire safety will help protect patients and personnel working in the operating room.

Every year, anesthesiologists must familiarize themselves with an increasing amount of medical and technical information to care for their patients. It is tempting to rely on technicians, equipment, and alarms for warnings about electrical safety in the operating room, but all operating room personnel should understand the basic concepts of electrical circuitry and the steps to take to protect patients and staff from electrical shocks or burns.

OPERATING ROOM ELECTRICAL SAFETY

Electrical Circuits, Grounding, and Shock

An electrical circuit is a closed loop consisting of a power source, wires, a load, and a switch. The wires take the electrons (which carry the electrical charge) to the device (often called a *load*) when the switch is activated, and the returning wires complete the circuit. In this circuit, electrons are continuously moving, thus powering the device until the switch cuts the flow. The motive force causing electrons to flow is measured in *volts*, and the rate at which the electrons travel in *amperes*. The more devices placed in a circuit, the larger the load and the greater the loss of energy from the circuit. An electrical device, or load, that offers resistance to the flow of electrons through the circuit is called a *resistor* and the amount of resistance is measured in *ohms*. In an electrical circuit, flow varies directly with voltage and inversely with resistance. This relationship is expressed as Ohm's law, in which amperes are calculated by dividing volts by ohms.

When multiple resistors are placed in a closed circuit, they can be connected either consecutively (series circuit) or by wires that branch off at a node and supply the resistors at the same time (parallel circuit). A complex circuit can have elements of both. If the electron flow in a circuit is always in the same direction, it is called direct current (DC). Battery-powered devices designed for household and hospital use typically use DC. In alternating current (AC), the voltage and flow reverse direction at regular intervals. In the United States, most household and hospital electrical outlets supply 120 volts of AC at a frequency of 60 Hertz (Hz), while 50 Hz is used in many other parts of the world. The voltage of AC is represented as a *sine wave* in which one complete oscillation occurs in 1/60 of a second, producing 60 cycles per second or 60 Hz. In an AC circuit, the opposition to flow called *impedance*, which is is the complex ratio of the voltage to the current. Impedance is determined by resistance, and also by the

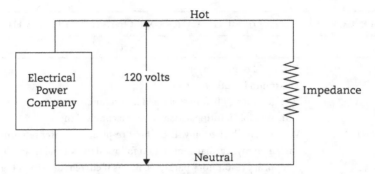

FIGURE 18.1: An alternating current (AC) circuit with 120 volts of potential difference between the hot and neutral side of circuit.

Reprinted with permission from Ehrenwerth J, Seifert HA. Electrical and fire safety. In: Barash PG, Cullen BF, Stoelting RK, eds. *Clinical Anesthesia.* 5th ed. Philadelphia: Lippincott Williams & Wilkins, 2006:151, fig. 3.

inductance and capacitance of each component in the circuit.

If the power company keeps the voltage at 120 volts, then the current flow will be inversely proportional to the impedance (Ohm's law). The electrical cord going to the device has two conductors. The hot conductor carries the current to the device, and the neutral conductor returns the current to the source. The electrical potential between the two is 120 volts (Figure 18.1).[1] According to Ohm's law, for a given voltage, if the impedance is low, then the current will be high. A short circuit results with almost no impedance and a high current flow.

With electrical power comes the risk of shock as we interact with an electrical circuit. Shock results when electricity flows through the body. The flow enters the body at one area and exits via contact with a grounded object or source, causing the body to become part of the electrical path (Figure 18.2).[1] The severity of the electrical shock depends on the amount of current passing through the body and the duration of contact with the body.

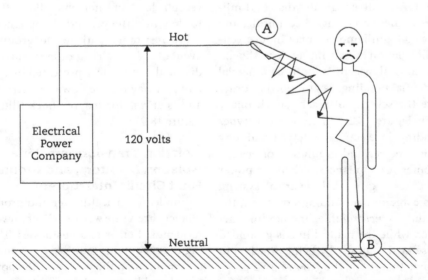

FIGURE 18.2: Completion of an electrical circuit through the body by touching a single hot wire (point A) while in contact with the ground (point B).

Reprinted with permission from Ehrenwerth J, Seifert HA. Electrical and fire safety. In: Barash PG, Cullen BF, Stoelting RK, eds. *Clinical Anesthesia.* 5th ed. Philadelphia: Lippincott Williams & Wilkins, 2006:152, fig. 4.

TABLE 18.1. EFFECTS OF 60-HZ CURRENT ON AN AVERAGE HUMAN

Current	Effect
1 mA	Threshold of perception
5 mA	Maximum harmless current
10–20 mA	"Let-go" current before sustained muscular contraction
50 mA	Pain, possible fainting, exhaustion, mechanical injury
100–300 mA	Ventricular fibrillation will start but respiratory center remains intact
6 A	Sustained myocardial contraction followed by normal heart rhythm. Temporary respiratory paralysis. Burns if current density is high.

The effects of a *macro-shock*, or a current of one milliampere (mA) or greater, are summarized in Table 18.1.[2] The longer the contact with the body, the more tissue damage results, as more energy is released. *Current density* describes the amount of current flowing through an area of tissue and is measured in amperes per unit area.

In an operating room, a patient with an implanted cardiac device, such as a pacemaker or saline-filled central line, may be susceptible to *micro-shock*, in which current passes directly through the heart, causing an arrhythmia. Because the current is delivered directly to the heart, 0.1 milliamperes can result in sufficient current density in the heart to injure the patient. Any current greater than 0.01 milliamperes is therefore considered unsafe, and as little as 0.1 milliamperes may induce ventricular fibrillation by causing a micro-shock.[3]

The electrical system in both commercial and residential buildings is grounded in order to reduce the severity of macro-shock injury (shown in Figure 18.2).[1] There are two types of grounding in electrical safety: grounding of electrical power and grounding of electrical equipment or appliances. When the power company uses a grounded electrical system, two lines come into a building's fuse box, the *hot* line and the *neutral* line. The hot line carries power, while the neutral line is grounded at the fuse box, typically by being attached to a metal pipe that enters the ground. In a properly grounded system, any leakage current (or fault current) is carried away harmlessly to the ground, so that only a small amount of current passes through an individual.

An appliance that is grounded is equipped with a three-wire cord and a three-pronged plug that is inserted into a matching outlet. The third wire and prong connect the metal frame or chassis of the appliance and a separate ground connection, frequently to a cold water pipe. The equipment's ground wire provides a low-impedance path for the fault current. Thus, if a frayed wire accidentally connects the frame to the hot side of the circuit, most of the electrical current goes to the ground wire and not the individual (Figure 18.3).[1]

An adapter plug (or "cheater" plug) should never be used to plug in a grounded appliance (one with a three-prong plug) into an electrical outlet with only two slots and no ground receptacle. A cheater plug allows the current to flow into the grounded appliance without a low-resistance pathway to ground. In the event of a short circuit or fault current, an individual is no longer protected by an alternative pathway for the flow of electrical current and is at risk for macro-shock (illustrated in Figure 18.2).[1]

Isolation Transformers, Line Isolation Monitors, and Ground Fault Circuit Interrupters

Grounded electrical power and grounded appliances are a safe way to deliver power in most residential homes and businesses. The operating room contains multiple electronic devices, power cords on the floor, and the potential for liquid puddles, creating many serious electrical hazards. In order to protect operating room personnel from the hazards posed by macro-shock, an electrically isolated power supply was

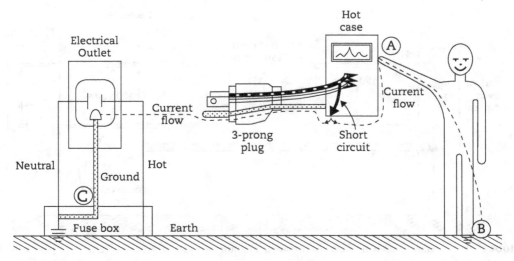

FIGURE 18.3: Grounded power and grounded equipment. Most of the fault current travels to the ground (point A to point C—lesser resistance) with only a small portion going through the individual (point A to point B— higher resistance).

Reprinted with permission from Ehrenwerth J, Seifert HA. Electrical and fire safety. In: Barash PG, Cullen BF, Stoelting RK, eds. *Clinical Anesthesia.* 5th ed. Philadelphia: Lippincott Williams & Wilkins, 2006:157, fig. 17.

developed. Isolated power supplies are used in many operating rooms because they protect patients and staff against macroshock. In an isolated circuit, both sides of the power supply are isolated from the ground. There is no hot or neutral side, so that 120 volts of electrical potential exist only between the two active wires, but not between the circuit and the ground. The wires are simply called line 1 and line 2.

Since the electrical power supply throughout the hospital is grounded, the supply to the operating room must be converted to an isolated system through an *isolation transformer*. An isolation transformer couples one circuit to another by using electromagnetic induction to provide a current on the isolated side of the transformer. Electrical power is supplied to the *primary winding* of the isolation transformer from the grounded power through a hot and a neutral wire. This creates a constantly changing magnetic field, which in turn induces an electrical current in the *secondary winding*. There is still a 120-volt electrical potential between line 1 and line 2 (just as there is between the hot and neutral wires on the primary side), but because neither side of the secondary winding is grounded, there is no potential between lines

1 and 2 and the ground. The electrical equipment used in the operating room still uses a ground wire (third prong), which goes directly back to ground on the primary side of the isolation transformer. The purpose of this ground wire is to protect against micro-shock and is discussed in the following paragraphs. A circuit with an isolation transformer is illustrated in Figure 18.4.[1]

In an operating room with isolated power (or the secondary side of an isolation transformer), an individual in contact with the current at line 1 or line 2 suffers no shock, even if he has firm contact with the ground. Since neither line 1 nor line 2 is grounded, the electrical circuit cannot be completed via the ground. The only way an individual in an operating room would receive a shock is if he came in contact with both line 1 and line 2 simultaneously. The probability of this dual contact is low. If either line 1 or line 2 is inadvertently connected to ground (e.g., a frayed wire that comes into contact with a metal equipment case), this results in a *first fault* condition. Essentially, the isolated power system has now been converted to a grounded system. In order for an individual to receive a shock, he or she would have to be

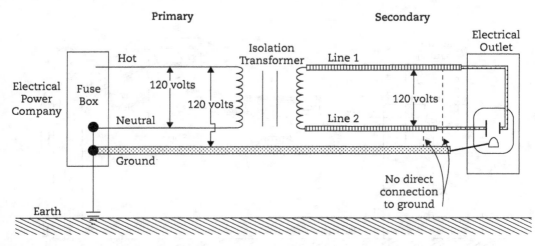

FIGURE 18.4: Diagram showing how the isolation monitor provides ungrounded electrical power to the secondary side.

Reprinted with permission from Ehrenwerth J, Seifert HA. Electrical and fire safety. In: Barash PG, Cullen BF, Stoelting RK, eds. *Clinical Anesthesia*. 5th ed. Philadelphia: Lippincott Williams & Wilkins, 2006:159, fig. 21.

connected to ground and come into contact with the other line. This adds another margin of safety and helps to prevent macro-shock.

An individual who is in a residence and comes into contact with a faulty appliance with a grounded power supply and a grounded device is protected because most of the current travels via the low-resistance ground wire, thus offering protection from a serious shock (shown in Figure 18.3).[1] If, however, the ground wire were broken or interrupted, the person would receive a potentially lethal shock. In an operating room with an isolated power system, however, an individual is not completing a circuit with the ground. He would still be safe from electrical shock, even if the grounded equipment is faulty. The isolated circuit on the secondary side of an isolation transformer therefore protects personnel from macro-shock.

Another safety feature of the isolated circuit is the circuit breaker. In the circuit breaker of an isolated power system, the ground wires are all connected at a common terminal, but line 1 and line 2 are connected at the circuit breaker to a completely different terminal. In the grounded power system, the neutral and ground wires are connected to the same terminal to provide an alternate flow to the ground. By separating line 1 and line 2 from the ground

terminal, a faulty piece of equipment will not activate the circuit breaker in the isolated circuit, even if a short circuit is present. Therefore, a faulty device or appliance in the operating room will not lose power. This feature is important if a device is life-critical (e.g., a cardiac bypass pump).

Each operating room with isolated power will have a *line isolation monitor* (LIM) that monitors the integrity of the isolated power system. The LIM continuously monitors the potential between line 1 and ground and line 2 and ground, which in an ideal isolated circuit would be 0 volts. All wires, cords, and devices that carry AC exhibit a small amount of capacitance that causes small "leakage currents" that are required to be less than 100 microamperes per device. Leakage current identified by the LIM may imply either a fault condition or a small amount of electromagnetic induction or capacitance within the powered devices, wires, and cords. If the LIM has a meter, it will display the total amount of "leakage" current in the operating room in mA. This indicates how much current could flow if either side of the isolated power system were connected to ground, and not how much current is actually flowing to ground.

If a faulty piece of equipment is plugged into the isolated power system, one side of the system becomes grounded, effectively reverting the circuitry to a grounded power system. This does not necessarily present a shock hazard because an individual touching the case does not necessarily complete a circuit. In order for a person to receive an electrical shock, he or she must come into contact with the opposite side of the power system (e.g., Line 2 if Line 1 were grounded). In that case, current would flow from Line 2, through the person, to ground, and then back to Line 1. This is called a *second fault* and results in electrical shock (Figure 18.3).[1]

Micro-shock is a potentially imperceptible electric current that is applied directly to the heart, disrupting normal cardiac function (i.e., by causing ventricular fibrillation). In order for a patient to receive a micro-shock, current must be applied either directly to the heart or to a saline-filled catheter or wire that terminates in the heart. In order for a patient to receive a macro-shock, his or her heart must be instrumented in some way, for example, during implantation of a pacemaker or while floating a pulmonary artery catheter. The risk of micro-shock is very low, but nearly all equipment used in the operating room is grounded in order to protect the patient against micro-shock caused by leakage current.

The LIM will not alarm unless it detects a *hazard current* (the amount of current that could flow between line 1 and ground or line 2 and ground) that is greater than a preset value, usually 2 mA or 5 mA, depending on the age and brand of the monitor.[4] Each piece of equipment causes a small amount of leakage current; the LIM monitors the total amount of leakage current in the room. Modern operating rooms have multiple electrical devices, and even when all equipment is functioning normally, the total leakage current may exceed 2 mA. Newer LIMs use a 5 mA alarm threshold, which is the maximum harmless current in a macro-shock. If an LIM alarms during a surgical procedure, this implies that a first fault condition exists, usually because a device with a faulty circuit has been added to the system. If it is safe to do so, unplug each device in the OR, beginning with the last device that was plugged in, until the LIM alarm stops. When the faulty device is found, it should be removed as soon as possible and sent for inspection and repair. Leaving the faulty device plugged in may not put anyone at risk, but if a second faulty device is added, there is potential for serious macro-shock injury.

A two-pronged or ungrounded electrical device does not have a ground wire, so a fault would not cause the LIM to alarm. Such equipment should be used in an operating room only if it meets the strict hospital standards designed to minimize the risk of micro-shock and macro-shock. Although the isolated power system would protect a person who comes into contact with this faulty device, a second fault condition would be created that increases the risk of a macro-shock injury. Moreover, leakage current might increase the risk of micro-shock. Biomedical engineering staff can usually test equipment to determine the effectiveness of its grounding system or the likelihood of creating a first-fault condition if a malfunction occurs.

Circuit breakers are another important means to increase electrical safety in both residential and healthcare settings. In the event of a short circuit, a large amount of current flowing through the circuit activates a solenoid that trips a switch, interrupting the flow of current. A ground fault circuit interrupter (GFCI) protects against macro-shock by interrupting the flow of current in the event of an imbalance between the hot and neutral lines. The GFCI is located in an individual special electrical safety outlet or in a distribution panel. It can be found in most modern construction where the risk for a short circuit is high, especially in areas with moisture such as bathrooms, kitchens, garages, crawl spaces, unfinished basements, and outdoors. When an electrical appliance is plugged into a GFCI outlet (Figure 18.5), the GFCI constantly monitors the amount of current flowing from hot to neutral. A GFCI is able to sense a mismatch in current flow as small as 4 mA to 5 mA and can react within 1/30 of a second. A GFCI uses a differential current transformer that surrounds, but is not electrically connected to, the hot and neutral lines. During normal operation, current flowing from the hot wire returns through neutral

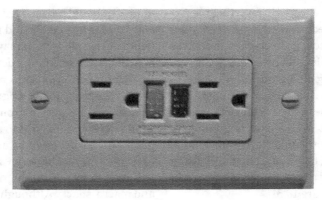

FIGURE 18.5: GFCI safety outlet found in one author's kitchen. The black is the TEST button; when pushed, it shuts off power if the device is working properly. The red is the RESET button; when pushed it returns the outlet to normal functioning after a test or if the GFCI has tripped the circuit. The smaller slot plug represents the hot side of the circuit; the larger slot, the neutral side. The circular hole connects the ground prong to the grounded circuit.

wire. Because the current on both sides is equal and flows in opposite directions, they cancel each other out. If, however, one side of the system is connected to ground, the imbalance creates a current in the differential transformer, which then causes power to be removed from a solenoid. This trips a switch that discontinues the flow of current.

GFCIs are complex devices that can be damaged by voltage surges or even from normal use over time. If the device is not working properly, it is not protecting people from the hazards of macro-shock. Therefore, it is recommended that these safety outlets be tested monthly.[5]

The use of GFCI safety outlets became popular in the 1980s, so hospitals newly constructed had a choice of going with isolated power systems or GFCIs in their operating rooms. Isolated power systems are more expensive, but they are commonly used in operating rooms because a fault will not result in the interruption of electrical power to life-support devices. If too many devices are plugged in (i.e., total leakage current exceeds the safe threshold) or one device has a fault, an LIM alarms, but electrical power remains on in the operating room. On the other hand, with a GFCI, any detection of an imbalance of electrical flow immediately cuts off power, protecting both patients and staff from shock hazards but at the cost of turning off potentially vital equipment during surgery.

By understanding the situations in which macro- and micro-shock are possible in grounded and isolated power systems, operating room personnel can help prevent electroshock hazards. It is crucial to know whether one is working in a GFCI or isolation transformer environment. In the latter, the location of the LIM and the type of alarm should be identified. In the former, the operating room team should have a plan of action if the GFCI cuts off power to the room. It is important that each critical service outlet be labeled with its circuit number and circuit breaker panel location; this will allow a quick return of service if the circuit is tripped.

OPERATING ROOM FIRES

Despite considerable research and publication in the area, operating room fires remain a serious problem that resists a comprehensive solution. While it is difficult to exactly quantify the number of operating room fires, estimates range from 200 to 650 fires per year; 20–30 result in serious injury, and 1 or 2 result in death.[6-8] Oxygen-enriched fires can cause a devastating and potentially lethal injury in a few seconds. Despite these sobering statistics, most operating room fires are often preventable. Anesthesia professionals can significantly reduce the risk of serious injury or death by minimizing the likelihood and amount of oxygen that reaches the surgical field or by

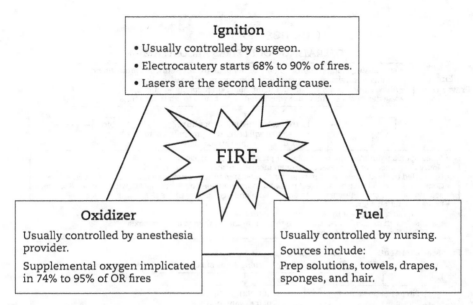

FIGURE 18.6: The fire triad. Usually oxidizing agents are controlled by the anesthesia professional, fuel sources by the nurse, and ignition sources by the surgeon.

responding quickly and appropriately during a fire in the operating room.

Anatomy of Operating Room Fires

The *fire triad* includes a fuel, a source of ignition, and an oxidizing agent (Figure 18.6). The removal of any one of these elements will prevent a fire from igniting or continuing to burn. Fuel sources in the operating room on or near the patient include alcohol-based prep solution; surgical gauze; drapes or towels; patient hair, skin, or tissue; or an airway device such as an endotracheal tube, supraglottic airway, nasal cannula, or a face mask. Sources of ignition in the operating room include lasers, electrocautery, and fiberoptic light bundles for laparoscopic surgical procedures. The oxidizing agent for nearly all fires is oxygen, but nitrous oxide can also act as an oxidizing agent. Many fuels found on or near the surgical field will burn slowly or not at all in 21% oxygen (i.e., room air), but will burn vigorously when exposed to a higher partial pressure of oxygen. A recently published Closed Claims analysis of operating room fires showed that supplemental oxygen was implicated in 95% of the fire claims analyzed. Although nitrous oxide will support combustion to the same degree as oxygen, it is not implicated in case reviews of operating room fires.

Fire Prevention by Education and Preparation

The American Society of Anesthesiologists (ASA) Practice Advisory for the Prevention and Management of Operating Room (OR) Fires makes specific recommendations to minimize the risk of operating room fires and to guide the response during a fire (Figure 18.7). The advisory recommends that anesthesia professionals receive fire safety education and that they participate in fire drills with the operating room team. The practice advisory recommends that, for each case, the anesthesia professional discuss the risk of fire with the procedure team (usually during the final verification or "time out"). A *high-risk procedure* is one in which an ignition source can come in proximity to an oxidizer-enriched atmosphere. If a high-risk situation is identified, the team should discuss ways to minimize fire risk and the role of each team member if a fire does occur.

The best way to avoid injury from an operating room fire is to prevent the fire from starting. It is important for all operating room

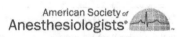

OPERATING ROOM FIRES ALGORITHM

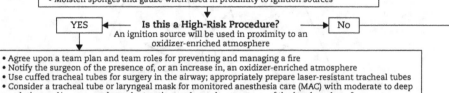

Fire Prevention:
- Avoid using ignition sources[1] in proximity to an oxidizer-enriched atmosphere[2]
- Configure surgical draps to minimixe the accumulation of oxidizers
- Allow sufficient drying time for flammable skin prepping solutions
- Moisten sponges and gauze when used in proximity to ignition sources

Is this a High-Risk Procedure?
An ignition source will be used in proximity to an oxidizer-enriched atmosphere

YES → / No →

- Agree upon a team plan and team roles for preventing and managing a fire
- Notify the surgeon of the presence of, or an increase in, an oxidizer-enriched atmosphere
- Use cuffed tracheal tubes for surgery in the airway; appropriately prepare laser-resistant tracheal tubes
- Consider a tracheal tube or laryngeal mask for monitored anesthesia care (MAC) with moderate to deep sedation and/or oxygen-dependent patients who undergo surgery of the head, neck, or face.
- *Before* an ignition source is activated:
  - *Announce* the intent to use an ignition source
  - *Reduce* th oxygen concentration to the minimum required to avoid hypoxia[3]
  - *Stop the* use of nitrous oxide[4]

Fire Management:

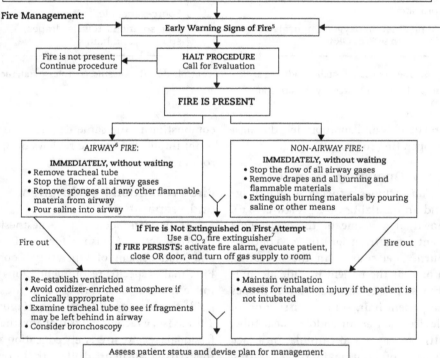

Early Warning Signs of Fire[5]

Fire is not present; Continue procedure

HALT PROCEDURE Call for Evaluation

FIRE IS PRESENT

AIRWAY[6] FIRE:

IMMEDIATELY, without waiting
- Remove tracheal tube
- Stop the flow of all airway gases
- Remove sponges and any other flammable materia from airway
- Pour saline into airway

NON-AIRWAY FIRE:

IMMEDIATELY, without waiting
- Stop the flow of all airway gases
- Remove drapes and all burning and flammable materials
- Extinguish burning materials by pouring saline or other means

Fire out

If Fire is Not Extinguished on First Attempt
Use a CO_2 fire extinguisher[7]
If FIRE PERSISTS: activate fire alarm, evacuate patient, close OR door, and turn off gas supply to room

Fire out

- Re-establish ventilation
- Avoid oxidizer-enriched atmosphere if clinically appropriate
- Examine tracheal tube to see if fragments may be left behind in airway
- Consider bronchoscopy

- Maintain ventilation
- Assess for inhalation injury if the patient is not intubated

Assess patient status and devise plan for management

[1] Ignition sources include but are not limited to electrosurgery or electrocautery units and lasers.

[2] An oxidizer-enriched atmosphere occurs when there is any increase in oxygen concentration above room air level, and/or the presence of any concentration of nitrous oxide.

[3] After minimixing delivered oxygen, wait a period of time (e.g., 1–3 min) before using an ignition source. For oxygen dependent patients, *reduce* supplemental oxygen delivery to the minimum repuired to avoid hypoxia. Monitor oxygenation with pulse oximetry, and if feasible, inspired, exhaled, and/or delivered oxygen concentration.

[4] After stopping the delivery of nitrous oxide, wait a period of time (e.g., 1–3 min) before using an ignition source.

[5] Unexpected flash, flame, smoke or heat, unusual sounds (e.g., a "pop," snap, or "foomp") or odors, unexpected movement of drapes, discoloration of drapes or breathing circuit, unexpected patient movement or complaint.

[6] In this algorithm, airway fire refers to a fire in the airway or breathing circuit.

[7] A CO_2 fire extinguisher may be used on the patient if necessary.

FIGURE 18.7: The American Society of Anesthesiologists algorithm to reduce operating room fires.

Reprinted with permission from the American Society of Anesthesiologists: Practice advisory for the prevention and management of operating room fires: an updated report by the American Society of Anesthesiologists Task Force on Operating Room Fires. *Anesthesiology* 2013;118:271–290.

personnel to understand the fire triad and to safely manage oxidizing agents, fuels, and ignition sources. Anesthesia professionals control oxidizing agents (oxygen and nitrous oxide) in the operating room. Nurses typically control fuels such as prep solutions, drapes, and towels, while surgeons control ignition sources.

Communication throughout the entire procedure is critical, especially if there is a chance that an oxidizer-enriched atmosphere may reach an ignition source. The 2013 closed claims analysis of operating room fires reported that 81% of fires occurred during monitored anesthesia care (MAC) cases and that an open oxygen-delivery system such as nasal cannula or a face mask was used in 84% of the claims.[7] The ASA practice parameters recommend using the minimum amount of supplemental oxygen required to prevent patient hypoxemia.

Controlling Oxidizing Agents

A fire can start if oxygen-enriched gases reach the surgical field, which contains fuel and a source of ignition. This is especially likely during surgery of the head, face, neck, and upper thorax. Surgical drapes should therefore be applied in a manner that minimizes the amount of oxygen that accumulates under the drapes or reaches the surgical field. This is especially important when an open oxygen source, such as nasal cannula, an oxygen mask, or an uncuffed endotracheal tube, is used. In this situation, the drapes should be applied in such a way as to direct oxygen away from the patient's face. If the drapes rest on or are close to the patient's face, a local atmosphere with a high oxygen concentration is created. The adhesive backing of the drape should be carefully applied to the patient's skin to create a barrier between the oxygen-enriched atmosphere near the patient's face and the surgical field.

If the patient is oxygen-dependent or will require moderate or deep sedation for a high-risk procedure, the anesthesia professional should consider securing the airway with a sealing device such as an endotracheal tube or supraglottic airway (SGA). These devices reduce the possibility that an oxygen-enriched atmosphere will reach the surgical field.

For surgery in the airway, the surgeon and the anesthesia professional should communicate before the use of an ignition source, such as a laser or electrocautery. The anesthesia professional can decrease the oxygen concentration and then ask the surgeon to wait 2–3 minutes before the laser or electrocautery device is used. If laser surgery is planned, a laser-resistant tube should be used, and the proximal cuff is filled with colored saline solution. Saline solution cools the cuff and reduces the chance of a fire (it will also help to extinguish a fire if one is started), and the indicator dye makes it easier for the surgeons to tell if the cuff has ruptured.

Controlling Fuel Sources

Most solutions used to prepare the skin for surgery contain a large proportion of isopropyl alcohol. Duraprep™ (3M,™ St. Paul, MN) is 74% isopropyl alcohol; ChloraPre® (CareFusion, San Diego, CA) contains 70% isopropyl alcohol. The package insert warns that after application of either product, a patient should not be draped or an ignition source used for 3 minutes on hairless skin; hair may take up to an hour to dry before the fire risk is minimized. The manufacturers recommend not allowing the solution to pool, and to avoid allowing the product to get into hair. Because hair can support combustion (especially if ignited in an oxygen-enriched atmosphere), the hair should be saturated with a water-based, sterile surgical lubricant such as Surgilube® (Fougera Pharmaceuticals, Melville, NY). Materials that are stained with prep solution should be removed from the prep area. This recommendation is especially important if a patient who is already draped is being prepped in a new area (e.g., for central line insertion after drapes are up). When skin is prepared in an area with surgical drapes or towels, an iodine-based solution that does not contain alcohol (e.g., povodine-iodine solution) should be considered.

Surgical drapes and towels usually do not support combustion in room air. However, surgical drapes may melt if exposed to a heat or an ignition source in room air and can burn vigorously if ignited in an oxygen-enriched atmosphere.

Controlling Ignition Sources

A study published by the Emergency Care Research Institute (ECRI) found that 68% of operating room fires were started by a cautery device. Lasers were the second most common source, accounting for 13% of fires.[8] Electrocautery was the ignition source in 90% of the 103 operating room fires reported in the Closed Claims analysis published in 2013. Electrocautery and other ignition sources should never be used in the presence of alcohol vapor from skin prep solution. The tip of the electrosurgical unit can remain hot enough to start a fire for a few seconds after use. For this reason, the unit should be placed in the provided holster after each use, rather than directly on the patient's skin or the surgical drape. Laser safety procedures should be followed, including keeping the laser on standby whenever the device is not in use. The tip of a fiberoptic light cable used for laparoscopic surgery can get hot enough to melt the surgical drape. For this reason, the light source intensity should be minimized until the cable has been attached to the laparoscopic instrument.

Response to an Operating Room Fire

Operating room fires may appear suddenly and may appear different from fires in other settings. Flames may be invisible, especially if alcohol or other volatile vapors are burning. Fire may present with a flash, an unusual sound (e.g., a "pop, snap, or foomp"), an unusual odor, or smoke or heat.[6] A sedated patient may report feeling hot. Combustion also may be concealed under surgical drapes. If an oxygen-enriched atmosphere is present, flames may propagate very quickly, and burning materials will produce more heat in less time than if the same material were burning in room air. The combination of these factors can lead to a serious burn injury in a short period of time. If an airway fire occurs, the patient may suffer an inhalation injury and poisoning from the toxic products of combustion, in addition to a local thermal injury around the area of the burning airway device.

If a fire is detected, the team should be informed of the fire, and the surgical procedure should stop as soon as possible. The anesthesia professional immediately stops the flow of all airway gasses. The team members complete their pre-assigned tasks, and each team member works independently, not waiting for other members to complete their tasks. Burning drapes must be removed immediately and extinguished away from the patient. If the patient is burning, the fire is extinguished by smothering it, or with a fire extinguisher, water, or saline. Carbon dioxide (CO_2) fire extinguishers offer dual benefits: they remove oxygen from the site of the fire, and since the discharging gas is cold, they cool thermally injured tissues, possibly minimizing the severity of the burn.

If the airway device is burning, it should be removed immediately. If the anesthesia professional cannot access the device (for example, if the operating room table is rotated), the surgeon is instructed to immediately remove the endotracheal tube or SGA. To prevent any oxidizer from reaching the burning airway device, the anesthesia professional may disconnect the breathing circuit from the anesthesia machine, which prevents the cycling of the ventilator from feeding the fire. After the burning airway device is removed, the airway is doused with saline. The airway is then suctioned and re-secured. After inspection of the airway for injury and residual foreign material, the patient will require supportive care. In most cases, the patient is admitted to the intensive care unit, and the airway should undergo serial evaluation to rule out injury.

If the burning material (e.g., drapes or operating table mattress) cannot be extinguished with a fire extinguisher, the patient and personnel are evacuated from the operating room, and the fire alarm is activated. The doors to the affected operating room are closed, and the supply of medical gasses to the involved operating room is shut off. Since the products of combustion can be highly toxic, it is recommended that only specially trained personnel or professional firefighters enter the room after it has been evacuated.

CONCLUSIONS

Virtually all anesthetizing locations contain dangerous electrical elements that can cause an electrical shock. All anesthesia professionals should appreciate the latent hazards of electrical equipment. Every year, anesthesiologists must familiarize themselves with an increasing amount of medical and technical information to care for their patients. It is tempting to rely on technicians, equipment, and alarms for warnings about electrical safety in the operating room, but all operating room personnel should understand the basic concepts of electrical circuitry and the steps to take to protect patients and staff from electrical shocks. Understanding the fundamentals of modern electrical systems will help protect patients and personnel working in the operating room.

Operating room fires are relatively rare, but their consequences can be devastating. It is important that all operating room personnel understand the importance of separating the fuel, oxidizer, and ignition elements of the fire triad. It is recommended that anesthesia professionals and other operating room team members receive fire education and participate in drills aimed at preventing and responding to fires. All fires are worsened by oxygen that we provide. It is incumbent upon us to separate oxygen from ignition sources.

Proper training, communication, and attention to safety measures will hopefully reduce the rate of serious operating room fires and the severity of injuries caused by them.

REFERENCES

1. Ehrenwerth J, Seifert HA. Electrical and fire safety. In: Barash PG, Cullen BF, Stoelting RK, eds. *Clinical Anesthesia*. 5th ed. Philadelphia: Lippincott Williams & Wilkins, 2006:149–174.
2. Leonard PF. Characteristics of electrical hazards. *Anesth Analg.* 1972;51:797–809.
3. Hull CJ. Electrocution hazards in the operating theatre. *Br J Anaesth.* 1978;50:647–657.
4. Bernstein MS. Isolated power and line isolation monitors. *Biomed Instrum Technol* 1990;24:221–223.
5. Electrical Safety Foundation International. Five easy steps to a safer home. *Electrical Safety Foundation International Newsletter*, March 2014.
6. American Society of Anesthesiologists Task Force on Operating Room Fires. Practice advisory for the prevention and management of operating room fires: an updated report by the American Society of Anesthesiologists Task Force on Operating Room Fires. *Anesthesiology* 2013;118:271–290.
7. Mehta SP, Bhananker SM, Posner KL, Domino KB. Operating room fires: a closed claims analysis. *Anesthesiology* 2013;118:1133–1139.
8. Emergency Care Research Institute (ECRI). New clinical guidance for surgical fire prevention. *Health Devices* 2009;38:1067–1075.

19

Disruptive Behavior

The Imperative for Awareness and Action

SHERI A. KEITZ AND DAVID J. BIRNBACH

INTRODUCTION

The operating room is a complex environment with rapidly evolving conditions, time pressures, and hierarchical gradients that can lead to anxiety and stress. It is therefore not surprising that a failure of communication in this often frenzied environment can lead to tension and interpersonal conflict. These conflicts often include some degree of disrespectful behavior, which can be caused by factors endogenous to the disruptive individual, such as threatened self-esteem, insecurity and anxiety, depression, narcissism, aggressiveness, prior victimization, and exogenous factors related to a stressful healthcare environment, such as unhealthy work culture, financial pressures, and productivity targets.[1] Studies have reported that as many as four "tense" communications occur between team members during each procedure, with some of these evolving into outright conflict.[2,3] It is clear that these conflicts can influence operating room team function,[4] cause adverse patient events,[5] and have a toxic impact on patient safety.[1] Furthermore, studies completed in other stressful environments, such as the aviation and military fields, have shown an association among high level of stress, teamwork failure, and impaired performance.[6]

SPECTRUM OF BEHAVIORS

There is a large body of evidence to suggest that conflicts and ensuing inappropriate, often escalating responses to aggressive behavior are relatively common in the operating room and that conflict management tools and educational programs should be embraced.[2] Ultimately, without proper preventive measures and effective leadership,[7] this hot bed of stress may lead to dysfunctional interpersonal interactions, which frequently cross over to a form of disruptive behavior.[8] While there is no single universally accepted definition of *disruptive behavior*, several similar definitions have been published. The AMA defines *disruptive behavior* as "[p]ersonal conduct, whether verbal or physical, that negatively affects or that potentially may negatively affect patient care constitutes disruptive behavior. (This includes but is not limited to conduct that interferes with one's ability to work with other members of the health care team.) However, criticism that is offered in good faith with the aim of improving patient care should not be construed as disruptive behavior."[9] More simply stated, disruptive behavior can be thought of as "any behavior that impairs the medical team's ability to achieve intended outcomes."[10] Examples of disruptive behavior include the use of profane, disrespectful, insulting, demeaning, or abusive language; boundary violations; gratuitous negative comments; passing severe judgment or censuring colleagues or staff in front of patients; outbursts of anger; and bullying.[11] In addition, jokes or non-clinical comments about race, ethnicity, religion, sexual orientation, age, physical appearance, or socioeconomic or education status should never be tolerated. Inappropriate actions, including throwing or breaking things, and the use or threat of unwarranted physical force must be dealt with immediately.[1]

Abuse does not need to be physical in order to have a major impact on outcome. Verbal abuse remains a persistent pattern, is endemic in the OR environment, and has many negative implications. It has been reported that uncivil experiences cause a decrease in employees' work effort, time on the job, productivity, and performance.[12]

Another real but seldom reported issue is that of institutional intimidation, which can manifest as subtle passive-aggressive breakdown in communication, gossip, or avoidance, resulting in a harsh, negative, or inflammatory environment. This phenomenon is not as overt as provider disruptive behavior, yet it occurs daily and continues because its nature is such that it is difficult to measure, and the victims often feel helpless. The perpetrators come from every level of the healthcare organization, including social workers, nursing assistants, housekeepers, administrators, and others who may not normally be perceived to be as essential to the flow of patient care. It has been postulated that this insidious intimidation chills communication, reduces morale, and ultimately harms patients.[13]

Disrespect, in any of its forms, is not always active. Passive disrespect consists of a range of uncooperative behaviors that are not malevolent or rooted in suppressed anger. As stated by Leape, "whether because of apathy, burnout, situational frustration, or other reasons, passively disrespectful individuals are chronically late to meetings, respond sluggishly to calls, fail to dictate charts or operating notes in a timely fashion, and do not work collaboratively or cooperatively with others."[1] Passive-aggressive behavior, defined by the American Psychiatric Association as a "pattern of negativistic attitudes and passive resistance to demands for adequate performance" can also be manifested and equally deleterious. It has been suggested that disruptive behaviors also include overt actions such as verbal outbursts and physical threats, as well as passive activities such as refusing to perform assigned tasks or quietly exhibiting uncooperative attitudes during routine activities.[14] All of these are representative of a broad set of disruptive behaviors summarized in Box 19.1.[15]

PREVALENCE

Numerous research studies have described the prevalence of disruptive behavior in healthcare across a spectrum of settings. Ninety-one percent of perioperative nurses have experienced at least one incidence of verbal abuse in the previous year.[16] In addition, 67% of nurses reported between one and five instances of disruptive behavior in the previous month,[17] and 64% of anesthesiologists have reported observing disruptive behavior in the perioperative setting.[18] In another study, 4 of 5 respondents reported that they had personally experienced disruptive behavior, and 73% also had observed a coworker who was the target of this behavior.[19] Evidence indicates that observing a disruptive behavior event can be as detrimental to the observer as it is to the target of the behavior.[19] Often, a component of this disruptive behavior is an environment that allows disrespect to flourish.

Inappropriate behavior is also found in the labor and delivery suite, with more than 60% of surveyed hospitals reporting disruptive behavior occurring in their obstetrical units.[20] This is no secret to hospital administrators and hospital leadership. In fact, more than 95% of physician executives reported knowledge of disruptive physician behavior within their organization.[21] The American College of Obstetricians and Gynecologists have addressed this issue in a Committee Opinion that identifies several contributing factors to a reluctance to systematically confront disruptive behavior, including financial concerns such as losing physician referrals, threats to takes one's practice to another hospital, and fear of retribution.[22] Box 19.2 highlights potential reasons for organizational reluctance to deal with disruptive behavior.

TRAINEES

Trainees, both medical students and resident physicians, are often involved in these behaviors, and due to the hierarchy seen in medicine, are often on the receiving end of disruptive behaviors from both attending physicians as well as nurses. Mistreatment of medical students has been documented by the Association of

BOX 19.1   EXAMPLES OF DISRUPTIVE BEHAVIORS

INAPPROPRIATE WORDS

- Profane, disrespectful, insulting, demeaning, or abusive language
- Shaming others for negative outcomes
- Demeaning comments or intimidation
- Inappropriate arguments with patients, family members, staff, or other care providers
- Rudeness
- Boundary violations with patients, family members, staff, or other care providers
- Gratuitous negative comments about another physician's care (orally or in chart notes)
- Passing severe judgment or censuring colleagues or staff in front of patients, visitors, or other staff
- Outbursts of anger
- Behavior that others would describe as bullying
- Insensitive comments about the patient's medical condition, appearance, situation, etc.
- Jokes or non-clinical comments about race, ethnicity, religion, sexual orientation, age, physical appearance, or socioeconomic or educational status.

INAPPROPRIATE ACTIONS/INACTION

- Throwing or breaking things
- Refusal to comply with known and generally accepted practice standards such that the refusal inhibits staff or other care providers from delivering quality care
- Use or threat of unwarranted physical force with patients, family members, staff, or other care providers
- Repeated failure to respond to calls or requests for information or persistent lateness in responding to calls for assistance when on call or expected to be available
- Repeated and unjustified complaints about a colleague
- Not working collaboratively or cooperatively with others
- Creating rigid or inflexible barriers to requests for assistance/cooperation

Reprinted with permission from College of Physicians and Surgeons of Ontario, Ontario Hospital Association. Guidebook for Managing Disruptive Physician Behavior. *Toronto: College of Physicians and Surgeons of Ontario; 2008.*

BOX 19.2   REASONS FOR ORGANIZATIONAL RELUCTANCE TO DEAL WITH DISRUPTIVE BEHAVIOR

- Cultural inertia
- History of tolerance
- Code of silence
- Fear of antagonistic physician reactions
- Organizational hierarchy
- Conflicts of interest
- Lack of organizational commitment
- Ineffective structure or policies
- Inadequate intervention skills

Reprinted with permission from Rosenstein AH. The quality and economic impact of disruptive behaviors on clinical outcomes of patient care. Am J Med Qual. 2011 Sep–Oct;26(5):372–379.

American Medical Colleges (AAMC) since 1991 through questions on the annual Medical School Graduation Questionnaire. Public humiliation is the most commonly reported form of mistreatment, with approximately one-third of all students reporting public belittling or humiliation. Sources of mistreatment included clinical faculty in the hospital (31%), residents or interns (28%), or nurses (11%).[23] These themes expand beyond medical students to graduate medical trainees. In a meta-analysis of 51 studies including 38,353 trainees, the pooled prevalence of harassment and discrimination was approximately 60%. Verbal abuse, gender discrimination, academic harassment, sexual harassment, and racial discrimination were common (Table 19.1).[24]

Interns report disruptive behavior at a greater rate than attending physicians, and they cite nurses as a frequent source. The behaviors most frequently reported by intern respondents include condescending behavior (74.6%), exclusion from decision-making (43.7%), yelling/raising voice (24.1%), inappropriate jokes (23.6%), and berating (20.3%) as commonly experienced behaviors.[25]

Residents and medical students indicate that they seldom report disrespectful acts because they are concerned about being seen as troublemakers and fear reprisal or vindictive retaliation, such as a lower grade, critical evaluation, or a poor recommendation for residency applications.[1] In the AAMC medical student questionnaire, only one-third of respondents who were mistreated reported incidents of mistreatment to their faculty or administrators, with nearly half citing fear of reprisal (48%) as the reason they did not report. Twenty-one percent of trainees reported a lack of clarity about what to do, and 37% of all respondents reported a sense of futility, stating that they felt reporting the incident would not be effective.[23]

Although much of the literature focuses on disruptive behavior being perpetrated on residents, they can also be the persons who are exhibiting disruptive behavior. A program director's management of disruptive and impaired physicians can be divided into four phases, including the discovery phase, decision/treatment phase, return to work phase, and finally, graduation and future employment.[26] Sanfey and colleagues have recommended steps for dealing with disrespectful behavior in residents, as highlighted in Box 19.3.[27]

CONSEQUENCE OF DISRUPTIVE BEHAVIORS

Disrespectful behavior threatens organizational culture and patient safety in many ways. In the immediate aftermath of an incident, the recipient may lose the ability to think clearly and may decrease focus and concentration, which can be associated with errors in decision-making or unsafe acts. Long-term effects on the work environment include decreased morale, high turnover, reduced team collaboration, failure to comply with system processes, and reduced information transfer (Box 19.4).[1,28]

Disruptive behavior has not only patient safety implications, but also financial impact. Disruptive behavior has negative impacts on nursing satisfaction and retention of healthcare personnel. This is a major issue in this era of nursing shortages and inability to recruit and retain adequate numbers of nurses.[29,30] Furthermore, disruptive behaviors have been shown to have a negative impact on work relationships and "process flow," which can have significant economic consequences.[26,30]

Disruptive behaviors also influence physician trainees, prompting some trainees to

---

TABLE 19.1. PREVALENCE OF HARASSMENT AND DISCRIMINATION AMONG MEDICAL STUDENTS AND RESIDENTS

Type of Harassment	% Students	% Residents
Harassment (overall)	59.6%	63.4%
Verbal abuse	68.8%	58.2%
Gender discrimination	49.8%	66.6%
Academic harassment	39.5%	27.7%
Sexual harassment	33.3%	36.2%
Racial discrimination	23.7%	26.3%
Physical harassment	9%	28.9%

Adapted from Fnais N, Soobiah C, Chen MH, Lillie E, Perrier L, Tashkhandi M, Straus SE, Mamdani M, Al-Omran M, Tricco AC. Harassment and discrimination in medical training: a systematic review and meta-analysis. *Acad Med.* 2014 May;89(5):817–827.

BOX 19.3   REMEDIATION STEPS FOR PROBLEM RESIDENTS

- Reflection
- Increase self-awareness through external and internal feedback
- Systems analysis: identifying features of residents' work environment that may trigger unprofessional behavior
- Punitive consequences
- Simulation activities
- Structured mentoring

Adapted from Sanfey H, Darosa DA, Hickson GB, Williams B, Sudan R, Boehler ML, Klingensmith ME, Klamen D, Mellinger JD, Hebert JC, et al. Pursuing professional accountability: an evidence-based approach to addressing residents with behavioral problems. Arch Surg. 2012 Jul;147(7):642–647.

---

consider leaving their current specialty training programs and influencing specialty choice, specifically in women trainees, who state that program rankings were influenced by gender discrimination and sexual harassment.[24]

SOLUTIONS

Inaction or ignoring these behaviors is not appropriate; it creates a culture of tolerance, which supports and reinforces disruptive behavior. Ultimately, inaction "poisons the well of collegiality and cooperation, undermines morale and inhibits transparency and feedback."[1] Disrespectful behavior threatens organizational culture and patient safety, and inaction has potentially dire consequences, as illustrated in Box 19.5.[30] The Joint Commission requires that a code of conduct be established in each

hospital, defining "disruptive and inappropriate" behaviors.[31,32] The Joint Commission also requires that a process for managing disruptive and inappropriate behaviors be created and implemented and that each medical staff member should acknowledge acceptance of the behavioral standards and the consequences of failure to comply with those standards at the time of appointment and reappointment. Box 19.6 highlights the Joint Commission recommendations for dealing with behaviors that undermine a culture of safety.[32]

Identification, Investigation, and Fair Peer Review

Any time behavior is reported that differs from institutional standards for respectful behavior, appropriate action should be taken by

---

BOX 19.4   WAYS IN WHICH DISRESPECTFUL BEHAVIOR THREATENS ORGANIZATIONAL CULTURE AND PATIENT SAFETY

- A sense of privilege and status can lead physicians to treat others with disrespect, creating barriers to open communication with the healthcare team.
- Dismissive treatment of patient and family members can impair communication and engagement as partners in safe care.
- A sense of physician autonomy can underlie resistance to following safe standardized practices, resulting in patient harm.
- Absence of respect undermines teamwork necessary to improve practice.

Adapted from Leape LL, Shore MF, Dienstag JL, Mayer RJ, Edgman-Levitan S, Meyer GS, Healy GB. Perspective: a culture of respect, part 1: the nature and causes of disrespectful behavior by physicians. Acad Med. 2012 Jul;87(7):845–852.

BOX 19.5   RISK OF INACTION

- Negative staff satisfaction and morale
- Staff turnover
- Compromises in patient safety
- Joint Commission noncompliance
- Negative hospital reputation
- Decreased patient satisfaction
- Increased liability and malpractice exposure
- Financial loss secondary to reimbursement penalties for adverse events and financial costs

Reprinted with permission from Rosenstein AH. The quality and economic impact of disruptive behaviors on clinical outcomes of patient care. Am J Med Qual. 2011 Sep–Oct;26(5):372–379.

---

clinical managers and supervisors, and leadership should be made aware and be involved in any ongoing plans. Leape and colleagues have suggested that the organization's leader is ultimately responsible for creating a culture of respect because only he or she can set the tone and initiate the process that will lead to change across the organization.[11] Characteristics of effective policies for managing disruptive behavior include fairness, consistency, graded response, restorative process, and the presence of surveillance mechanisms. Furthermore, others within the institution need to share in any lessons learned. It has been shown that to change culture, it is necessary to create awareness of the problem in order to motivate others to take action and to create a sense of urgency around doing so.[33]

Under the umbrella of a respectful culture that is set by the organization's leadership, department and unit leaders and managers need to implement that culture through day-to-day management of individual people and individual incidents. Protocols should be put in place and implemented when a concern is raised about a disruptive physician. The first step in any process must be swift, fair, and thorough review of the allegation, which obtains all perspectives of the situation, including that of the alleged disruptive individual, without taking sides. Input should be sought from relevant supervisors and multidisciplinary team members, including nursing, administration, and staff. This will allow everyone involved to feel that his or her right to respectful treatment is honored.

Following unbiased data collection, a synthesis of findings should allow the reviewer to assess whether these findings support or refute allegations that were made, or whether there were insufficient findings to draw conclusions. Also, any immediate threats to patient or staff safety should be identified and addressed. Supervisor input should be sought to identify prior behaviors to determine whether a more sustained pattern emerges that may modify interpretation of the current incident. The results of the fair, thorough, and unbiased review should be vetted against institutional rules, policies, and any potential legal standards that may apply. General counsel or institutional officials in human resources or the office of faculty affairs may be of assistance. At this point, potential interventions, consequences, and next steps would be discussed to address the disruptive behavior or incident being reviewed. A document outlining the steps of review, findings, relevant policies, and chosen actions should be created for the faculty file and for the faculty member, if appropriate. A final step should always be to focus on institutional learning; specifically, institutional opportunities to remove barriers, improve systems, or educate team members should be identified and acted upon in a continuous improvement framework.

Disruptive behavior is not always as it appears. Sometimes disruptive behavior can be

---

BOX 19.6   JOINT COMMISSION RECOMMENDATIONS FOR DEALING WITH BEHAVIORS THAT UNDERMINE A CULTURE OF SAFETY

1. Educate all team members on appropriate behavior defined by the organization's code of conduct.
2. Enforce the code of conduct consistently and equitably among all staff.
3. Develop and implement policies that address
   * Zero tolerance for disruptive behavior
   * Complementary policies for physicians and non-physicians
   * Reduce fear of intimidation or retribution with policies, including clear non-retaliation clauses
   * Empathic responses to patients and or families who experience or witness disruptive behavior
   * How and when to begin disciplinary actions.
4. Develop an interdisciplinary process for addressing disruptive behavior with input from medicine, nursing, administration, and other employees.
5. Provide skills-based training and coaching for leaders and managers in conflict resolution.
6. Assess staff perceptions of disruptive behavior and threat to patient safety.
7. Develop a reporting/surveillance system for identifying disruptive behavior.
8. Support surveillance with tiered nonconfrontational strategies that begin informally and move toward escalating disciplinary actions if pattern persists.
9. Conduct interventions with a commitment to well-being of all staff and with resources to support individuals whose behavior is caused or influenced by physical or mental health problems.
10. Encourage inter-professional dialogues across a variety of forums as a proactive way to address ongoing conflicts and moving toward collaboration and communication.
11. Document all attempts to address intimidating and disruptive behaviors.

Adapted from Joint Commission recommendations available at http://www.jointcommission.org/assets/1/18/ SEA_40.PDF (accessed November 2, 2014).

---

a sign of medical disease (cognitive decline, depression, uncontrolled diabetes), and other times it might signal alcohol or substance abuse.[34] In addition, it is possible that physicians who appear to be guilty of abusive or disruptive behavior are actually innocent of such behavior. It has been suggested that the label of *disruptive physician* has been used by hospitals to control physician behavior and perform "economic credentialing." Zbar and colleagues reported that "because of the hemorrhaging of revenue, some hospital administrators have taken the easy route of labeling surgeons who remove better paying cases to private ambulatory surgery centers as disruptive."[35] The need to protect providers who respectfully and appropriately identify concerns or call for

institutional improvement is directly referenced in the second part of the AMA definition of disruptive behavior: "However, criticism that is offered in good faith with the aim of improving patient care should not be construed as disruptive behavior."[9]

Department leaders or unit managers will need to obtain the facts that surround the allegation, usually involving interviews of the claimant and the alleged disruptive individual as well as witnesses, if appropriate. Written documents such as e-mails, texts, or incident reports may also be reviewed when relevant. Knowledge of institutional policies and procedures pertaining to allegations is critical. At many organizations, a member of the human resources team or an office of faculty affairs may assist in the investigation, including data collection and synthesis of facts in management of the circumstance.

Reviews involving disruptive physicians may have legal implications and should be undertaken with meticulous attention to fairness, documentation, and due process. Organizational leadership, frequently including a chief medical officer or leader of the practice group, may engage input from the general counsel's office if revocation or non-renewal of clinical privileges is being considered. General counsel's guidance will also be critical, for example, if there is a question as to whether a physician's behavior and institutional management have to be reported to a state medical board. Central to any potential legal review, the organization's own policies and procedures should be followed and documented, consistent with the organization's bylaws. When direct patient care is involved, the peer review process should be engaged as a basic component of institutional safety and quality assurance programs intended to assess and maintain standards of care. Guiding principles for hospitals' peer review process of an alleged disruptive physician include the following:[36]

- They must operate with a reasonable belief that they are improving the quality of patient care.
- They must only make their decision to revoke or refuse renewal of staff privileges after a reasonable effort to obtain the facts.
- They must provide a fair hearing.

Effective Management of Disruptive Behavior

Once a full set of facts are collected, leaders will need to assess which, if any, behavioral violations occurred. If an individual was determined to have been disruptive, a process should be engaged for feedback and, when necessary, escalating disciplinary action. The response and action should be graded to be proportional to the nature of the incident, as well as mindful of prior behavioral patterns.

The intent of the management process is awareness and behavior change to restore the clinical environment to one that is safe and highly functioning and should include a mechanism for surveillance.[11] Hickson and colleagues have recommended the following four graduated interventions:[10]

1. Informal conversations for single incidents;
2. Nonpunitive "awareness" interventions when data reveal patterns;
3. Leader-developed action plans if patterns persist;
4. Imposition of disciplinary processes if the plans fail.

Creating a culture in which such reviews can take place and interventions can be successful involves a multifaceted approach. The reporting of disruptive incidents is a crucial part of the process. Traditional obstacles to reporting are the reluctance to report a coworker, the fear that reporting will lead to retaliation, or previous experiences of reporting and never seeing any action or improvements.[37] Therefore, educational programs must also deal with the importance of timely and accurate reporting.

On a positive note, the AAMC focus on medical student mistreatment has brought visibility to these issues, and there was increasing medical student awareness of institutional policies on mistreatment, from 50% in the 2000 survey to nearly 90% in 2011.[23] Such awareness programs are critical because the most effective surveillance tools for detecting unprofessional behavior are the eyes and ears of patients, visitors, and healthcare team members.

Characteristics of effective policies for managing disruptive behavior are summarized in Box 19.7.[11]

Proactive Measures

While most organizations are at the stage of seeking to create a culture of respect and to define processes for the management of disruptive behaviors, the best organizations are working to establish programs and paradigms in which the code of conduct is understood and

---

BOX 19.7   CHARACTERISTICS OF EFFECTIVE POLICIES FOR MANAGING DISRUPTIVE BEHAVIOR

- *Fair:* process for managing breaches in the code of conduct must be perceived by all to be fair; there should be an explicit link to code of conduct, well-described process for investigation of allegations, and clearly described progressive disciplinary actions, as well as consequences for failure to adhere.
- *Consistent:* responsive to all complaints without regard to status or level of individuals accused.
- *Graded:* response to a complaint should be proportional to the nature of the incident.
- *Restorative process:* the goal of the process is successful behavior change and restoration of productive, meaningful role for the provider in the health system; disciplinary action should be reserved for those refractory to intervention or situations that threaten staff or patient safety.
- *Surveillance mechanisms:* mechanisms for safe reporting of concerns to identify individuals and circumstances that need review, including proactive strategies such as "360-degree" evaluations.

Adapted from Leape LL, Shore MF, Dienstag JL, Mayer RJ, Edgman-Levitan S, Meyer GS, Healy GB. Perspective: a culture of respect, part 1: the nature and causes of disrespectful behavior by physicians. Acad Med. 2012 Jul;87(7):845–852.

---

actions are taken to proactively prevent disruptive behaviors. It has been suggested that educational programs focusing on professionalism and disruptive behavior should be interactive to stimulate discussion and self-reflection.[38]

A recurrent theme in teamwork literature is the need for effective communication in order to reduce difficulties. When that communication fails, disruptive behaviors may ensue. Therefore it is not surprising that many of the interventions reported in the literature focus on communication skills training. For example, a 2-day communication skills training program in Kansas increased perioperative nurses' perceived self-efficacy to address disruptive physician behavior. In addition, participants reported an improved ability to address disruptive physician behavior.[8] Maimonides Medical Center in Brooklyn, New York, implemented a broad sweeping initiative to create a code of mutual respect that requires respectful behavior, as well as steps to implement the code. Implementation involved training to provide skills for "code advocates" and for mediating conflicts, plans to identify and address operational systems issues, and an accountability and measurement process.[39]

High-fidelity simulation is a promising method to enhance teamwork and communication among OR personnel and to thereby reduce potential friction that may occur as a result of difficulty in communication and in understanding each other's roles.[40] It has been reported[41] that using high-fidelity medical simulation is more representative of clinical care and is the "proper paradigm in which to perform teamwork training." One particular area that can be improved through simulation-based learning is acquiring adaptive behaviors and trust among team members.[42]

PUTTING IT INTO PRACTICE

Case Scenarios 19.1–19.3 are intended to provide examples of types of circumstances that arise within all healthcare organizations. These representative cases highlight practical tips that can be applied locally in all organizations.

CASE SCENARIO 19.1

You are contacted by the nurse manager for the OR to discuss a concern about an incident that occurred earlier today during a urology case. She states that Dr. Jones (the surgeon) became angry when the patient briefly became hypotensive and he did not feel that the anesthesiologist was responding quickly enough to the changing clinical situation. She states that the physician threw a sponge stick across the table while shouting, "Does the patient need to be dead to get your attention?" Once the patient's blood pressure stabilized, he calmed down and stated, "You know—I wouldn't have to behave in this way if all of you were competent."

You are also told that the procedure was done with neuraxial blockade, rather than general anesthesia. Thus the patient was awake during this interaction.

Dr. Jones is the chief of the division of urology within the department of surgery. Your first call is to his direct supervisor (his department chair) to ask whether there is a pattern of behavior. The chair responds, "The OR staff are oversensitive—this only happens when there is a critical clinical situation and people need to pay attention to Dr. Jones. Every time this happens, I tell them to focus on how the OR staff can prevent these problems. It is clear they don't like Dr. Jones, but he is a great surgeon with very high volumes and they just need to get over it."

Case Discussion

Tip #1: Don't jump to conclusions. Always start with a fair and thorough review of facts, including the perspective of the individual accused of disruptive behaviors. Remember that when you have heard one side of the story, you have heard one side of the story.

Your initial review of the situation includes gaining information from the OR staff, collecting facts as to the sequence of events. You confirm that multiple individuals were present and directly observed the following behaviors by Dr. Jones: loud voice, angry tone, disrespectful and demeaning language to the staff and a physical manifestation of anger when he threw a sponge stick. In your interviews, you are careful to direct the conversation to behaviors (e.g., loud voice, throwing of an instrument), rather than judgments (e.g., he was behaving like a jerk; he is always a hothead). This is best done with questioning focused on specific observations and a timeline of facts (e.g., What did you see? What did you hear? When did he enter the room?).

Your review includes a witnessed interview with Dr. Jones to gain his perspective. You open the conversation with an open-ended and non-judgmental invitation for his perspective (e.g., we want your input on what happened in the OR last week; we have received feedback that there was an incident in the OR that made some people feel uncomfortable). He is initially defensive, but quickly confirms the basic facts, including acknowledgment that he threw an instrument. He does not take responsibility for his actions, but rather continues to blame the OR team for "making him" behave in an angry way.

Tip #2: Seek supervisory input and assess for prior incidents and patterns of behavior.

Your discussion with Dr. Jones's supervisor, the chair of surgery, is concerning for confirmation of recurrent behaviors. Furthermore, the department chair is dismissive of concerns raised by staff, supporting Dr. Jones in blaming the staff, rather than focusing on the need for a respectful environment and holding Dr. Jones accountable for his behaviors. You point out to the department chair that Dr. Jones is in a supervisory role as a division chief, which adds additional weight to his disruptive behavior. While all faculty members are expected to behave respectfully, leaders are expected to role model behaviors consistent with the organization's expected code of conduct. In your conversation to debrief with the dean of faculty affairs, you identify the department chair's perspective as one that may need direction from more senior leadership.

Tip #3: Look for red flags that suggest a more difficult problem and assess for safety.

Red flags that signal a higher level of problem with this surgeon include recurrent behaviors, the creation of an unsafe environment, including physical threat by throwing an instrument, and lack of insight and accountability for these actions. Red flags that signal an unhealthy work culture include the department chair's dismissal of allegations, blame orientation, and normalization of disrespectful, bullying, and unsafe behaviors.[43] Given that a patient is reported to have been awake during this interaction, you seek guidance from risk management, and the nurse manager reaches out to the patient and family. In addition, the nurse manager intervenes to reassure the staff that the incident is being taken seriously and is under review.

Tip #4: Review relevant policies and seek guidance from institutional partners such as human resources, general counsel, and your faculty affairs office.

Given that this provider created an unsafe environment and does not appear to have insight, you are advised to put him on an administrative leave during the review period. This will allow a "cooling off" period and a period of time for the assessment of other stressors, including physical illness, substance use, or psychosocial stressors. This is done with the engagement of the department chair.

Case Resolution

Working with the office of faculty affairs, general counsel, and the chief medical officer, as well as his department chair, you agree that this is serious behavior that jeopardizes this clinician's career at this organization. Following a witnessed meeting with Dr. Jones to provide follow-up and verbal counseling, you create a behavioral contract and require anger management intervention as conditions for his return to the work environment. This is in addition to written final warning that, if the behavior does not stop, consequences will escalate up to and including termination. As a part of the discussion, general counsel guidance is necessary as to whether there is any required reporting to the state medical board. This is a delicate area with final recommendations requiring knowledge of both chosen actions for the licensed provider and also state legal and licensing regulations.

This case also identifies that there are serious cultural barriers to a safe, respectful work environment that will need to be addressed at an organizational level. Separate from this process, the senior associate dean for faculty affairs and the medical school dean had a discussion with the surgical department chair to discuss his role as an institutional leader, in setting the tone of the department and holding his leaders accountable. The importance of the dean and department chair's agreement with the plan of action and endorsement and signature on the behavioral contract cannot be overstated. Unless leadership embraces a culture of safety, it is unlikely that success can be achieved.[44,45]

Tip #5: Always close the loop.

You circle back to the nurse manager for closure. You transparently report that there was an in-depth review and appropriate actions are being taken. You request that the OR team swiftly report any recurrent behaviors. At the same time, you maintain confidentiality for the faculty member and reiterate to all involved that confidentiality is expected. Specific details of an intervention for a disruptive physician are confidential HR matters that are handled by department leaders, clinical supervisors, and the clinician.[44]

While acknowledging the importance of respect and confidentiality, remember that failure to close the loop may result in the other individuals involved (providers and staff) making assumptions that no actions were taken or that respect is not prioritized by leadership. Watching disrespectful behaviors go unaddressed is disheartening and discouraging to those who follow the rules and model professional, respectful behaviors. You can preface your conversation to close the loop with an opening disclaimer such as, "I know you understand that the particular details of the review of Dr. Jones's behavior are confidential. However, it is important for you to know that fair and thorough review is complete and appropriate actions are being taken. Please let us know right away if there are new concerns that arise."

Finally, following discussion between the dean and the two department chairs, there is an agreement that the departments of surgery and anesthesiology will do a shared Grand Rounds presentation on the relationship between a respectful operating room environment, quality of care, patient safety and satisfaction, and engagement in the work environment.

CASE SCENARIO 19.2

You are rounding in the ICU on a postop patient and stop at the nursing station to answer a call. While standing at the station you observe one of the nurses verbally berating the unit clerk. Her voice is raised and she shouts, "Are you an idiot? I have never seen such incompetence in my entire life. A monkey could do a better job!" She storms off, bumping into the unit clerk and several other bystanders as she passes muttering audibly, "What a #$@%-ing moron."

Case Discussion

Tip #6: All members of the healthcare team need to be held accountable to the same appropriate code of conduct.

Disruptive behaviors are not limited to physicians, or the OR. They can occur in any setting and by any member of the healthcare team. An effective policy for managing disruptive behaviors in staff or nursing is a Joint Commission requirement and should provide a fair and consistent approach to such behavior, with intent to restore the clinical environment to a safe and functional state. All team members need to be held equally accountable for modeling and embracing desirable behaviors.[46] As you observed these behaviors directly, you can start with a conversation with the nurse manager in which you report what you saw and what you heard.

Tip #7: Focus on the behaviors; the "why" doesn't matter.

Although we do not know what happened to trigger this outburst, profane, insulting, or demeaning language is always inappropriate. Furthermore, bumping, touching, or pushing behaviors represent another very serious dimension, beyond verbal aggression. It is common for persons exhibiting these behaviors to attempt to focus the interview on the "reasons" for their behavior, including frustrations or inefficiencies in the clinical environment. It is the job of a skilled interviewer to respectfully listen and acknowledge process inefficiencies and frustrations that may exist, but then swiftly and definitively redirect the focus to the unacceptable behaviors.

The skilled interviewer might say, "I appreciate that there are frustrations for us all in the work environment, and they are extremely important to address. However, that is not what we are here to talk about today; right now, we need to focus on your behaviors. It is never acceptable to shout, use profanity, or abruptly push into people in the clinical environment."

Tip #8: Safe reporting is a necessary first step.

Creating an environment in which witnessed events can be safely reported is necessary. Organizations should have multiple mechanisms for reporting, including direct reporting to managers or supervisors, confidential reporting systems, and mechanism for recording incident reports.

Case Resolution

The nurse manager reviews this nurse's performance record and does not identify prior outbursts. However, in speaking with the nurse, she discovers that there are significant stressors in her home situation, as her spouse has just been laid off, which leaves her as sole wage earner for her family of four. In addition, she has a special needs child, which has placed further strain on her family. The nurse is referred to the employee assistance program for support and is also provided coaching on stress management in the clinical setting. She is advised to seek assistance if she feels overwhelmed or out of control and is reminded that it is never acceptable to use profanity or aggression in the work environment, and that repeat behaviors will result in escalation of consequences that can jeopardize her career with the organization. She is also asked to accept responsibility and apologize to the person who was on the receiving end of her vitriolic outburst.

Tip #9: You must balance support and understanding with accountability.

Support for healthcare team members in difficult circumstances is appropriate and humane. However, it must be balanced with accountability and does not absolve responsibility for disrespectful behavior. Ultimately, if this nurse is unable to control her behaviors, her career will be at risk.

CASE SCENARIO 19.3

An anesthesiology resident reaches out to the residency program director to inform her of an incident that occurred in the preoperative holding area. The resident reported that he saw the attending physician, who is well known for abusive comments and angry outbursts, berate one of the medical students after he asked a question about a patient. "I have more knowledge in my little finger than you will ever have!" as he raised his fist angrily in the air. "If you ever question me again in front of a patient, I promise you will never get a residency, in this program or anywhere else!" The medical student was visibly shaken. She is applying for anesthesiology residency and asked the resident what she should do. She is now afraid that, if she complains, the attending physician will retaliate and undermine her residency application. The resident is similarly worried since she is currently applying for a fellowship and knows that this faculty member is well known and connected in the anesthesiology community.

Case Discussion

Students, residents, and other trainees both witness and experience disrespectful treatment from disruptive physicians with alarmingly high frequency. However, they seldom report disrespectful or unprofessional acts for fear of retaliation or being seen as troublemakers and not team players. Concerns about grades, recommendations, and undermining future career opportunities are all barriers to reporting. In this case, the program director thanks the resident for making her aware of the incident and reaches out to the student, both to seek perspective and provide reassurance of the priority of a respectful environment. She also explicitly states that retaliation from faculty members who have been reported for unprofessional behavior is never tolerated and that the student should reach out to her directly for any specific or follow-up concerns.

The program director next seeks input and perspective from the division chief of this faculty member, who confirms that this is not the first time such behavior has been reported. The program director and division chief decide to jointly meet with the faculty member to seek understanding of perspective and to clarify expectations for appropriate respectful behavior. Following review, the attending is given a written warning and behavioral contract outlining both expectations and potential consequences of continued behaviors.

The program director also communicates with medical school leadership to provide assurance of fair and respectful assistance to the student in her residency applications. The chair is involved to assure that no negative comments will be made regarding the corroborating resident who is applying for fellowship. Leaders discuss communication with medical students reinforcing safe mechanisms to report concerns to medical school and residency program leadership.

Tip #10: We have a training imperative and are responsible for being proactive.

We have an obligation to teach our trainees about professionalism and how to recognize, report, and manage disruptions in the work environment. Interactive programs, role play, and simulations (using both high-fidelity mannequins and standardized patients) can all be used not only to highlight recognition of inappropriate behaviors, but also to provide strategies for responding to situations in which there are violations of the code of conduct. In the most optimistic view of the new training paradigm in which professionalism is prioritized, we are teaching a new generation of physicians how to handle their cool in the heat of the moment.

Case Discussions: The Bigger Picture

Each of these cases highlights responses to individual incidents and demonstrates that swift management is critical to ensuring a safe and respectful environment. The cases have many features in common, occur in every healthcare setting, and are greatly facilitated in settings such as the operating room with a pressure cooker environment. All members of the healthcare team must learn to identify and report behaviors when they occur as the first step in management.

However, managing each incident in a vacuum is necessary but not sufficient. Organizations need to set institutional culture, leaders must be role models for professional behavior, and tools need to be in place for building the communication and management skill sets that will support and sustain respect.[47]

REFERENCES

1. Leape LL, Shore MF, Dienstag JL, Mayer RJ, Edgman-Levitan S, Meyer GS, Healy GB. Perspective: A culture of respect, part 1: the nature and causes of disrespectful behavior by physicians. *Acad Med*. 2012 Jul;87(7):845–852.

2. Rogers DA, Lingard L, Boehler ML, Espin S, Mellinger JD, Schindler N, Klingensmith M. Surgeons managing conflict in the operating room: defining the educational need and identifying effective behaviors. *Am J Surg*. 2013 Feb;205(2):125–130.

3. Lingard L, Reznick R, Espin S, Regehr G, DeVito I. Team communications in the operating room: talk patterns, sites of tension, and implications for novices. *Acad Med*. 2002 Mar;77(3):232–237.

4. Lingard L, Garwood S, Poenaru D. Tensions influencing operating room team function: does institutional context make a difference? *Med Educ*. 2004 Jul;38(7):691–699.

5. Christian CK, Gustafson ML, Roth EM, Sheridan TB, Gandhi TK, Dwyer K, Zinner MJ, Dierks MM. A prospective study of patient safety in the operating room. *Surgery*. 2006 Feb;139(2):159–173.

6. Piquette D, Reeves S, LeBlanc VR. Stressful intensive care unit medical crises: How individual responses impact on team performance. *Crit Care Med*. 2009 Apr;37(4):1251–1255.

7. Suliman A, Klaber RE, Warren OJ. Exploiting opportunities for leadership development of surgeons within the operating theatre. *Int J Surg*. 2013;11(1):6–11.

8. Saxton R, Hines T, Enriquez M. The negative impact of nurse-physician disruptive behavior on patient safety: a review of the literature. *J Patient Saf*. 2009 Sep;5(3):180–183.

9. Opinion 9.045—Physicians with disruptive behavior; c2000. http://www.ama-assn.org/ama/pub/physician-resources/medical-ethics/code-medical-ethics/opinion9045.page#. Accessed October 31, 2014.

10. Hickson GB, Pichert JW, Webb LE, Gabbe SG. A complementary approach to promoting professionalism: identifying, measuring, and addressing unprofessional behaviors. *Acad Med*. 2007 Nov;82(11):1040–1048.

11. Leape LL, Shore MF, Dienstag JL, Mayer RJ, Edgman-Levitan S, Meyer GS, Healy GB. Perspective: a culture of respect, part 2: creating a culture of respect. *Acad Med*. 2012 Jul;87(7):853–858.

12. Brewer CS, Kovner CT, Obeidat RF, Budin WC. Positive work environments of early-career registered nurses and the correlation with physician verbal abuse. *Nurs Outlook*. 2013 Nov-Dec;61(6):408–416.

13. Zimmerman T, Amori G. The silent organizational pathology of insidious intimidation. *J Healthc Risk Manag*. 2011;30(3):5,6, 8–15.

14. Leiker M. Sentinel events, disruptive behavior, and medical staff codes of conduct. *WMJ*. 2009 Sep;108(6):333–334.

15. *Guidebook for Managing Disruptive Physician Behavior*. Toronto: College of Physicians and Surgeons of Ontario; 2008.

16. Cook JK, Green M, Topp RV. Exploring the impact of physician verbal abuse on perioperative nurses. *AORN J*. 2001 Sep;74(3):317, 320, 322–327, 329–331.

17. Sofield L, Salmond SW. Workplace violence: a focus on verbal abuse and intent to leave the organization. *Orthop Nurs*. 2003 Jul–Aug;22(4):274–283.

18. Rosenstein AH, O'Daniel M. Impact and implications of disruptive behavior in the perioperative arena. *J Am Coll Surg*. 2006 Jul;203(1):96–105.

19. Walrath JM, Dang D, Nyberg D. An organizational assessment of disruptive clinician behavior: Findings and implications. *J Nurs Care Qual*. 2013 Apr–Jun;28(2):110–121.

20. Veltman LL. Disruptive behavior in obstetrics: a hidden threat to patient safety. *Am J Obstet Gynecol*. 2007 Jun;196(6):587.e1, 4; discussion 587.e4–5.

21. Weber DO. Poll results: doctors' disruptive behavior disturbs physician leaders. *Physician Exec*. 2004 Sep–Oct;30(5):6–14.

22. ACOG committee opinion no. 508: disruptive behavior. *Obstet Gynecol*. 2011 Oct;118(4):970–972.

23. Mavis B, Sousa A, Lipscomb W, Rappley MD. Learning about medical student mistreatment from responses to the medical school graduation questionnaire. *Acad Med*. 2014 May;89(5):705–711.

24. Fnais N, Soobiah C, Chen MH, Lillie E, Perrier L, Tashkhandi M, Straus SE, Mamdani M, Al-Omran M, Tricco AC. Harassment and

discrimination in medical training: a systematic review and meta-analysis. *Acad Med.* 2014 May;89(5):817–827.

25. Mullan CP, Shapiro J, McMahon GT. Interns' experiences of disruptive behavior in an academic medical center. *J Grad Med Educ.* 2013 Mar;5(1):25–30.

26. Rawson JV, Thompson N, Sostre G, Deitte L. The cost of disruptive and unprofessional behaviors in health care. *Acad Radiol.* 2013 Sep;20(9):1074–1076.

27. Sanfey H, Darosa DA, Hickson GB, Williams B, Sudan R, Boehler ML, Klingensmith ME, Klamen D, Mellinger JD, Hebert JC, et al. Pursuing professional accountability: an evidence-based approach to addressing residents with behavioral problems. *Arch Surg.* 2012 Jul;147(7):642–647.

28. Halverson AL, Neumayer L, Dagi TF. Leadership skills in the OR: part II: recognizing disruptive behavior. *Bull Am Coll Surg.* 2012 Jun;97(6):17–23.

29. Rosenstein AH. Original research: nurse-physician relationships: impact on nurse satisfaction and retention. *Am J Nurs.* 2002 Jun;102(6):26–34.

30. Rosenstein AH. The quality and economic impact of disruptive behaviors on clinical outcomes of patient care. *Am J Med Qual.* 2011 Sep–Oct;26(5):372–379.

31. *2015 Comprehensive Accreditation Manual for Hospitals: The Patient Safety Systems Chapter*; c2014. http://www.jointcommission.org/assets/1/6/PSC_for_Web.pdf. Accessed October 31, 2014.

32. The Joint Commission. Sentinel event alert, issue 40: behaviors that undermine a culture of safety; c2008.http://www.jointcommission.org/sentinel_event_alert_issue_40_behaviors_that_undermine_a_culture_of_safety/. Accessed November 1, 2014.

33. Kotter J. Leading change: why transformation efforts fail. 1995:59.

34. Hughes PH, Brandenburg N, Baldwin DC, Jr, Storr CL, Williams KM, Anthony JC, Sheehan DV. Prevalence of substance use among US physicians. *JAMA.* 1992 May 6;267(17):2333–2339.

35. Zbar RI, Taylor LD, Canady JW. The disruptive physician: righteous maverick or dangerous pariah? *Plast Reconstr Surg.* 2009 Jan;123(1):409–415.

36. Grogan MJ, Knechtges P. The disruptive physician: a legal perspective. *Acad Radiol.* 2013 Sep;20(9):1069–1073.

37. Rosenstein AH, Naylor B. Incidence and impact of physician and nurse disruptive behaviors in the emergency department. *J Emerg Med.* 2012 Jul;43(1):139–148.

38. McLaren K, Lord J, Murray S. Perspective: delivering effective and engaging continuing medical education on physicians' disruptive behavior. *Acad Med.* 2011 May;86(5):612–617.

39. Kaplan K, Mestel P, Feldman DL. Creating a culture of mutual respect. *AORN J.* 2010 Apr;91(4):495–510.

40. Hunt EA, Shilkofski NA, Stavroudis TA, Nelson KL. Simulation: translation to improved team performance. *Anesthesiol Clin.* 2007 Jun;25(2):301–319.

41. Shapiro J, Whittemore A, Tsen LC. Instituting a culture of professionalism: the establishment of a center for professionalism and peer support. *Jt Comm J Qual Patient Saf.* 2014 Apr;40(4):168–177.

42. Burke CS, Salas E, Wilson-Donnelly K, Priest H. How to turn a team of experts into an expert medical team: guidance from the aviation and military communities. *Qual Saf Health Care.* 2004 Oct;13 Suppl 1:i96–104.

43. Jacobs GB, Wille RL. Consequences and potential problems of operating room outbursts and temper tantrums by surgeons. *Surg Neurol Int.* 2012;3(Suppl 3):S167–173.

44. Richter JP, McAlearney AS, Pennell ML. The influence of organizational factors on patient safety: examining successful handoffs in health care. Health Care *Manage Rev.* 2014 Jul 15.

45. Auer C, Schwendimann R, Koch R, De Geest S, Ausserhofer D. How hospital leaders contribute to patient safety through the development of trust. *J Nurs Adm.* 2014 Jan;44(1):23–29.

46. Leape LL, Fromson JA. Problem doctors: is there a system-level solution? *Ann Intern Med.* 2006 Jan 17;144(2):107–115.

47. Samenow CP, Swiggart W, Spickard A, Jr. A CME course aimed at addressing disruptive physician behavior. *Physician Exec.* 2008 Jan–Feb;34(1):32–40.

20

Managing Adverse Events

The Aftermath and the Second Victim Effect

SVEN STAENDER

INTRODUCTION

The focus of anesthesiologists' training and activities concern the management of critically ill patients and the avoidance of catastrophe, rather than management of the aftermath.[1] We spend years acquiring technical expertise, and there are checklists for dealing with complications. Anesthesiologists have accumulated an immense knowledge in physiology, pathophysiology, and pharmacology, but there is little understanding of how to deal with the overwhelming emotions that occur after a severe complication. Death or severe harm to a patient under our care may be rare events, but can significantly impact our ability to care for patients and may also affect life outside the hospital.

PROBABILITY OF EXPERIENCING A PERIOPERATIVE CATASTROPHE

Death attributable solely to anesthesia is an extremely rare event. Large-scale studies suggest an incidence of about 0.5–0.8 per 100,000 cases.[2,3] Death in the perioperative period may be much more common, however, occurring after up to 1 in 500 anesthetics. Nearly every member of the perioperative care team will experience a perioperative death at some point in his or her career[4], and any death (e.g., after severe trauma) may have a significant psychological impact upon the involved team members.

A perioperative death may also be detrimental to the future career, especially if the complication was avoidable or was associated with an error. For example, an average of 149.7 serious errors and 80.5 adverse events occur every 1000 patient days in a university intensive care unit; 45% of these were prevetable.[5] In a 2012 national survey among members of the American Society of Anesthesiology (ASA), 62% reported to have been involved in at least one perioperative catastrophe over the course of the previous 10 years.[6] Every healthcare professional must therefore recognize that he or she will encounter some sort of adverse event or medical error at some point during his or her career.

EMOTIONAL CONSEQUENCES: THE "SECOND VICTIM" SYNDROME

It has been widely shown that healthcare professionals who are involved in a maloccurrence can experience their own emotional reactions, which may lead to a personal crisis.[7-10] One study of general practitioners in the United States found that 81% experienced a sense of compassion toward the patient, 79% encountered anger directly toward themselves, 72% a sensation of personal guilt, and 60% a feeling of inadequacy.[10] A Norwegian study reported that 17% of physicians who were involved in an adverse event experienced emotional problems that affected their private lives, and that emotional distress sufficient to impair their ability to continue working occurred in 11% of physicians who were involved in a severe medical error.[7] Waterman et al. found that physicians who have been involved in a severe adverse event experienced increased anxiety when managing a similar situation in the future (61% out of 3171 physicians in the US and Canada), 42% reported sleep disturbances, and 13% reported a perceived decrease in professional reputation.[9]

Gazoni explored the emotional impact of such cases among anesthesiologists. In their study, 73% of respondents reported feeling anxiety and guilt. Between 48% and 63% felt depression, sleeplessness, anger, and self-doubt.[6] A white paper of the Association of Anaesthetists of Great Britain and Ireland (AAGBI) listed the feelings that would affect an individual who has been involved in an intra-operative catastrophe (www.aagbi.org):

- Reliving the event
- Shock
- Restlessness
- Feelings of doom and gloom
- Anger
- Fear
- Guilt
- Physical reactions such as tiredness, headaches, and palpitations.

Each of these responses may be detrimental to a physician's ability to care for a patient, and the time required for recovery is variable: 21% of physicians in Gazoni's study reported a time to emotional recovery of 1 week after an adverse event, while 16% reported needing 1 month of recovery; 10% of physicians required 6 months, and 8% took over a year to completely recover.[6]

White and Akerele surveyed anesthetists in England regarding their experiences with intra-operative death, asking specifically about whether a return to clinical duty immediately after the event was appropriate, and, if not, how much time should be given to the responsible physician. The majority of the respondents agreed that it was reasonable for medical staff to be relieved from duty for 24 hours after an intra-operative death.[11] These answers must, however, be put into perspective: intra-operative death can occur under a variety of circumstances.

Patients who require emergency surgery and who are not expected to live after multiple traumatic injuries elicit a different reaction than would a patient who dies during elective surgery, for example after an anesthetic or surgical error. Children, colleagues, or other high-profile patients who are injured or killed may elicit a stronger reaction than would a patient who was previously unknown to the anesthesiologist. This is consistent with White and Akerele's data; 77% of survey respondents did not feel that their ability to care for their patients after a critical event had been impaired.[11] This was similar to a study of orthopedic surgeons in which 81% continued to operate, and none admitted to a diminished operating capability.[12]

It is now widely accepted that physicians experience emotional distress after catastrophic events, but there is a paucity of data to guide abstinence from clinical activities. Every anesthesia group should, however, have a policy in place that allows affected personnel to refrain from clinical care until he or she has recovered, taking the subjective wishes of the individuals involved into account.[11] These recommendations are dictated by good clinical governance and are included as part of a departmental or institutional risk management strategy.[13]

MANAGING THE PERIOD AFTER A CATASTROPHIC EVENT

The Involved Patient and Relatives

Patient Expectations and the Effect of Open Disclosure

What are the expectations of patients and their relatives after an adverse event has occurred? Gallagher et al. organized focus groups that included only adult patients or academic and community physicians, and three groups that included both physicians and patients.[14] Analysis of the transcripts focused on the need for disclosure of adverse events, the content of information being disclosed, and the necessity to address the emotional needs of both patients and physicians. Both patients and physicians had unmet needs after adverse events and medical errors.

Patients who have been the victims of an adverse event expected full disclosure of everything that caused harm. They also want information about what happened and why. They expect to know how the error's consequences will be dealt with, if there is something that can be learned from the error, and how future occurrences might be prevented. Physicians agreed that harmful errors should be openly disclosed but felt that one should "choose one's words carefully" when discussing adverse events and errors with patients. Patients sought emotional comfort from their physicians after an adverse event, including an apology for what had happened, if appropriate. In contrast, physicians were worried that such an apology might constitute an admission of legal liability.

Hospital risk managers demonstrate more favorable attitudes with regard to open disclosure of errors to patients but are less prepared to provide a full apology.[15,16] A study from 2004 surveying 958 adults showed that non-disclosure of adverse events was associated with higher levels of patient dissatisfaction, less trust in the physician, and a stronger adverse emotional response.[15,17] Again, patients wanted a clear explanation of the events that transpired and reassurance that something has been learned as a consequence. Patients want to know that their suffering was not in vain, and that future patients might benefit from lessons that were learned.[18] Interestingly, financial compensation was not usually mentioned by patients as being their principal goal after an adverse incident. Four principal reasons for litigation were identified in a survey of patients and relatives who initiated lawsuits: accountability, the desire for an explanation of what had happened, learning for standards of care, and compensation for their injury or loss. The need for compensation was cited as the primary reason to initiate litigation in only a few cases, whereas the desire for a full explanation was a major concern.[19]

Recommendations for Open Disclosure

The first and most important component of managing an adverse incident is the safe continuation of patient care. With regard to the provision of anesthesia, the same team should continue to provide the patient's care. If there is a supervising anesthesiologist, he or she should be informed immediately. The complexity of tasks and decisions that must be made after an adverse event may require an experienced physician to develop and oversee a care strategy.[18] Each team member who was involved in the adverse event should record a detailed narrative as soon as possible, and all supplies, equipment, and drugs should be kept for potential further investigation. This is important for two reasons: first, to not mask important details for a legal workup; and second, as the personal notes of the physician. It is not unusual that detailed investigations of such cases take years to be handled. Then it might prove important to be able to remember the details of what has happened. Such personal notes do not necessarily have to be part of the patient's history but are the personal notes of the involved physician.

After rescuing the patient and recording the facts of what happened, the next step is to disclose the events to the patient or his or her relatives. This meeting should be led by the most senior and experienced physician available and should take place in a private location. This conversation should focus on the events that transpired and indicate the next steps to be taken. Patients should be offered the opportunity to request a change of the physician responsible for their care, and an apology should be offered as appropriate.[18]

The Involved Physicians and Teams
What Do Physicians Need After an Adverse Event and What Do They Get?

The manner in which the institution, senior management, and colleagues respond to an adverse event seems to be an important determinant of the involved physicians' recovery.[20,21] Enabling healthcare professionals to accept responsibility for an error can lead to important lessons being learned, and ultimately to an improvement in an individual's performance. Talking to dependable colleagues about errors is an important aspect of dealing with adverse events.[22] Physicians reported that establishing a dialogue with a trusted colleague to discuss a critical incident was one of the most important means to overcome the emotional burden associated with an adverse event.[6]

CURRENT CONCEPTS OF DEALING WITH ADVERSE EVENTS IN HOSPITALS

Morbidity and mortality conferences offer a forum in which adverse events can be openly discussed and learned from. The discussions should consist of an open and truthful dialogue among experienced professionals and should avoid a culture of blame, accusation, and punishment.[22] Responsibly conducted morbidity and mortality conferences allow young residents to learn how to talk about errors in patient care. This also permits residents to identify reliable and trustworthy senior faculty whom they might approach if they have been directly involved in an adverse incident.

A debriefing session that includes the entire team was reported as the second most important factor in a study by Gazoni (89%), but only 53% of the respondents received some type of formal debriefing.[6] White and Akerele report that fewer than one-third of involved anesthetists participated in any form of debriefing. Only 7% of the respondents in Gazoni's study were given time away from clinical duties.[6,11]

ORGANIZATIONAL APPROACHES FOR THE SUPPORT OF STAFF AFTER A MEDICAL ERROR HAS OCCURRED

Recommendations by the Anesthesia Patient Safety Foundation

See the Anesthesia Patient Safety Foundation's (APSF) adverse event protocol, "The Basic Plan."[23]

Upon recognition of a major adverse event:

- Call for help.
- The primary caregiver should continue and direct patient care, except in very unusual circumstances.
- An "incident supervisor" should be assigned who assumes overall direction and control of the event, organizes and

assigns tasks to all in the operating room (OR), verifies the event has ended, involves consultants and advisors as indicated, coordinates and facilitates communications (with the surgical team in the OR, then with the surgeon and anesthesiologist, and, if appropriate, with the patient and/or family).

- Close the OR for the day. If any equipment needs to be tested, do so. Discard nothing.
- Contact the facility's risk manager.
- Arrange immediate comfort and support for the patient and/or family. Share as much information as possible.
- Designate a follow-up supervisor (who may or may not be the same as the incident supervisor) who will verify that the elements of the protocol have been applied, consider whether to organize team debriefing, maintain ongoing communication with all caregivers involved, coordinating and facilitating as much integration as possible, and pursue the accident investigation in conjunction with involved quality assurance and risk management systems and personnel.
- Document everything.
- Try to review formal reports submitted by the institution to the authorities.
- Continue involvement after the event when the patient survives: talk to the surgeons about care and make suggestions as indicated, be visible, supportive and not defensive with all involved, communicate as much as possible.

Recommendations by the Association of Anaesthetists of Great Britain and Ireland (Catastrophes in Anaesthetic Practice–dealing with the aftermath. The Association of Anaesthetists of Great Britain and Ireland, 21 Portland Place, London W1B 1PY, 2005)

- The majority of anesthetists are likely to be involved with an anesthetic catastrophe at some point in their careers.

- The psychological impact on staff following death or serious injury to a patient should not be underestimated.
- It is vital that members of the anesthetic department support the anesthetist, and a senior colleague or mentor should be assigned to this role.
- Contemporaneous records of the event must be kept.
- The clinical commitment of the anesthetist concerned should be reviewed immediately by the clinical director.
- A team approach should be adopted to breaking bad news with relatives. This should not be done over the telephone.
- The task of breaking bad news should not be carried out by a trainee or staff grade or associate specialist (SAS) doctor without a consultant present.
- Each hospital must have a procedure for dealing with and investigating catastrophic events.
- Critical incident stress debriefing by trained facilitators with further psychological support may assist individuals to recover from the traumatic event.
- Anesthetists are strongly advised to be a member of a medical defense organization.

Recommendations by the Swiss Foundation for Patient Safety

The Swiss Foundation for Patient Safety[21] has published guidelines describing the actions to take after an adverse event has occurred (for details, see www.patientensicherheit.ch).[24]

The following recommendations are a condensed summary of the advice offered by the Swiss Foundation for Patient Safety. These recommendations are separated in recommendations for senior staff members, for colleagues of involved team members, and for directly involved healthcare professionals.

1. Recommendations for senior staff members
   - A severe medical error is an emergency and must be treated as such (by being given absolute priority). It can have a severe emotional impact for the team involved.
   - Confidence between the senior staff and the involved professional, as well as empathic leadership, is an important prerequisite for the workup of that situation.
   - Involved professionals need a professional and objective discussion, as well as emotional support with peers in their department.
   - Seniors should offer support for the disclosing conversation with the patient and/or the relatives and for further clinical work in cases where involved professionals might feel insecure in their daily work.
   - A professional workup of that case, based on facts, is important for analysis and learning from medical error.
2. Recommendations for colleagues
   - Be aware that such an adverse event could happen to you.
   - Offer time to discuss the case with your colleague. Listen to what your colleague wants to tell and support him or her with your professional expertise.
   - Address any culture of blame either directly from within the team or by any other colleagues.
   - Take care of your colleague and be mindful of any feelings of isolation or withdrawal he or she may be experiencing.
3. Recommendations for healthcare professionals directly involved in an adverse event
   - Do not suppress any feelings of emotion you may encounter after your involvement in a medical error.
   - Talk through what has happened with a dependable colleague or senior member of staff. This is not weakness. This represents appropriate professional behavior.
   - Take part in a formal debriefing session. Try to draw conclusions and learn from this event.

- If possible, talk to your patient and/or their relatives and engage with them in open disclosure conversations.
- If you experience any uncertainties regarding the management of future cases, seek support from colleagues or seniors.

REFERENCES

1. Aitkenhead AR. Anaesthetic disasters: handling the aftermath. *Anaesthesia.* 1997;52:477–482.
2. Gibbs N, Borton CL. Safety of anaesthesia in Australia: a review of anaesthesia related mortality 2000–2002. Australian and New Zealand College of Anaesthetists: 2006.
3. Lienhart A, Auroy Y, Pequignot F, Benhamou D, Warszawski J, Bovet M, Jougla E. Survey of anesthesia-related mortality in France. *Anesthesiology.* 2006;105:1087–1097.
4. Pearse RM, et al. EuSOS: European surgical outcomes study. *Eur J Anaesth.* 2011;28(6): 454–456.
5. Rothschild JM, Landrigan CP, Cronin JW, Kaushal R, Lockley SW, Burdick E, Stone PH, Lilly CM, Katz JT, Czeisler CA, Bates DW. The Critical Care Safety Study: the incidence and nature of adverse events and serious medical errors in intensive care. *Crit Care Med.* 2005;33:1694–1700.
6. Gazoni FM, Amato PE, Malik ZM, Durieux ME. The impact of perioperative catastrophes on anesthesiologists: results of a national survey. *Anesth Analg.* 2012;114:596–603.
7. Aasland OG, Forde R. Impact of feeling responsible for adverse events on doctors' personal and professional lives: the importance of being open to criticism from colleagues. *Qual Saf Health Care.* 2005;14:13–17.
8. Delbanco T, Bell SK. Guilty, afraid, and alone: struggling with medical error. *N Engl J Med.* 2007;357:1682–1683.
9. Waterman AD, Garbutt J, Hazel E, Dunagan WC, Levinson W, Fraser VJ, Gallagher TH. The emotional impact of medical errors on practicing physicians in the United States and Canada. *Jt Comm J Qual Patient Saf.* 2007;33:467–476.
10. Wu AW, Folkman S, McPhee SJ, Lo B. Do house officers learn from their mistakes? *Qual Saf Health Care.* 2003;12:221–226.
11. White SM, Akerele O. Anaesthetists' attitudes to intraoperative death. *Eur J Anaesthesiol.* 2005; 22:938–941.
12. Smith IC, Jones MW. Surgeons' attitudes to intraoperative death: questionnaire survey. *BMJ.* 2001;322:896–897.
13. Seifert BC. Surgeons' attitudes to intraoperative death: anaesthetic departments need action plans to deal with such catastrophes. *BMJ.* 2001;323:342.
14. Gallagher TH, Waterman AD, Ebers AG, Fraser VJ, Levinson W. Patients' and physicians' attitudes regarding the disclosure of medical errors. *JAMA.* 2003;289:1001–1007.
15. Loren DJ, Garbutt J, Dunagan WC, Bommarito KM, Ebers AG, Levinson W, Waterman AD, Fraser VJ, Summy EA, Gallagher TH. Risk managers, physicians, and disclosure of harmful medical errors. *Jt Comm J Qual Patient Saf.* 2010;36:101–108.
16. Wears RL, Wu AW. Dealing with failure: the aftermath of errors and adverse events. *Ann Emerg Med.* 2002;39(3):344–346.
17. Mazor KM, Simon SR, Yood RA, Martinson BC, Gunter MJ, Reed GW, Gurwitz JH. Health plan members' views on forgiving medical errors. *Am J Manag Care.* 2005; 11: 49–52
18. Manser T, Staender S. Aftermath of an adverse event: supporting health care professionals to meet patient expectations through open disclosure. *Acta Anaesthesiol Scand.* 2005; 49: 728–734
19. Vincent C, Young M, Phillips A. Why do people sue doctors? A study of patients and relatives taking legal action. *Lancet.* 1994;343:1609–1613.
20. Engel KG, Rosenthal M, Sutcliffe KM. Residents' responses to medical error: coping, learning, and change. *Acad Med.* 2006;81:86–93.
21. Staender SE, Manser T. Taking care of patients, relatives and staff after critical incidents and accidents. *Eur J Anaesthesiol.* 2012;29:303–306.
22. Pierluissi E, Fischer MA, Campbell AR, Landefeld CS. Discussion of medical errors in morbidity and mortality conferences. *JAMA.* 2003;290:2838–2842.
23. Eichhorn J. Organized response to major anesthesia accident will help limit damage. *APSF Newsl.* 2006;21:11–13.
24. Schwappach D, Hochreutener MA, von Laue N, Frank O. Täter als Opfer. *Schriftenreihe 3.* January 10, 2010. Zürich: Stiftung für Patientensicherheit Schweiz.

INDEX